Hypothyroidism - Causes, Screening and Therapeutic Approaches

Edited by Robert Gensure

Published in London, United Kingdom

Hypothyroidism - Causes, Screening and Therapeutic Approaches
http://dx.doi.org/10.5772/intechopen.1000408
Edited by Robert Gensure

Contributors
Adina Mariana Ghemigian, Aisyah Elliyanti, Amanda Merck, Amirreza Rafiei Javazm, Athanasios Notopoulos, Corina Risca (Popazu), Cristiana Voineag, Dan Mircea Cheta, Dilek Yazıcı, Emily Beckett, Evangelia Zaromytidou, Huiwen Tan, Kalaipriya Gunasekaran, Mohab Elmubarak, Muzaffer Serdar Deniz, Ngiap Chuan Tan, Nicoleta Dumitru, Nitya Virippil, Oana-Andreea Parliteanu, Octavian Alexe, Palacios-Bayona Karen Lorena, Sarah Exley, Sawsan A. Omer, Sedat Carkit, Selin Çakmak Demir, Sumita Cholekho, Udaya Kabadi, Vincent C.S. Lee, Xinyu Zhang, Yuke Liu

First published in London, United Kingdom, 2025 by IntechOpen
IntechOpen is the global imprint of INTECHOPEN LIMITED, registered in England and Wales, registration number: 11086078, 167-169 Great Portland Street, London, W1W 5PF, United Kingdom

For EU product safety concerns: IN TECH d.o.o., Prolaz Marije Krucifikse Kozulić 3, 51000 Rijeka, Croatia, info@intechopen.com or visit our website at intechopen.com.

British Library Cataloguing-in-Publication Data
A catalogue record for this book is available from the British Library

Hypothyroidism - Causes, Screening and Therapeutic Approaches
Edited by Robert Gensure
p. cm.
Print ISBN 978-0-85466-584-6
Online ISBN 978-0-85466-583-9
eBook (PDF) ISBN 978-0-85466-585-3

If disposing of this product, please recycle the paper responsibly.

Meet the editor

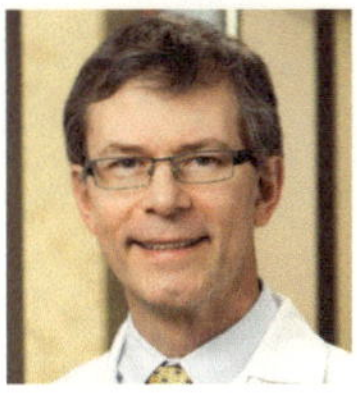

Robert Gensure, M. D./Ph.D. is a physician-scientist with significant experience in basic science and clinical research, and in clinical practice of pediatric endocrinology. He has authored 46 publications on topics including parathyroid hormone function, vitamin D supplementation, and inherited disorders of bone and mineral metabolism. He is currently serving as chief of pediatric endocrinology at Dartmouth Health Children's in Lebanon, NH, USA.

Contents

Preface

Hypothyroidism is a long-recognized clinical condition. It is often of insidious onset, with affected individuals feeling slow loss of energy, increasing need for sleep, and progressive weight gain despite having a low appetite. It can affect individuals of all ages, including newborns. There are special concerns for children with hypothyroidism, as children with hypothyroidism will also cease growing in stature. Importantly, thyroid hormone is essential for brain development in the first 2 years of life.

Because of its insidious onset and nonspecific symptoms, hypothyroidism may take years to come to clinical attention. This has led to the development of screening recommendations, and given the dire consequences to newborns with untreated hypothyroidism, all newborns are screened for hypothyroidism at birth as part of the newborn screening programs.

As we've learned more about thyroid hormone production and the pathophysiology of the various forms of hypothyroidism, screening and treatment recommendations have evolved. Synthetic defects, maldevelopment of the thyroid gland, pituitary disorders, or resistance syndromes can cause hypothyroidism in newborns. Given the diverse etiologies, screening recommendations have centered on measuring thyroid hormone rather than screening for root causes. Outside the newborn period, hypothyroidism is overwhelmingly the result of an autoimmune disorder. Since autoimmunity falls in clusters, individuals with related autoimmune disorders (i.e. type 1 diabetes mellitus) are routinely screened for hypothyroidism. The propensity to develop autoimmune disorders is hereditary, so individuals with a family history placing them at risk are also often routinely screened. Antibodies to the thyroid gland will often precede frank hypothyroidism, so individuals with positive thyroid antibodies are usually routinely screened.

As thyroid hormone has long been available in synthetic form, levothyroxine has become the mainstay for the treatment of hypothyroidism. Some individuals with impaired conversion to the more potent form, T3, may receive combined therapy with both agents. Thyroid hormones have a very long half-life, so daily oral dosing is sufficient to maintain blood levels similar to those achieved by the steady production of thyroid hormones by the thyroid gland itself. Synthetic thyroid hormone is chemically identical to endogenously produced thyroid hormone, so there are no idiosyncratic reactions to therapy. Adequate monitoring of therapy can achieved with annual blood tests in most adults.

While treatment with synthetic thyroid hormone can adequately replace thyroid hormone in individuals with hypothyroidism, the treatment does not address any of the root causes of hypothyroidism, and the medication must, therefore, be taken lifelong. With an improved understanding of the pathophysiology of various causes of hypothyroidism, in particular autoimmune disease, there are now efforts to block the immune response to the thyroid gland and restore normal thyroid function. As more specific immune modulator therapies become available, this treatment strategy holds promise for curing autoimmune thyroid disease.

This manuscript provides a comprehensive review of our current knowledge base regarding hypothyroidism. Screening recommendations and treatment strategies are discussed in detail. There is a thorough review of the pathophysiology of the various forms of hypothyroidism and a discussion about new treatment strategies in development to prevent or cure hypothyroidism.

Robert Gensure, M.D./Ph.D.
Dartmouth Health Childre,
Lebanon, NH, USA

Section 1

Introduction/Pathophysiology

Chapter 1

Causes and Management of Hypothyroidism

Sawsan A. Omer and Mohab Elmubarak

Abstract

Hypothyroidism is common. It could be due to a primary disorder within the thyroid gland or secondary to pituitary or hypothalamic disease. The clinical presentation of hypothyroidism depends on the duration and severity of the disease. Since thyroid hormones affect the metabolism and function of virtually all nucleated cells, it has diverse clinical manifestations. The most important diagnostic test is the thyroid function test (TFT). Screening for thyroid function is recommended for neonates and elderly patients. Replacement therapy with levothyroxine is indicated. Sickle cell anemia (SCA) is an inherited hemoglobinopathy that frequently causes hypothyroidism. One study conducted among patients with SCA who have high serum ferritin levels assessed the association between gonadal and thyroid hormones with iron indices; it was found that there was a significant relation between serum ferritin level and free T3 and free T4. This was probably due to endocrine dysfunction secondary to high ferritin levels and iron overload.

Keywords: hypothyroidism, causes, clinical features, screening, management, sickle cell anemia, endocrine, thyroid hormones

1. Introduction

Hypothyroidism is one of the commonest endocrine disorders following obesity and diabetes mellitus [1]. The prevalence of thyroid disorders in mountain areas like the Himalayas where iodine deficiency is common exceeds 10%, and 4% of females aged 20–50 years in the UK have thyroid disorder [2]. The metabolism of almost all tissues is virtually controlled by thyroid hormones [1]. Endocrine disorders present in many different ways with nonspecific symptoms or with asymptomatic biochemical abnormalities. For example, thyroid disorders, which are common occurring in 5% of population and mainly affect females, has diverse clinical manifestations [2]. Hypothyroidism is commonly due to primary disorder within the thyroid gland itself but could be secondary to pituitary disease. Primary hypothyroidism is one of the commonest endocrine disorders, with a prevalence of over 2% in women in the UK but less than 0.1% in men, and lifetime prevalence increases with age, with 9% for women and 1% for men around 60 years. The prevalence of subclinical hypothyroidism varies from 1 to 10% worldwide [2]. Patients with sickle cell anemia with chronic anemia and frequent blood transfusion will have iron overload and other factors like vaso-occlusive occlusion, infraction, or hypoxia associated with chronic anemia, and this could be responsible for endocrine dysfunction in such patients. Thyroid disorders were frequently reported in patients with sickle cell anemia. So, these patients need frequent screening for serum ferritin level and hormonal assays including thyroid hormones [3].

Since hypothyroidism is a common condition and may present with nonspecific symptoms with different varieties of causes and clinical presentation, in this chapter, elaboration of causes, clinical presentation, screening, diagnosis, and therapeutic approach for hypothyroidism will be discussed in addition to the relation between sickle cell anemia and endocrine disorders including thyroid disorders.

2. Anatomy

The thyroid gland lies in the anterior part of the neck; it consists of two lobes connected by an isthmus. It is closely attached to the thyroid cartilage and to the upper end of the trachea and hence moves with swallowing. It has rich blood supply from superior and inferior thyroid arteries. Histologically, the thyroid gland consists of follicles surrounded by basement membrane. Each follicle is lined by cuboidal epithelioid cells that contain the colloid (the iodinated glycoprotein thyroglobulin), which is synthesized by the follicular cells [1]. Between the follicles lie the parafollicular cells that secrete calcitonin, which has no apparent physiological effect on the human body [2].

3. Physiology

3.1 Synthesis

The thyroid synthesizes two hormones: triiodothyronine (T3), which acts at the cellular level, and L-thyroxine (T4), which is the prohormone. T4 is produced more than T3, but in some peripheral tissues like liver, kidney, and muscles, it is converted to the more active T3 [1]. The follicular epithelial cells synthesize thyroid hormones by incorporating iodine into the amino acid tyrosine on the surface of thyroglobulin, a protein secreted into the colloid of the follicle. Iodide is essential for thyroid hormone synthesis, and the daily requirement should be around 100 μg/day to maintain normal thyroid function [2]. In plasma, more than 99% of T3 and T4 is bound to thyroxine-binding globulin (TBG), thyroid-binding prealbumin (TBPA), and albumin. The free T3 and T4 hormones diffuse in tissues and exert different metabolic effects in tissues, so in assessment of thyroid function, free T3 and T4 levels should be measured because they are not affected by changes of binding proteins levels in the plasma. For example, if TBG is increased by estrogen (in contraceptive pills), this will lead to a false increase in total T3 and T4 levels. The secretion of thyroid hormones by the thyroid gland is a continuous process. T4 has a half-life of 7–10 days, while T3's half-life is 6–10 hours, with little variation in level all the time. The secretion of thyroid hormones is controlled by the hypothalamic-pituitary-thyroid axis (shown in **Figure 1**), where thyrotropin-releasing hormone (TRH), a peptide hormone produced by the hypothalamus, stimulates the anterior pituitary gland to secrete thyroid-stimulating hormone (TSH). TSH stimulates the growth and activity of thyroid follicular cells

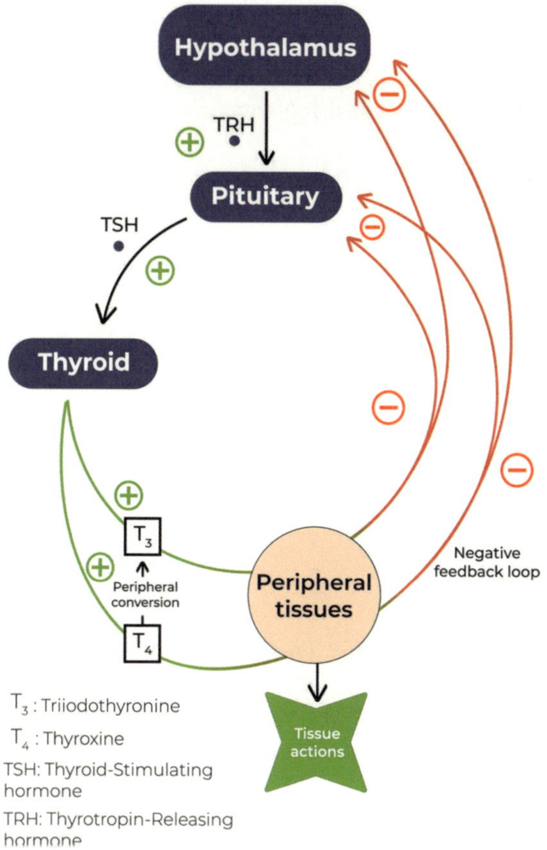

Figure 1.
The hypothalamic-pituitary-thyroid axis.

via G-protein coupled with TSH membrane receptors, and the secreted T3 and T4 hormones are released in the circulation, and they exert negative feedback on the pituitary and hypothalamus. In primary hypothyroidism, low levels of T3 and T4 will stimulate the secretion of TSH, and its level will be elevated [1, 2].

3.2 Effects of thyroxine

The effects of thyroxine include the following [1, 2]:

- Increases the heart rate and cardiac output.
- Increases bone turnover and resorption.
- Maintains normal hypoxic and hypercapnic drive in the respiratory center.
- Increases gut motility.
- Increases oxygen release to tissues by increasing 2,3-biphospoglycerate (2,3-BPG).

- Increases speed of muscle contraction and relaxation and muscle protein turnover.
- Increases hepatic gluconeogenesis/glycolysis and intestinal glucose absorption.
- Increases lipolysis and cholesterol synthesis and degradation.
- Increases catecholamine activity.
- Decreases cardiac α-adrenergic receptors.

4. Causes of hypothyroidism

Hypothyroidism results from an insufficient production or action of thyroid hormones that leads to decreased metabolism in almost all tissues [4]. The causes could be as follows (shown in **Table 1**).

4.1 Primary hypothyroidism

It is due to a disease process in the thyroid gland leading to a loss of negative feedback mechanism and subsequent elevation in the thyroid-stimulating hormone from the anterior pituitary gland [1]. Primary hypothyroidism is the most common form and can be subdivided into neonatal or acquired hypothyroidism [4].

Causes of hypothyroidism		
Primary causes	Neonatal	Thyroid gland aplasia hypoplasia or failure to descend
		Inability to synthesize hormones
		Peripheral resistance to thyroid hormone action
		Anti-thyroid drugs or iodine during pregnancy
	Acquired	Hashimoto's disease
		Iodine deficiency
		Treatment of hyperthyroidism (radioactive iodine, subtotal thyroidectomy, etc.)
		Drugs like amiodarone or lithium carbonate or antithyroid
		Subacute thyroiditis
Secondary causes	Anterior pituitary gland disease	Pituitary adenoma
		Surgery for pituitary tumors
		Postpartum pituitary necrosis (Sheehan syndrome)
		After head/neck injury
		Infiltration of the pituitary by amyloidosis or sarcoidosis
Tertiary causes	TRH deficiency	Hypothalamic lesions

Table 1.
Causes of hypothyroidism.

4.1.1 Neonatal hypothyroidism

It results from thyroid gland aplasia, hypoplasia, or failure to descend during embryonic development or from the inability of the thyroid gland to synthesize hormones as a result of inherited defects. Peripheral resistance to thyroid hormone action could be a very rare cause of neonatal hypothyroidism. The use of anti-thyroid drugs or iodine during pregnancy may result in neonatal hypothyroidism. Endemic cretinism may occur in areas where there is iodine deficiency [4].

4.1.2 Acquired hypothyroidism

Chronic autoimmune thyroiditis (Hashimoto's disease) is the most common cause of acquired hypothyroidism. Other causes include iodine deficiency in endemic areas, treatment of hyperthyroidism with radioactive iodine, subtotal thyroidectomy for nodular goiter, excessive intake of iodides in radiocontrast dyes, or drugs like amiodarone or lithium carbonate or anti-thyroid. Subacute thyroiditis may rarely cause hypothyroidism [2, 4].

4.2 Secondary hypothyroidism

There is an inappropriate low level of TSH due to anterior pituitary gland disease, leading to low circulating levels of T3 and T4 [1]. This may be caused by hypopituitarism due to pituitary adenoma, surgery for pituitary tumors, postpartum pituitary necrosis (Sheehan syndrome), or after head/neck injury. It can also be caused by infiltration of the pituitary glands by amyloidosis or sarcoidosis [2, 4].

4.3 Tertiary hypothyroidism

This occurs due to decreased level of TRH because of hypothalamic lesions [4].

4.4 Hashimoto's thyroiditis

It is also known as autoimmune thyroiditis and is the most common cause of hypothyroidism and goiter in children and young adults in areas with no iodine deficiency. There is a rare variant of chronic thyroiditis know as Riedel thyroiditis, which causes fibrous destruction of the thyroid cells, causing a firm mass in the thyroid with retrosternal extension extending outside the gland. It may be confused with thyroid cancer.

4.4.1 Pathogenesis of Hashimoto's thyroiditis

It is an autoimmune disorder causing lymphocytic destruction of the thyroid tissues with increased titers of thyroid peroxidase antibodies in the plasma with increased thyroglobulin antibodies and TSH receptor antibodies. The female-to-male ratio prevalence of Hashimoto's thyroiditis is 4:1, respectively. It may be associated with autoimmune polyglandular diseases like Addison's disease, diabetes mellitus type 1, and so on. The common clinical presentation of Hashimoto's thyroiditis is diffused painless goiter. Patients are usually euthyroid or have only mild hypothyroidism but may suffer from severe hypothyroidism in case of severe destruction of the thyroid gland.

5. Clinical features of hypothyroidism

Prevalence of hypothyroidism is around 5%, and females are affected approximately six times more frequently than males [2].

The clinical presentation of hypothyroidism depends on the duration and severity of the disease. Patients who have developed complete thyroid failure insidiously may present with many of the clinical features of hypothyroidism that are mentioned below. Prolonged hypothyroidism results in the infiltration of many body tissues by the mucopolysaccharides hyaluronic acid, and chondroitin sulphate, resulting in many clinical features like a low-pitched voice, poor hearing, slurred speech due to a large tongue (macroglossia), and compression of the median nerve at the wrist (carpal tunnel syndrome). Infiltration of the dermis gives rise to non-pitting edema (myxedema), which is most marked in the skin of the hands, feet, and eyelids [2].

5.1 Neonatal hypothyroidism

It is manifested as poor feeding, respiratory difficulty, cyanosis, jaundice, hypotonia, muscle weakness, umbilical hernia, and growth retardation [4]. In the Pendred syndrome, neonates have goiter, deafness, and mental retardation. In infants, muscle involvement may result in the Kocher-Debré-Sémélaigne syndrome or "infant Hercules" [5].

5.2 Hypothyroidism in children

Clinical features include growth and mental retardation, a puffy face and hands, retardation in bone maturation, and neurological signs of pyramidal and extrapyramidal tract abnormalities [4].

5.3 Hypothyroidism in adults

The common symptoms include chronic fatigue, inability to concentrate, coldness, weight gain, constipation, and menstrual irregularities. In addition to periorbital swelling, swollen hands and feet (non-pitting oedema), a hoarse voice, and a thickening of the tongue, patients may complain of paraesthesia, muscle cramps, and muscle weakness [4] as well as hypothermia, bradycardia, dry skin with yellow tone (carotenemia), and deafness. Features of other autoimmune endocrinopathies may also be found [5, 6]. The best single clinical indicator for hypothyroidism is delayed relaxation of ankle jerk (Woltman's sign), and patients may have goiter. In adults, the presence of painful myopathy and myotonia with myxedema is known as Hoffmann syndrome [5].

Severe form of hypothyroidism leads to myxedema coma, which is associated with decreased level of consciousness, profound hypothermia, hypoventilation, hypotension, striking bradycardia, and pleural and pericardial effusions [6].

5.4 Differential diagnosis

Differential diagnosis of hypothyroidism includes the following conditions: (**Table 2**) [2, 6].

Clinical features of hypothyroidism	
Neonates	Poor feeding
	Respiratory difficulty
	Cyanosis
	Jaundice
	Hypotonia
	Muscle weakness
	Umbilical hernia
	Growth retardation
Children	Growth and mental retardation
	Retardation in bone maturation
	Puffy hands
	Neurological signs of pyramidal and extrapyramidal abnormalities
Adults	Chronic fatigue
	Slurred speech
	Inability to concentrate
	Cold intolerance
	Weight gain
	Constipation
	Menstrual irregularities
	Periorbital swelling
	Non-pitting oedema (Myxedema)
	Carpal tunnel syndrome
	Paraesthesia
	Muscle cramps
	Muscle weakness
	Hypothermia
	Bradycardia
	Dry skin with yellow tone
	Deafness
	Delayed relaxation of ankle jerk
	Features of other autoimmune endocrinopathy

Table 2.
Clinical features of hypothyroidism.

- Chronic fatigue syndrome
- Congestive heart failure
- Primary amyloidosis

- Depression
- Exposure hypothermia
- Parkinson's disease.

6. Diagnosis of hypothyroidism

Anemia may be microcytic or macrocytic due to impaired hemoglobin synthesis or impaired intestinal absorption of iron, folic acid, or due to pernicious anemia (in association with other polyglandular autoimmune disease) [4]. Hyponatremia and hyperprolactinemia with elevated serum cholesterol and creatinine kinase levels may be detected [5].

The most important diagnostic test is thyroid function test (TFT). TSH and free T4 and free T3 are measured by immunoassay technique at any time since there is no circadian rhythm for thyroid hormone secretion. In primary hypothyroidism, there is an elevated serum TSH level (>10 mIU/L) with low free T4; serum triiodothyronine (T3) concentrations are a poor indicator of hypo-thyroid state [5]. In secondary hypothyroidism, free T4 will be low, and TSH is also low normal or subnormal. Thyroid autoantibodies (peroxidase antibodies) will be found in autoimmune thyroiditis. MRI brain for the pituitary gland is needed if secondary hypothyroidism is suspected [4]. Isolated elevation of TSH may be detected in cases of mild (subclinical) hypothyroidism and use of some medications like amiodarone and lithium [5].

In severe hypothyroidism, ECG changes in form of bradycardia, with low voltage complex and ST segment and T-wave abnormalities, are found [2].

In severely ill patients, there is low total and free T4 and T3 serum levels with a normal or low normal TSH level (sick euthyroid' syndrome); this change is probably mediated by interleukins IL-1 and IL-6. TFT should be repeated after the patient illness is resolved to exclude hypothyroidism [1].

The occurrence of hypothyroidism with autoimmune alopecia and transient acantholytic dermatosis is known as Grover's disease [5].

7. Screening for hypothyroidism

Increased threshold for suspicion of hypothyroidism is the best screening test for hypothyroidism; however, elderly people especially female should be screened after the age of 50 years. The mean average age at diagnosis was 58–59 years, and the probability of developing hypothyroidism increased steadily with age. Screening for congenital hypothyroidism is essential since it is relatively common (1:4000 births); blood sample from heel prick is taken for TSH assessment. Serious results may occur from delay in diagnosis of congenital hypothyroidism such as brain damage with mental and physical retardation [7].

Screening of inpatient for hypothyroidism is ineffective because the nonspecific effect of acute illness on thyroid function test corrected itself after recovery [7].

7.1 Screening in special groups

Hypothyroidism occurs after all types of treatment for hyperthyroidism, for example, iodine therapy or thyroidectomy, so such patients need annual checkup for

Indications for screening for hypothyroidism
Elderly patients
For congenital hypothyroidism
Following treatment of hyperthyroidism
Neck irradiation
Pituitary surgery or irradiation
Patients on medications like lithium or amiodarone
Females with type 1 diabetes
Female over 40 with nonspecific complaints
Unexplained infertility
Patients with post-partum thyroiditis
Thyroiditis
Bipolar disorder with frequent cycling
Autoimmune Addison's disease
Turner's syndrome and Down's syndrome
Patients with dementia
Patients with sickle cell anemia
Patients with breast cancer

**Screening is not indicated for ill patients.*

Table 3.
Indications for screening for hypothyroidism.

thyroid function. Patients taking lithium or amiodarone are at risk for both hypothyroidism and hyperthyroidism and need regular monitoring of thyroid function as well as female patients with type 1 diabetes mellitus or unexplained infertility. Also, women who have had postpartum thyroiditis should be screened annually for thyroid function since 25% of these women will develop overt hypothyroidism within the next 5 years. Patients with Turner's and Down's syndromes have a high prevalence of hypothyroidism than the general population and should be screened. Patients with bipolar affective disorder with recurrent cycling of refractory depression should be screened for hypothyroidism. Patients with dementia may be worth screening for thyroid function. It is uncertain whether patients with breast cancer may benefit from screening for hypothyroidism or not, because there is uncertain association between breast cancer and autoimmune (Hashimoto's) thyroiditis, with a threefold increase in the prevalence of thyroid antibodies [7]. Patients with sickle cell anemia need testing for thyroid function because SCA results in sickling of erythrocytes that cause micro-vascular obstruction leading to acute complications and chronic organ damage, and endocrine glands are commonly affected. Thyroid disorders were frequently reported in patients with SCA [3]. Indications for screening for hypothyroidism are shown in **Table 3** [3, 7].

8. Treatment of hypothyroidism

Treatment for hypothyroidism is thyroid hormone replacement therapy for life, with levothyroxine starting with a low dose of 50 μg once per day for 3 weeks and increasing gradually until patients become euthyroid with a maintenance dose of

100–150 μg per day; it should be taken on empty stomach. In younger patients, levothyroxine can be started in a dose of 100 μg for rapid response and normalization of TFT [2, 5, 6]. Dose adjustment should be done every 3 weeks depending on clinical response and suppression of the elevated TSH level [5]. Response to treatment occurs within 2–3 weeks. Reduction in weight and periorbital puffiness occurs quickly, but resolution of effusions and restoration of hair and skin texture may take 3–6 months [2]. If there is no response to thyroxine therapy, patient compliance should be assessed; alternative diagnosis should be ruled out underlying psychiatric disorder, presence of pernicious anemia, or association with other endocrine disorders such as Addison's disease. In pregnant ladies who are known to have hypothyroidism, the dose of levothyroxine should be increased to up ~50% in the first half of pregnancy because inadequate treatment of hypothyroidism during pregnancy may result in impaired cognitive development in the fetus. Elderly patients or patients with ischemic heart disease should be started with low dose thyroxine (25 μg) to avoid development of angina [2, 5].

9. Myxedema coma

This is a very rare presentation of severe hypothyroidism and is a medical emergency where there is decreased level of consciousness usually in an elderly patient with severe hypothyroidism and myxedema. It is also associated with hypothermia (body temperature may be 25°C), and convulsions are not uncommon. Mortality rate is very high and may reach up to 50%. Early recognition is essential for proper treatment. Suspected cases should be treated before laboratory confirmation of diagnosis [2]. Rewarming of the patient is essential as the first measure of treatment. Intravenous levothyroxine is given, and intravenous hydrocortisone may be added if adrenal insufficiency is suspected [6].

Liothyroine in a dose of 20 μg is given, then injections of 20 μg three times daily until the patient improves clinically. The body temperature rises in the first 24 hours, and after 2–3 days, the patient can be shifted to a dose of 50 μg levothyroxine once per day. If the patient is not known to have primary hypothyroidism, thyroid failure should be suspected to be secondary to pituitary or hypothalamic disease, and treatment with intramuscular hydrocortisone in form of 100 mg three times a day until the biochemical results of TFT and cortisol is obtained [2].

10. Subclinical hypothyroidism

In this condition, serum TSH is elevated with low normal serum levels of T3 and T4. This may persist for many years, and there is risk for conversion to overt hypothyroidism especially if thyroid antibodies are present or if TSH is above 10 mIU/L. Such patients should be treated with levothyroxine. Patients with nonspecific symptoms and with laboratory findings of subclinical hypothyroidism should be treated with levothyroxine, and the dose should be sufficient to make TSH serum level within normal [2].

11. Sickle cell anemia and hypothyroidism

Sickle cell anemia is an inherited hemoglobinopathy resulting in sickling of erythrocytes that cause micro-vascular obstruction, leading to acute complications and chronic organ damage. Adults with SCA have endocrine complications and metabolic alterations. A study was conducted among patients with SCA who have high serum ferritin level to assess the association between gonadal and thyroid hormones with iron indices. It was found that there was a significant relation between serum ferritin level in patients with sickle cell who have high serum ferritin level and the following: serum iron, TIBC, serum testosterone, LH, prolactin, free T3, and free T4. This was most likely due to endocrine dysfunction secondary to high ferritin level and iron overload. The explanation of endocrine dysfunction is due to vaso-occlusion secondary to polymerization of red blood cells, leading to microcirculation and endocrine organ damage. In addition, the damage to endocrine system in SCA could be indirect *via* anemia, tissue hypoxia, and iron overload. Endocrine system dysfunction was reported as the most common and earliest complication of sickle cell disease. Thyroid disorders were frequently reported in patients with SCA. So, such patients need regular clinical monitoring with frequent checkup for serum ferritin level and hormonal assays, including test for thyroid hormones [3]. However further studies are recommended to detect if the severity of sickle cell disease affects hormonal levels in these patients.

12. Conclusions

In conclusion, hypothyroidism is a common condition and has a variety of causes and needs high clinical suspicion for diagnosis and screening because it has diverse clinical manifestations. Screening for neonates, elderly, and special groups of population (patients who have had treatment of hyperthyroidism or neck irradiation, etc.) is recommended. TFT is the diagnostic test for hypothyroidism, and the definitive treatment is hormone replacements for life. Patients with SCA need frequent checkup for hypothyroidism as it is one of the most frequent complications of SCA.

Acknowledgements

Special thanks to my son, Mohab Abdallhameed, for helping me with this book chapter and for being there for me throughout all of my other publications. No matter how much I write I cannot thank him enough. I'd also like to thank my family for their tremendous support and endless love despite being displaced from home because of the war in Sudan. Hoping that the disastrous war will end soon and I, along with my Sudanese brothers and sisters will return safely to our homes and we will meet once again soon.

Conflict of interest

The authors declare no conflict of interest.

Thanks

I'd like to thank Mr. Dorian Salatic, the publishing process manager of Intechopen for his help and support and my thanks extends to all the team of Intechopen.

Author details

Sawsan A. Omer[1*] and Mohab Elmubarak[2]

1 Faculty of Medicine, Department of Internal Medicine, University of Gezira, Sudan

2 University of Gezira, Sudan

*Address all correspondence to: sawsanomer63@yahoo.co.uk

References

[1] Kumar P, Clark ML. Kumar and Clark's Clinical Medicine. 8th ed. UK: Elsevier Health Sciences; 2012. p. 940, 959-961

[2] Ralston SH, Penman ID, SMW J, Hobson RP. Davidson's Principles and Practice of Medicine. London: Elsevier; 2018. pp. 634-642

[3] Mostafa GG, Zahran FE, Omer SA, Ibrahim A, Elhakeem H. The effect of serum ferritin level on gonadal, prolactin, thyroid hormones, and thyroid stimulating hormone in adult males with sickle cell anemia. Journal of Blood Medicine. 2020;**11**:27-32. DOI: 10.2147/jbm.s232562

[4] Siegenthaler W. Differential Diagnosis in Internal Medicine. Stuttgart: Thieme; 2007. pp. 484-489

[5] Baliga RR. 250 Cases in Clinical Medicine. Edinburgh: Elsevier/Saunders; 2012. pp. 516-520

[6] Tierney LM, Saint S, Whooley MA. Essentials of Diagnosis & Treatment. 2nd ed. New York: Lange Medical Books/McGraw Hill; 2002. p. 179

[7] Weetman AP. Fortnightly review—Hypothyroidism: Screening and subclinical disease. BMJ. 1997;**314**:1175-1178

Chapter 2

Hypothyroidism: Pathophysiology and Management

Nitya Virippil, Amanda Merck, Emily Beckett, Sarah Exley and Udaya Kabadi

Abstract

The thyroid plays an essential role in the homeostasis of the human body. Its hormones, thyroxine (T4) and triiodothyronine (T3), affect nearly every cell by regulating basal metabolism, protein synthesis, and growth and development. Hypothyroidism is a result of thyroid hypofunction. It can be described as a primary or central disorder. Primary disorders are dysfunctions of the thyroid gland itself, whereas central disorders occur due to disruptions in the HPT axis. Primary hypothyroidism has a higher incidence compared to central. It is predicted that 4.6% of Americans have hypothyroidism without knowing. Therefore, it is integral for healthcare providers to recognize and treat hypothyroidism to prevent morbidity. Clinical manifestations are nonspecific but play a role in determining the diagnosis, severity, and treatment strategies. Diagnosis is made with TSH and serum free T4 levels. Through adequate treatment, patients can achieve symptom resolution and euthyroidism. This chapter describes the epidemiology, etiology, pathophysiology, clinical manifestations, and treatments of hypothyroidism.

Keywords: hypothyroidism, thyroid, HPT axis, hypothalamic-pituitary-thyroid axis, TSH, thyroid stimulating hormone, T3, T4, thyroxine, triiodothyronine, thyroid disorders

1. Introduction

The thyroid plays an essential role in maintaining homeostasis of the body. Its function is regulated by the hypothalamic-pituitary-thyroid (HPT) axis and the associated feedback loops. The hypothalamus synthesizes and secretes thyrotropin-releasing hormone (TRH) which activates the release of thyroid-stimulating hormone (TSH) by pituitary thyrotrophs. TSH binds to the receptor on the thyroid gland and stimulates the synthesis and secretion of thyroid hormones (TH). The thyroid is composed of two main endocrine cell types, follicular cells and parafollicular C-cells. C-cells produce calcitonin which couples with parathyroid hormone to maintain serum calcium. However, this will not be discussed further as it is beyond the scope of this review of hypothyroidism [1]. The follicular cells are responsible for producing both inactive thyroxine (T4) and active triiodothyronine

(T3) with a circulating T4:T3 ratio of 13:1–16:1 [2]. Serum TSH levels are determined by TRH stimulation, negative feedback with T3, temperature, and diurnal pulse secretion. About 80% of T3 is generated in peripheral tissues via conversion of T4 by deiodinase enzymes, and it is considered the active hormone due to its ten-fold greater affinity for thyroid hormone receptors compared to T4 [3]. TH influences almost every cell in the body to regulate basal metabolism, protein synthesis, as well as growth and development [4].

Thyroid dysfunction is categorized as primary or central. Primary disorders result from dysfunction of the thyroid gland itself, whereas central disease states occur due to disruption of the hypothalamic-pituitary-thyroid axis [3]. Alternatively, thyroid disorders may be classified as physiologic, anatomical, and mixed.

According to the American Thyroid Association (ATA), it is estimated that 20 million Americans have a thyroid disorder with almost 60% being unaware of the presence. The ATA estimates that 1 in 8 women are likely to manifest a thyroid disease during their lifetime. Epidemiology estimates predict women are 5–8 times more prone than men to present with a thyroid disorder. Therefore, it is important for primary healthcare providers to be familiar with common thyroid disorders for early recognition and treatment options to prevent further morbidity associated with thyroid dysfunction.

Screening recommendations for thyroid dysfunction in asymptomatic adults vary wildly [5]. The American Academy of Family Physicians (AAFP) recommends screening subjects ≥60 years of age. Alternatively, the ATA recommends screening both women and men >35 years of age every 5 years. The American Association of Clinical Endocrinologists (AACE) recommends screening older patients without a specific age guideline, especially women. Lastly, the American College of Physicians (ACP) recommends screening in women ≥50 years of age with symptoms suggestive of thyroid disease [6]. Additionally, several organizations suggest assessment of thyroid function in pregnant women [7]. Utilizing any of the screening guidelines may be appropriate with good clinical judgment based on history, especially the presence of thyroid disorder in a family member, and a physical examination. Screening should be initiated in the presence of other manifestations including dyslipidemia, dementia, mental status changes, menstrual irregularities, atrial fibrillation, etc.

This review describes the epidemiology, etiology, pathophysiology, and clinical manifestations of hypothyroidism.

2. Epidemiology/etiology

Hypothyroidism is defined as high serum TSH in the presence of low serum-free T4. Hypothyroidism's prevalence varies between 0.1% and 2.0%. However, it's predicted around 4.6% of people in the United States have hypothyroidism without them knowing [8]. Women are up to 8-times more likely to have hypothyroidism compared to men. Other risk factors include personal or family history of autoimmune diseases, increased age, anti-thyroid peroxidase antibodies (TPOAb), genetic diseases like Down Syndrome or Turner Syndrome, and Caucasian and Asian ethnicities [8–13]. The main cause of hypothyroidism in iodine-sufficient areas is Hashimoto's thyroiditis, a chronic autoimmune disorder characterized by the formation of autoantibodies against the thyroid, leading to its destruction [14]. Other causes include excessive treatment of hyperthyroidism, the presence of a goiter, iodine deficiency or excess, and certain medications [15].

DOI: http://dx.doi.org/10.5772/intechopen.1004851

3. Clinical manifestations

Symptoms of hypothyroidism are nonspecific but can play a role in determining the diagnosis, severity, and treatment strategies of hypothyroidism [15]. See **Table 1** for clinical signs and symptoms.

4. Diagnosis

TSH levels must be drawn to make the clinical diagnosis since symptoms are nonspecific. High serum TSH above the upper limit of normal (ULN) with low serum T4 levels are seen in patients with hypothyroidism. The ULN depends on the laboratory but is commonly referenced as 4–5 miU/L. If a patient has hypothyroid symptoms, but normal TSH levels and low serum free T4 levels even after repeat, it may be due to central hypothyroidism [6]. TPOAb and thyroglobulin antibodies (TgAb) are positive in most patients with hypothyroidism due to Hashimoto's thyroiditis [6]. TPOAb is not routinely measured to determine the diagnosis, however, situations that may be helpful to measure TPOAb include patients with a goiter in the absence of hypothyroidism, subclinical hypothyroidism, painless thyroiditis, or postpartum thyroiditis, as is discussed below. This can help predict the chance of progressing to overt hypothyroidism [6].

Organ system	Hypothyroidism	Hyperthyroidism
Constitutional	Fatigue, weight gain, cold intolerance	Heat intolerance, weight loss, goiter, fatigue
Skin	Dry or coarse skin, hair loss	Sweating, warm skin, onycholysis, softening of nails, hyperpigmentation, pruritis, thinning of hair
Neuromuscular	Muscle weakness, cramps, arthralgia, increased creatine kinase	Tremor, weakness
Cardiovascular	Decreased cardiac output, bradycardia, decreased contractility, decreased exercise capacity	Palpitations, tachycardia, systolic hypertension, cardiomyopathy, atrial fibrillation, mitral valve prolapse
Gastrointestinal	Decreased gut motility, constipation, decreased taste sensation, gastric atrophy, nonalcoholic fatty liver disease, ascites (rare)	Anorexia, vomiting, hyperdefecation, dysphagia due to goiter, increased liver function tests, abdominal tenderness
Metabolic	Hyponatremia, reversible serum creatin increases, hyperlipidemia	Osteoporosis, hyperglycemia, reduced HDL, gynecomastia in men
Hematologic	Pernicious anemia	Normochromic, normocytic anemia, increased clotting factors
Genitourinary	Menstrual irregularities, oligomenorrhea, amenorrhea, hypermenorrhea-menorrhagia, sexual dysfunction, decreased fertility	Urinary frequency, amenorrhea, reduced libido, decreased fertility
Neuropsychiatric	Slowed mentation, poor concentration, mood impairment	Agitation, depression, anxiety, confusion, poor concentration, nervousness, disturbed sleep

Table 1.
Signs and symptoms of hypo- and hyperthyroidism [16–19].

5. Management

The goals of treatment are symptoms resolution and to achieve euthyroidism. First line treatment for hypothyroidism is synthetic T4, levothyroxine. Most patients can meet their goals with T4 monotherapy. This results in fewer cardiovascular side effects compared to T3 and T4 therapy combined. Levothyroxine's normal starting dose is 1.6 mcg/kg per day for adults. However, patients >60 years old or patients with coronary artery disease should be initiated at a lower dose of 12.5–25 mcg/day [20]. Additional situations that would call for lower doses are weight loss >10% of body weight and initiation of androgen therapy [20]. Alternatively, patients being treated with estrogen therapy or who are pregnant will require higher doses than usual patients. Patients with celiac or Crohn's disease or a history of bariatric surgery may require higher doses as well due to decreased absorption [9].

Appropriate administration of thyroid hormone is important in achieving appropriate therapeutic levels. Levothyroxine should be taken on an empty stomach 30–60 minutes before breakfast around the same time each day. It is recommended to avoid changing between generic or brand name equivalents for levothyroxine due to variations in formulations in terms of potency and bioavailability.

Medications that can decrease levothyroxine absorption should be separated by 4 hours before or after administration [21]. **Table 2** lists common medications that can impact levothyroxine levels [21, 22]. If administration habits are changed or a medication is added or discontinued, evaluating TSH levels and adjusting doses is necessary. Encouraging patients to let their providers know if medications have been added, stopped, or doses adjusted will also allow for better disease state management.

Most patients taking levothyroxine tolerate it without adverse effects [20]. Headache, palpitations, and anxiety are common side effects, but they may be mitigated by starting at a lower dose and titrating slowly. Some major adverse effects that can occur with overcorrecting thyroid levels include atrial fibrillation and osteoporosis. In patients with dye hypersensitivity, the 50 mcg tablets can be used to avoid allergic reactions [20].

The idea of using combination therapy with both T4 and T3 is to mimic the normal 13:1–16:1 ratio in physiologic circulation [20]. The combination may be beneficial in patients in whom conversion of T4 to T3 in peripheral tissues is inhibited secondary to chronic illness, diets, or drugs. However, combination therapy is not currently recommended by either the ATA or AACE guidelines for most patients. There is a lack of evidence supporting the superiority of combination therapy compared to T4 monotherapy, even in patients who are still symptomatic on levothyroxine therapy [16, 20]. Certain situations may be appropriate to trial combination therapy, but patients should be closely monitored to avoid inducing hyperthyroidism. This includes patients on T4 monotherapy who are still symptomatic after a thyroidectomy or ablative therapy with radioiodine or have a serum T3 level that is subnormal. Combination therapy is better avoided in the elderly, pregnant patients, and anyone with the presence of cardiovascular disease [20].

Desiccated thyroid, also known as thyroid extract, is not a preferred treatment for hypothyroidism. It has not been shown to be superior to levothyroxine and there are clinical concerns with thyroid extracts. The ratio of T4 to T3 in desiccated thyroid is 4.2:1 compared to the ~14:1 secreted by the normal thyroid gland. The ratio poses the risk of supraphysiologic levels, and the shorter half-life causes greater fluctuations of T3 throughout the day. This can increase the risk of thyrotoxicosis if not carefully monitored [20].

DOI: http://dx.doi.org/10.5772/intechopen.1004851

Decreases absorption	• Bile acid sequestrants (cholestyramine, colestipol, colesevelam) • Sucralfate • Cation exchange resins (Kayexelate) • Oral bisphosphonates • Proton pump inhibitors • Multivitamins (containing ferrous sulfate or calcium carbonate) • Ferrous sulfate • Phosphonate binders (sevelamer, aluminum, hydroxide) • Calcium salts (carbonate, citrate, acetate) • Chromium picolinate • Charcoal • Orlistat • Ciprofloxacin
Increases clearance	• Phenobarbital • Primidone • Phenytoin • Carbamazepine • Oxcarbazepine • Rifampin • Growth hormone • Sertraline • Tyrosine kinase inhibitors • Quetiapine • Stavudine
Peripheral metabolism	• Amiodarone: impair conversion of T4 to T3 • Glucocorticoids and some beta-blockers at high doses: impair conversion of T4 to T3 (may not be clinically relevant)

Table 2.
Medications that Impact Levothyroxine [6, 21] (derived from ATA/AACE Guidelines for Hypothyroidism).

Steady-state concentrations may not be achieved until 6 weeks of levothyroxine use; however, symptoms should improve within 2 weeks of therapy. It is recommended to measure serum TSH 6–8 weeks after initiating treatment and levothyroxine be titrated by 12.5–25 mcg depending on the TSH levels and subsequently rechecked after an additional 4–6 weeks [20]. Thereafter, follow-up visits at 6–12 month intervals suffice for monitoring. Assessing TSH sooner may be necessary with changes in the patient's overall health status or if interacting medications are initiated or discontinued [20]. However, determining TSH alone may be counterproductive in patients with unreliable compliance. Determination of free T4 is helpful in assessing compliance, appropriate administration, as well as gastrointestinal absorption. It is important to note that after starting treatment for hypothyroidism, the metabolism of other medications may be increased and should be monitored closely as well, especially high-risk medications.

6. Pregnancy

Pregnancy increases the demands of thyroid hormone for proper development of the fetus. Overt hypothyroidism in pregnancy is defined as an elevated TSH and a decreased T4 outside of the trimester-specific normal ranges. Normal ranges as defined by the institutional laboratory should be adhered to for diagnosis of thyroid dysfunction. Serum TPOAb should be determined as its presence has been documented to increase the risk of pregnancy-related adverse outcomes [7].

Hypothyroidism in pregnancy increases the risk of several adverse outcomes including premature birth, low birth weight, decreased fetal neurocognitive development, and pregnancy loss. Therefore, prompt treatment of hypothyroidism is recommended. Evidence of treatment for subclinical hypothyroidism is not well defined. However, subjects with subclinical hypothyroidism and positive TPOAb are prone to increased risk of complications, and levothyroxine supplementation has been documented to improve outcomes [7].

Levothyroxine is the thyroid hormone of choice for hypothyroid treatment in pregnancy as well. T3 or desiccated thyroid must not be used due to an increased risk of attaining supraphysiologic levels of T3 and the inability of T3 to cross the fetal central nervous system. In patients already on levothyroxine, increases in doses may be required within 4–6 weeks of pregnancy. Levothyroxine requirements increase through 16–20 weeks due to a rise in thyroid hormone binding globulin caused by increasing circulating estrogen levels as well as enhanced renal clearance. According to the American Thyroid Association, a dose increase of 20–30% should be prescribed preemptively once pregnancy is confirmed prior to further testing. Monitoring TSH every 4 weeks until midgestation and at least once around 30 weeks is recommended [7]. The daily dose frequently declines over 3–4 weeks postpartum.

7. Subclinical hypothyroidism

Subclinical hypothyroidism is defined as elevated TSH with T4 levels in the normal range. Prevalence of this is greater than overt hypothyroidism with a rate of 4.3% in the National Health and Nutrition Examination Survey (NHANES III) and 8.5% in the Colorado Thyroid Prevalence Study [6]. Prevalence is higher in adults aged 65 years or older at a rate of 8–18% and it is more commonly seen in women compared to men [23]. Common causes include medications, thyroiditis, thyroid infiltration, and TSH gene mutation.

Treatment is controversial if TSH levels are 4.5–10 miU/L, but is usually recommended if >10 miU/L. The rationale for treatment includes prevention of progression to overt hypothyroidism and development of cardiovascular events, whereas consensus against treatment is based on the absence of data showing long-term progression in many patients, risk of overtreatment including hyperthyroid manifestations and complications such as arrhythmia and osteoporosis especially in the elderly, as well as the cost and commitment of lifelong therapy [24]. Levothyroxine is the preferred agent for subclinical hypothyroidism with similar monitoring as overt hypothyroidism but with a lower initiating dose. Depending on the TSH elevation, a daily dose of 25–75 mcg may be appropriate [6]. A randomized, double-blinded control trial looked for potential benefits of treating older adults with subclinical hypothyroidism. They found no difference in thyroid symptoms or a tiredness score between patients receiving treatment versus placebo at 6–8 weeks of treatment. Cardiovascular events were not measured since it was underpowered to determine this outcome [23]. However, several recent studies recommend attaining a serum TSH level between 5 and 10 miU/L in elderly patients as survival is longer with this TSH level in comparison to subjects achieving normal TSH concentrations [24–29].

The presence of TPOAb can help decide whether to treat or not. It was found that patients with subclinical hypothyroidism and positive TPOAb levels have a 4.6% rate per year of progression to overt hypothyroidism compared to those with negative levels at 2.6% per year [6]. Overall, deciding to treat a patient or not should be based on the risks, benefits, patient preference, and clinical decision-making.

8. Hashimoto's thyroiditis

Hashimoto's thyroiditis is a chronic autoimmune disease that causes the destruction of the thyroid gland. It is the most common cause of hypothyroidism in iodine-sufficient areas [14, 30]. The clinical manifestations are similar to classic hypothyroidism symptoms. It is rare to have pain associated with Hashimoto's thyroiditis [30].

Autoantibodies attack the thyroid gland causing it to lose function over time, leading to hypothyroidism. However, it is important to note that these autoantibodies may not be present in all cases. Checking TSH, TPOAb, and TgAb along with analyzing a thyroid ultrasound will help determine a Hashimoto's thyroiditis diagnosis [30].

There is not one specific cause of Hashimoto's thyroiditis, but it is more so thought to be due to both genetic and environmental factors. Specific genes that play a role in T cell function, thyroid development, and thyroid hormone enzymes have been identified among patients with Hashimoto's. Other precipitating factors include high iodine intake, stress, radiation exposure, sex steroids, and infection [30].

The primary treatment of Hashimoto's thyroiditis is targeted towards replenishing thyroid hormone since it causes destruction of the thyroid [30].

9. Conclusions

The thyroid is integral to the body's ability to maintain homeostasis. Through the release of thyrotropin-releasing hormone (TRH) from the hypothalamus and thyroid-stimulating hormone (TSH) by the pituitary gland, thyroid hormones regulate basal metabolism, protein synthesis, and growth and development. Hypothyroidism is a thyroid gland disorder that can occur at the level of the thyroid or within the hypothalamic-pituitary-thyroid axis. Clinical manifestations of hypothyroidism include fatigue, weight gain, cold intolerance, hair loss, muscle cramps, constipation, menstrual irregularities, and slowed mentation.

Diagnosis cannot be made with symptoms only as they are nonspecific. With primary hypothyroidism, patients typically have high serum TSH and low serum T4 laboratory values. If a patient has hypothyroid symptoms, normal TSH, and low serum T4, it may be due to central hypothyroidism. Antibodies to thyroid peroxidase (TPOAb) or thyroglobulin (TgAb) indicate Hashimoto's Thyroiditis, which is hypothyroidism due to the autoimmune destruction of the thyroid gland.

Treatment of hypothyroidism is focused on achieving euthyroidism. The first-line treatment for hypothyroidism is levothyroxine, which is a synthetic T4. T4 monotherapy is favored over T3 and T4 combination due to fewer cardiovascular side effects.

Many medications affect the absorption, clearance, or metabolism of levothyroxine, and therefore should be noted while prescribing the medication. Pregnancy causes increased demands for thyroid hormones to support the proper development of the fetus. Therefore, prompt treatment of hypothyroidism is recommended.

Primary care physicians should utilize any of the screening guidelines along with maintaining good clinical judgment based on history, physical exam, and laboratory values. Following the initiation of medication, serum TSH levels should be measured 6–8 weeks later to ensure adequate treatment.

Conflict of interest

The authors declare no conflict of interest.

Author details

Nitya Virippil[1*], Amanda Merck[2], Emily Beckett[3,4], Sarah Exley[3] and Udaya Kabadi[3,4]

1 Des Moines University, West Des Moines, Iowa, United States of America

2 VA Salt Lake Health Center, Salt Lake City, Utah, United States of America

3 Broadlawns Medical Center, Des Moines, Iowa, United States of America

4 University of Iowa, Iowa City, Iowa, United States of America

*Address all correspondence to: nitya.virippil@gmail.com

References

[1] Armstrong M, Asuka E, Fingeret A. Physiology, Thyroid Function. Treasure Island, FL: StatPearls Publishing; 2020. Available from: https://www.ncbi.nlm.nih.gov/books/NBK537039/

[2] Wiersinga WM, Duntas L, Fadeyev V, Nygaard B, Vanderpump MP. 2021 ETA Guidelines: The use of L-T4 + L-T3 in the treatment of hypothyroidism. European Thyroid Journal. 2012;**1**(2):55-71

[3] Ortiga-Carvalho TM, Chiamolera MI, Pazos-Moura CC, Wondisford FE. Hypothalamus-pituitary-thyroid axis. Comprehensive Physiology. 2016;**6**(3):1387-1428

[4] General Information/Press Room. American Thyroid Association. Prevalence and Impact of Thyroid, are unaware of their condition. 2020. Available from: https://www.thyroid.org/media-main/press-room/#:~:text [Accessed: June 22, 2020]

[5] LeFevre M et al. Screening for thyroid dysfunction: U.S. preventive services task force recommendation statement. Annals of Internal Medicine. 2015;**162**:641-650

[6] Garber J. Clinical practice guidelines for hypothyroidism in adults: Cosponsored by the American association of clinical endocrinologists and the American Thyroid Association. Endocrine Practice. 2012;**18**(6):988-1028

[7] Alexander EK, Pearce EN, Brent GA, et al. 2017 guidelines of the American Thyroid Association for the diagnosis and management of thyroid disease during pregnancy and the postpartum. Thyroid. 2017;**27**(3):315-389

[8] Tunbridge WM, Evered DC, Hall R, et al. The spectrum of thyroid disease in a community: The Whickham survey. Clinical Endocrinology. 1977;**7**(6):481-493

[9] Vanderpump MP, Tunbridge WM, French JM, et al. The incidence of thyroid disorders in the community: A twenty-year follow-up of the Whickham survey. Clinical Endocrinology. 1995;**43**(91):55-68

[10] Vanderpump MP, Tunbridge WM. The epidemiology of thyroid diseases. In: Braverman LE, Utiger RD, editors. The Thyroid: A Fundamental and Clinical Text. 8th ed. Philadelphia: Lippincott Williams and Wilkins; 2000. p. 467

[11] Canaris GJ, Manowitz NR, Mayor G, Ridgway EC. The Colorado thyroid disease prevalence study. Archives of Internal Medicine. 2000;**160**(4):526-534

[12] Aoki Y, Belin RM, Clickner R, Jeffries R, Phillips L, Mahaffey KR. Serum TSH and total T4 in the United States population and their association with participant characteristics: National Health and Nutrition Examination Survey (NHANES 1999-2002). Thyroid. 2007;**17**(12):1211-1223

[13] American Thyroid Association. Hypothyroidism a Booklet for Patients and their Families. 2013. Available from: https://www.thyroid.org/wp-content/uploads/patients/brochures/Hypothyroidism_web_booklet.pdf.

[14] American Thyroid Association. Hashimoto's Thyroiditis (Lymphocytic Thyroiditis). n.d. Available from: https://www.thyroid.org/hashimotos-thyroiditis/#:~:text=There%20are%20many%20possible%20causes,chronic%20inflammation%20of%20the%20thyroid

[15] Haugen BR. Drugs that suppress TSH or cause central hypothyroidism. Best Practice & Research. Clinical Endocrinology & Metabolism. 2009;**23**(6):793-800

[16] Chaker L, Bianco AC, Jonklaas J, Peeters RP. Hypothyroidism. Lancet. 2017;**390**(10101):1550-1562

[17] De Leo S, Lee SY, Braverman LE. Hyperthyroidism. Lancet. 2016;**388**:906-918

[18] Nordyke RA, Gilbert FI Jr, Harada AS. Graves' disease: Influence of age on clinical findings. Archives of Internal Medicine. 1988;**148**:626

[19] Woeber KA. Thyrotoxicosis and the heart. The New England Journal of Medicine. 1992;**327**:94

[20] Jonklaas J, Bianco AC, Bauer AJ, et al. Guidelines for the treatment of hypothyroidism: Prepared by the American thyroid association task force on thyroid hormone replacement. Thyroid. 2014;**24**(12):1670-1751

[21] Levothyroxine® [package insert]. Caguas. Puerto Rico: Neolpharma, Inc; 2017

[22] Dong BJ. How medications affect thyroid function. The Western Journal of Medicine. 2000;**172**(2):102-106

[23] Stott DJ, Rodondi N, Kearney PM, et al. Thyroid hormone therapy for older adults with subclinical hypothyroidism. The New England Journal of Medicine. 2017;**376**(26):2534-2544

[24] Biondi B, Cappola AR, Cooper DS. Subclinical hypothyroidism: A review. Journal of the American Medical Association. 2019;**322**(2):153-160

[25] Ross DS. Treating hypothyroidism is not always easy: When to treat subclinical hypothyroidism, TSH goals in the elderly, and alternatives to levothyroxine monotherapy. Journal of Internal Medicine. 2022;**291**(2):128-140

[26] Biondi B, Cappola AR. Subclinical hypothyroidism in older individuals. The Lancet Diabetes and Endocrinology. 2022;**10**(2):129-1414

[27] Duntas LH, Yen PM. Diagnosis and treatment of hypothyroidism in the elderly. Endocrine. 2019;**66**(1):63-69

[28] Effraimidis G, Watt T, Feldt-Rasmussen U. Levothyroxine therapy in elderly patients with hypothyroidism. Frontier in Endocrinology (Lausanne). 2021;**12**:641560. Published March 12, 2021

[29] Calissendorff J, Falhammar H. To treat or not to treat subclinical hypothyroidism, what is the evidence? Medicina (Kaunas). 2020;**56**(1):40. Published January 19, 2020

[30] Ragusa F, Fallahi P, Elia G, et al. Hashimoto's thyroiditis: Epidemiology, pathogenesis, clinic and therapy. Best Practice & Research. Clinical Endocrinology & Metabolism. 2019;**33**(6):101367

Chapter 3

Hypothyroidism and Gut Microbiota

Amirreza Rafiei Javazm

Abstract

The complex interplay between hypothyroidism and gut microbiota is investigated, particularly focusing on how minerals such as iodine, selenium, and iron affect thyroid function and the involvement of gut bacteria in their absorption and processing. The mechanisms by which gut microbiota regulate mineral absorption and thyroid hormone metabolism are clarified, emphasizing their importance in hypothyroidism management and treatment outcomes. Furthermore, the influence of sex hormones and age on gut microbiota composition is analyzed, suggesting a potential role in hypothyroidism development. Additionally, while probiotics hold promise for managing hypothyroidism, conflicting evidence from clinical trials highlights the need for further research to ascertain their efficacy.

Keywords: hypothyroidism, gut microbiota, probiotics, iodide, levothyroxine

1. Introduction

Hypothyroidism is a prevalent medical condition often diagnosed due to its substantial impact on various physiological aspects such as metabolic rate, growth, fertility, and cognitive functions [1]. Minerals play a crucial role in thyroid function and can significantly influence the development and management of hypothyroidism. Among these minerals, iodine is a key component of thyroid hormones T4 and T3, essential for regulating metabolism, growth, and development. Inadequate iodine intake can lead to iodine deficiency, a primary cause of hypothyroidism, particularly in regions with low dietary iodine levels. Selenium acts as a cofactor for enzymes involved in the conversion of T4 to T3, thus ensuring proper thyroid hormone synthesis and metabolism. Deficiencies in selenium have been associated with impaired thyroid function and may exacerbate hypothyroidism symptoms. Iron is necessary for thyroid hormone production and plays a critical role in the synthesis and secretion of these hormones. Insufficient iron levels can impair thyroid hormone synthesis and lead to hypothyroidism, highlighting the importance of adequate iron intake for maintaining thyroid health [2–4].

In the human intestine, a complex ecosystem comprising bacteria, fungi, viruses, and various other microorganisms collectively forms the intestinal microbiota. Among these microorganisms, aerobic and anaerobic bacteria predominantly constitute the microbial community. In typical conditions, the reciprocal relationship between the intestinal microbiota and the host sustains a dynamic equilibrium.

However, when the self-regulatory capacity of the human micro-ecosystem is exceeded, the resulting state of intestinal dysbiosis may precipitate the onset of disease [5]. There is evidence indicating a correlation between the makeup of the gut microbiota and the levels of thyroid hormones [6].

The gut microbiota wields a multifaceted influence over mineral absorption and thyroid hormone metabolism, operating through a spectrum of mechanisms. These intestinal bacteria play a pivotal role in modulating the bioavailability of essential minerals such as iodine, selenium, and iron, which are integral to thyroid function [7–9]. Additionally, the composition and activity of the gut microbiota can impact the efficiency and effectiveness of medications prescribed for thyroid disorders. These intestinal bacteria have the potential to modulate the absorption, metabolism, and distribution of thyroid medications, thereby influencing their therapeutic outcomes. Furthermore, alterations in gut microbiota composition induced by various factors such as diet, lifestyle, and medication use can further complicate thyroid medication management by potentially altering drug metabolism and bioavailability [10].

2. Iodine and gut microbiota

There are three primary forms of iodine:

1. Iodide (I^-)

2. Iodate ($IO3^-$), typically added to salt for iodization

3. Naturally bound iodine found in food.

The majority of ingested iodide is absorbed within the duodenum, the initial segment of the small intestine. Upon ingestion of iodate, it undergoes reduction to iodide within the gastrointestinal tract before being assimilated by the body. Conversely, when iodine is bound to other food constituents, the digestive process liberates iodide for subsequent absorption [2, 7, 11]. Iodide absorption in the gut involves the sodium/iodide symporter (NIS) on enterocyte membranes, along with other carriers such as sodium multivitamin transporter (SMVT) and cystic fibrosis transmembrane conductance regulator (CFTR) [12–14]. And through molecular mechanisms, iodide enters the bloodstream [7]. So, iodide plays a pivotal role in the synthesis of thyroid hormones, as it is actively concentrated by the thyroid gland through specialized transporters and serves as the critical raw material for hormone production [15].

The function of the gut microbiota is crucial, as it can control the metabolism of iodine. Gut bacteria contribute to this process by releasing compounds such as lipopolysaccharides (LPS) and short-chain fatty acids (SCFAs) [16]. Lipopolysaccharide (LPS), commonly referred to as endotoxin, is a constituent found in the outer cell wall of Gram-negative bacteria, with the gut microbiota being the primary origin of LPS in humans. Its well-known function involves triggering conditions such as sepsis, septic shock, and multiple organ failure [17]. LPS interferes with thyroid homeostasis through several mechanisms.

In one of these LPS mechanisms, it has been demonstrated that LPS boosts the activity of the TSH-stimulated TG gene at the transcriptional level in thyroid follicular cells [18]. Furthermore, LPS has the potential to influence the function of the NIS gene, responsible for encoding the sodium/iodide symporter protein. This protein

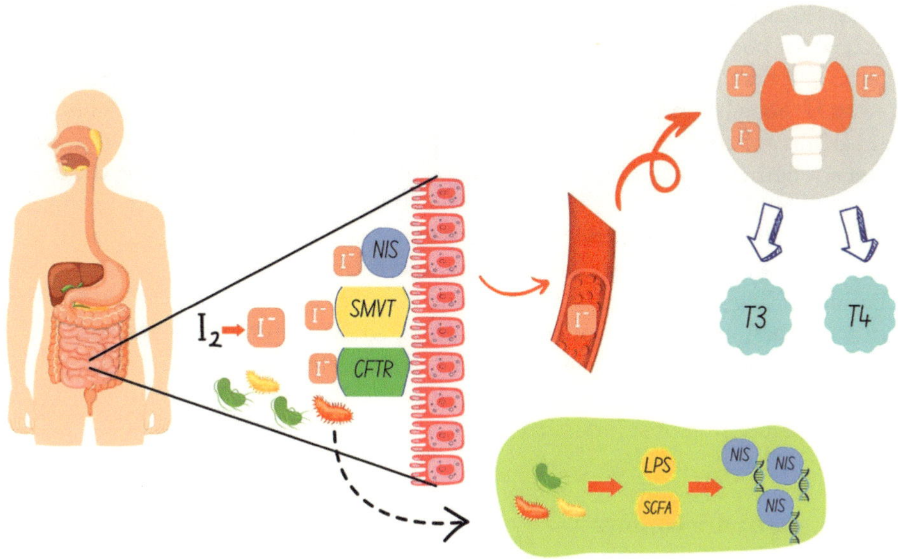

Figure 1.
The influence of gut microbiota on thyroid function.

plays a critical role in transporting iodine into thyroid cells, a crucial step in thyroid hormone synthesis. Thus, by elevating NIS gene expression, LPS can augment the thyroid cells' capacity to absorb iodine, thereby impacting thyroid hormone production and function [19].

In the thyroid gland, the signaling pathway involving nuclear factor kappa-B (NF-κB) is vital for the survival of thyrocytes and the expression of key thyroid markers such as Nis, Ttf1, Pax8, Tpo, and thyroglobulin. This transcription factor is indispensable for preserving normal thyroid function. Research indicates that lipopolysaccharide (LPS) acts as a facilitator in activating nuclear factor kappa-B (NF-κB) through toll-like receptor 4 (TLR-4) on thyroid cells. This highlights the importance of LPS in NF-κB activation, which plays a critical role in controlling thyroid cell function [20].

Similarly, SCFAs, produced by gut bacteria, are pivotal in regulating NIS expression in thyroid cells. Notably, SCFAs such as butyric acid inhibit histone deacetylation, reactivating the NIS gene in thyroid cancer cells, thus assisting in restoring their typical functions and facilitating iodine absorption. This intriguing finding was not exclusive to thyroid cancer cells; it was also observed in various other cancer cell types such as MCF-7, Hep-G2, and MKN-7. This implies that altering SCFAs to promote histone acetylation and increase NIS expression might enhance tumor cells' sensitivity to radioactive iodine. However, further research is needed for a comprehensive understanding of this phenomenon (**Figure 1**) [16].

3. Selenium and gut microbiota

In the thyroid gland, selenium plays a crucial role in acting as an antioxidant and aiding in the metabolism of thyroid hormones. Selenium is essential for transforming T4 into T3. Numerous studies suggest that a lack of selenium is linked to a higher occurrence of thyroid disorders. Individuals with insufficient selenium intake may develop hypothyroidism [3]. As discussed earlier, the composition of the gut microbiota influences how the body absorbs vital thyroid nutrients. Animal research revealed that when bacterial outer membrane LPS attaches to thyroid cells' TLR-4, it triggers the NF-κB pathway, ultimately binding with PAX8, a key regulator of NIS expression. Additionally, Lactobacillus enhances the absorption of essential micronutrients like selenium, which further strengthens the binding and activation of PAX8, thereby promoting the transcription of NIS [8]. Additionally, Calomme et al. showed that Lactobacillus bacteria can change sodium selenite inside cells into selenocysteine and selenomethionine. This process helps the body absorb selenium as organic selenium [21].

Besides aiding in selenium absorption and influencing thyroid function, selenium also contributes to gut flora health. Inadequate selenium intake may lead to a gut microbiota phenotype prone to colitis and *Salmonella typhimurium* infection. Conversely, sufficient or high selenium levels in the diet can improve gut microflora, offering protection against intestinal issues and chronic diseases [22].

4. Iron and gut microbiota

Iron is a crucial element for the growth of bacteria, meaning that its availability can impact the types of bacteria that thrive in the gut. Conversely, the composition of the gut microbiota can also influence the availability of iron. Since iron plays a significant role in the efficient utilization of iodine and the synthesis of thyroid hormones, any disturbances in its levels could lead to thyroid disorders. For instance, insufficient iron levels could impair the synthesis, storage, and secretion of thyroid hormones, ultimately affecting thyroid function and potentially leading to thyroid-related health issues. Therefore, maintaining proper iron levels is essential for supporting thyroid health and overall well-being [4].

A recent laboratory study revealed that *Lactobacillus fermentum*, a bacterium commonly found in the human gut, possesses the ability to reduce ferric iron due to its secretion of p-hydroxyphenyllactic acid. This action aids in the absorption of iron in the digestive system. Furthermore, the gut microbiota has been observed to enhance the availability of dietary iron by converting ellagic acid (EA) into urolithin A (UA), which remains active without the need to bind to Fe^{3+}. UA functions to suppress the production of reactive oxygen species, offering protection against oxidative stress and inflammation.

In instances of low iron levels within the body, there is an increase in the expression of divalent metal transporter 1 (DMT1), promoting greater absorption and release of iron into the bloodstream through the action of ferroportin—a protein found in duodenal epithelial cells, among other locations. Conversely, during periods of iron overload, absorption is reduced, and excess iron is stored within enterocytes by binding to ferritin, the principal protein responsible for storing iron. Furthermore, a deficiency in dietary iron leads to a decline in populations of beneficial intestinal bacteria, such as *Roseburia*, *Bacteroides*, and *Eubacterium rectale*, while promoting the growth of strains like *Lactobacillus* and *Enterobacteriaceae* [9].

5. The association between intestinal bacteria and hypothyroidism

Previous research has highlighted the connection between hypothyroidism and gastrointestinal functionality, indicating that hypothyroidism often accompanies impaired gastrointestinal motility. This reduced motility sets the stage for the colonization and excessive proliferation of intestinal bacteria. Consequently, this bacterial overgrowth can compound issues with the neuromuscular function of the gastrointestinal tract, worsening chronic gastrointestinal symptoms in hypothyroid patients. Notably, hypothyroidism notably diminishes the motility of the gastroesophageal region. Therefore, it is advisable to evaluate thyroid function in patients exhibiting dyspeptic symptoms. Gastroesophageal scintigraphy, a noninvasive and straightforward method, can effectively assess the motility of the esophagogastric region. These evaluations offer valuable insights to clinicians in devising suitable treatment approaches for individuals with hypothyroidism [23].

The recent study conducted by Su et al. aimed to characterize the gut microbiome in individuals with primary hypothyroidism. A cohort of 52 primary hypothyroidism patients and 40 healthy controls were enrolled in the study. Significant variations in both the diversity and composition of gut microbiota were noted between hypothyroid patients and their healthy counterparts. Four specific types of intestinal bacteria emerged as potential indicators for discerning untreated hypothyroid patients from those who are healthy. The study revealed alterations in the microbial composition and function among individuals with primary hypothyroidism, with *Veillonella*, *Paraprevotella*, *Neisseria*, and *Rheinheimera* showing promise as distinguishing markers for the condition. These findings underscore a connection between primary hypothyroidism and shifts in the gut microbiome, presenting potential avenues for probiotic-based interventions in its management [24].

6. How gut microbiota interacts with hypothyroidism medications

The microbiome influences several aspects related to thyroid hormone metabolism and the effectiveness of certain medications used in thyroid disorders. The enterohepatic circulation refers to the continuous recycling of substances between the liver and the intestines. In the context of thyroid hormones, this process involves the secretion of thyroid hormones, such as thyroxine (T4), into the bloodstream by the thyroid gland. A portion of these hormones is then metabolized by the liver and excreted into the bile. In the intestines, gut bacteria may interact with bile components and metabolize thyroid hormones before they are reabsorbed back into circulation. This process, known as enterohepatic cycling, can affect the overall levels of thyroid hormones in the body and their physiological effects.

Levothyroxine is a synthetic form of the thyroid hormone thyroxine (T4) commonly used in the treatment of hypothyroidism. The bioavailability of levothyroxine refers to the proportion of the medication that reaches the systemic circulation and is available for physiological action. The gut microbiota may influence the absorption, distribution, metabolism, and excretion of levothyroxine within the gastrointestinal tract. Changes in gut microbiota composition or function can potentially alter the bioavailability of levothyroxine, impacting its effectiveness in managing hypothyroidism [10].

Furthermore, oral administration of levothyroxine necessitates its passage through the intestinal barrier to enter systemic circulation. The intestinal microbiota seems to regulate the expression of tight junction proteins, influencing intestinal permeability as well as the morphology of enterocytes and the structure of the mucus layer, which is integral to the barrier function [6]. Studies on animals indicate that germ-free mice exhibit diminished absorptive surface area in the intestines, primarily due to reduced villus height and crypt depth, along with compromised permeability leading to impaired transport of essential nutrients and ions, as well as a thinner mucus layer, impacting the absorption of medications. Certain gastrointestinal conditions can alter the composition of the microbiome, potentially increasing the need for oral levothyroxine supplementation [25].

Studies by Virili et al. [26] and Cellini et al. [27] noted an increased demand for levothyroxine in individuals with untreated celiac disease and gastrointestinal issues. For instance, in a retrospective cohort study conducted in 2017, Brechmann et al. explored various factors, including oral levothyroxine replacement therapy, in relation to the development of small intestinal bacterial overgrowth (SIBO). They discovered that both hypothyroidism itself and the use of levothyroxine were the primary factors associated with an increased risk of SIBO development [28].

In another study, Yao and colleagues looked at how the bacteria in the gut relate to the medication levothyroxine in people with a condition called subclinical hypothyroidism. They studied 117 patients and split them into groups based on their lipid profile levels. These groups were then divided into two: One group was taking levothyroxine pills, and the other group was not taking any medication. Among the patients taking levothyroxine, they further divided them into three smaller groups based on how much medication they were taking: low, medium, or high doses. The researchers found that the types of bacteria called *Odoribacter* and *Enterococcus* varied depending on how much levothyroxine the patients were taking. The medium-dose group had the most of these bacteria, while the high-dose group had the least. When they looked at all the patients taking levothyroxine compared to those not taking any medication, they found that a type of bacteria called *Ruminococcus*, which is common in the gut, was more abundant in the group not taking medication. They saw similar results with other types of bacteria called *Alistipes* and *Anaerotruncus*. The research showed that the differences in L-thyroxine doses needed to keep the TSH level stable in patients with subclinical hypothyroidism might be linked to the varied compositions of gut bacteria among individuals. This potential mechanism could be associated with the differences in how the gut metabolizes thyroxine [29].

Overall, there is an intricate relationship between the gut microbiome and thyroid hormone metabolism, with potential implications for the effectiveness of medications used in thyroid disorders such as hypothyroidism. Further research is needed to elucidate the specific mechanisms by which gut microbiota impact these processes and to explore potential therapeutic interventions targeting the gut microbiome for improved management of thyroid disorders.

7. The impact of sex hormones and age on gut microbiota

A systematic review was conducted to examine the correlation between sex hormones (estrogen and testosterone) and the makeup and variety of the gut microbiota. The review indicates a notable interaction and link between estrogen and testosterone levels and the composition and diversity of microbial populations. Specifically, it acknowledges the increasing research dedicated to understanding how estrogen influences gut microbiota, revealing a strengthening connection between estrogen and microbial structure. These findings extend not only to individuals in good health but also to those with medical conditions. However, it underscores the limited number of studies exploring the impact of testosterone on the gut microbiota compared to those centered on estrogen. Nevertheless, existing evidence suggests that testosterone also holds significance in shaping the diversity and makeup of microbial communities [30].

The makeup and variety of gut microbiota exhibit notable transformations as individuals age, as evidenced by research revealing distinct microbial profiles between older adults and younger individuals. Elderly subjects tend to harbor a greater abundance of Bacteroides species and display unique distributions of Clostridium groups compared to their younger counterparts. Moreover, centenarians often showcase shifts in the Firmicutes population alongside an enrichment in facultative anaerobes, reflecting age-related alterations in microbial composition. Similarly, studies in rodent models have linked aging with changes in gut microbiota, with aged rats exhibiting heightened levels of specific microbial groups such as Ruminococcaceae and Lachnospiraceae, recognized for their role in butyrate production.

Furthermore, gender hormones exert a pivotal influence on the gut microbiota, beginning in the early developmental stages. Investigations involving germ-free mice have shed light on the sex-specific impacts of early-life microbiota status on serotonin production, hinting at a complex interplay involving the microbiota, gender hormones, and neurodevelopment. Moreover, alterations in gonadal hormones during puberty have lasting effects on sexually dimorphic brain development, which may not be entirely reversible through hormone replacement in adulthood. Additionally, human studies have demonstrated that early-life adversities affect gut microbiota differently depending on gender, underscoring the intricate interrelationship between gender hormones, microbial composition, and host physiology [31].

In summary, both age and gender hormones wield considerable influence over the composition and diversity of the gut microbiota. Delving into the dynamic interplay between age-related changes, gender hormones, and the gut microbiota may yield valuable insights into age-related health issues and gender-specific disparities in disease susceptibility. However, further research is warranted to unravel the underlying mechanisms driving these associations and their implications for human health across different stages of life. Based on the correlation between thyroid hormones and gut microbiota, it can be inferred that sex hormones and age may play a notable role in hypothyroidism by influencing changes in gut microbiota composition. Further investigation into this relationship is warranted in future studies.

8. Using probiotics to manage hypothyroidism

Probiotics, which are live microorganisms that confer health benefits when consumed, have been investigated for their potential effects on hypothyroidism. In a clinical trial in which 60 individuals diagnosed with hypothyroidism participated, researchers conducted a randomized, double-blind, placebo-controlled study to examine the impact of synbiotic supplementation on thyroid function. The synbiotic capsules provided to the participants contained a blend of seven freeze-dried probiotic strains, including *Lactobacillus casei*, *Lactobacillus acidophilus*, *Lactobacillus rhamnosus*, *Lactobacillus bulgaricus*, *Bifidobacterium breve*, *Bifidobacterium longum*, and *Streptococcus thermophilus*. The findings from the study revealed that after an 8-week period of synbiotic supplementation, there was a significant decrease observed in the concentration of thyroid-stimulating hormone (TSH) among individuals with hypothyroidism [32].

However, in the clinical trial conducted by Spaggiari and colleagues, which utilized a combination of Lactobacilli and Bifidobacteria, there were no discernible variations noted in thyroid function when comparing the intervention group to the control group. Despite the supplementation of Lactobacilli and Bifidobacteria, which are commonly recognized as beneficial probiotic strains, the study did not reveal any significant alterations in thyroid function parameters between the two groups under investigation [33].

Additionally, a systematic review and meta-analysis study conducted in 2023 aimed at examining the advantages of probiotics, prebiotics, and synbiotics in managing thyroid diseases. The findings of this study revealed low-certainty evidence derived from two randomized trials, indicating that the regular use of probiotics, prebiotics, or synbiotics might offer minimal to no discernible benefit for individuals diagnosed with primary hypothyroidism. Despite the growing interest in the potential therapeutic role of gut microbiota modulation in thyroid disorders, the results of these trials underscore the need for further investigation and refinement of probiotic interventions to establish their efficacy in effectively managing primary hypothyroidism. Such insights gleaned from systematic reviews and meta-analyses contribute valuable evidence for guiding clinical decision-making and shaping future research endeavors aimed at optimizing treatment strategies for thyroid diseases [34].

Author details

Amirreza Rafiei Javazm
Department of Nursing, University of Social Welfare and Rehabilitation Sciences, Tehran, Iran

*Address all correspondence to: amirrezarafie@yahoo.com

References

[1] Chaker L, Bianco AC, Jonklaas J, Peeters RP. Hypothyroidism. Lancet. 2017;**390**(10101):1550-1562

[2] Zimmermann MB. Iodine deficiency. Endocrine Reviews. 2009;**30**(4):376-408

[3] Ventura M, Melo M, Carrilho F. Selenium and thyroid disease: From pathophysiology to treatment. International Journal of Endocrinology. 2017;**2017**:1297658

[4] Knezevic J, Starchl C, Tmava Berisha A, Amrein K. Thyroid-gut-axis: How does the microbiota influence thyroid function? Nutrients. 2020;**12**(6):1769

[5] Zhu X, Zhang C, Feng S, He R, Zhang S. Intestinal microbiota regulates the gut-thyroid axis: The new dawn of improving Hashimoto thyroiditis. Clinical and Experimental Medicine. 2024;**24**(1):39

[6] Virili C, Centanni M. "With a little help from my friends" - the role of microbiota in thyroid hormone metabolism and enterohepatic recycling. Molecular and Cellular Endocrinology. 2017;**458**:39-43

[7] De la Vieja A, Santisteban P. Role of iodide metabolism in physiology and cancer. Endocrine-Related Cancer. 2018;**25**(4):R225-Rr45

[8] Leoni SG, Sastre-Perona A, De la Vieja A, Santisteban P. Selenium increases thyroid-stimulating hormone-induced sodium/iodide symporter expression through thioredoxin/apurinic/apyrimidinic endonuclease 1-dependent regulation of paired box 8 binding activity. Antioxidants & Redox Signaling. 2016;**24**(15):855-866

[9] Skrypnik K, Suliburska J. Association between the gut microbiota and mineral metabolism. Journal of the Science of Food and Agriculture. 2018;**98**(7):2449-2460

[10] Fröhlich E, Wahl R. Microbiota and thyroid interaction in health and disease. Trends in Endocrinology and Metabolism. 2019;**30**(8):479-490

[11] Alexander WD, Harden RM, Harrison MT, Shimmins J. Some aspects of the absorption and concentration of iodide by the alimentary tract in man. The Proceedings of the Nutrition Society. 1967;**26**(1):62-66

[12] Ravera S, Reyna-Neyra A, Ferrandino G, Amzel LM, Carrasco N. The sodium/iodide symporter (NIS): Molecular physiology and preclinical and clinical applications. Annual Review of Physiology. 2017;**79**:261-289

[13] Quick M, Shi L. The sodium/multivitamin transporter: A multipotent system with therapeutic implications. Vitamins and Hormones. 2015;**98**:63-100

[14] Strong TV, Boehm K, Collins FS. Localization of cystic fibrosis transmembrane conductance regulator mRNA in the human gastrointestinal tract by *in situ* hybridization. The Journal of Clinical Investigation. 1994;**93**(1):347-354

[15] Rousset B, Dupuy C, Miot F, Dumont J. Thyroid Hormone Synthesis and Secretion. South Dartmouth (MA): MDText.com, Inc.; 2015

[16] Jiang W, Lu G, Gao D, Lv Z, Li D. The relationships between the gut microbiota and its metabolites with thyroid diseases.

Frontiers in Endocrinology (Lausanne). 2022;**13**:943408

[17] An L, Wirth U, Koch D, Schirren M, Drefs M, Koliogiannis D, et al. The role of gut-derived lipopolysaccharides and the intestinal barrier in fatty liver diseases. Journal of Gastrointestinal Surgery. 2022;**26**(3):671-683

[18] Vélez ML, Costamagna E, Kimura ET, Fozzatti L, Pellizas CG, Montesinos MM, et al. Bacterial lipopolysaccharide stimulates the thyrotropin-dependent thyroglobulin gene expression at the transcriptional level by involving the transcription factors thyroid transcription factor-1 and paired box domain transcription factor 8. Endocrinology. 2006;**147**(7):3260-3275

[19] Nicola JP, Nazar M, Mascanfroni ID, Pellizas CG, Masini-Repiso AM. NF-kappaB p65 subunit mediates lipopolysaccharide-induced Na(+)/I(−) symporter gene expression by involving functional interaction with the paired domain transcription factor Pax8. Molecular Endocrinology. 2010;**24**(9):1846-1862

[20] Nicola JP, Vélez ML, Lucero AM, Fozzatti L, Pellizas CG, Masini-Repiso AM. Functional toll-like receptor 4 conferring lipopolysaccharide responsiveness is expressed in thyroid cells. Endocrinology. 2009;**150**(1):500-508

[21] Calomme M, Hu J, Van den Branden K, Vanden Berghe DA, Seleno-lactobacillus. An organic selenium source. Biological Trace Element Research. 1995;**47**(1-3):379-383

[22] Zhai Q, Cen S, Li P, Tian F, Zhao J, Zhang H, et al. Effects of dietary selenium supplementation on intestinal barrier and immune responses associated with its modulation of gut microbiota. Environmental Science & Technology Letters. 2018;**5**(12):724-730

[23] Yaylali O, Kirac S, Yilmaz M, Akin F, Yuksel D, Demirkan N, et al. Does hypothyroidism affect gastrointestinal motility? Gastroenterology Research and Practice. 2009;**2009**:529802

[24] Su X, Zhao Y, Li Y, Ma S, Wang Z. Gut dysbiosis is associated with primary hypothyroidism with interaction on gut-thyroid axis. Clinical Science (London, England). 2020;**134**(12):1521-1535

[25] Natividad JM, Verdu EF. Modulation of intestinal barrier by intestinal microbiota: Pathological and therapeutic implications. Pharmacological Research. 2013;**69**(1):42-51

[26] Virili C, Bassotti G, Santaguida MG, Iuorio R, Del Duca SC, Mercuri V, et al. Atypical celiac disease as cause of increased need for thyroxine: A systematic study. The Journal of Clinical Endocrinology and Metabolism. 2012;**97**(3):E419-E422

[27] Santaguida MG, Virili C, Del Duca SC, Cellini M, Gatto I, Brusca N, et al. Thyroxine softgel capsule in patients with gastric-related T4 malabsorption. Endocrine. 2015;**49**(1):51-57

[28] Brechmann T, Sperlbaum A, Schmiegel W. Levothyroxine therapy and impaired clearance are the strongest contributors to small intestinal bacterial overgrowth: Results of a retrospective cohort study. World Journal of Gastroenterology. 2017;**23**(5):842-852

[29] Yao Z, Zhao M, Gong Y, Chen W, Wang Q, Fu Y, et al. Relation of gut microbes and L-thyroxine through altered thyroxine metabolism in subclinical hypothyroidism subjects. Frontiers in Cellular and Infection Microbiology. 2020;**10**:495

[30] d'Afflitto M, Upadhyaya A, Green A, Peiris M. Association between

sex hormone levels and gut microbiota composition and diversity-a systematic review. Journal of Clinical Gastroenterology. 2022;**56**(5):384-392

[31] Yoon K, Kim N. Roles of sex hormones and gender in the gut microbiota. Journal of Neurogastroenterology and Motility. 2021;**27**(3):314-325

[32] Talebi S, Karimifar M, Heidari Z, Mohammadi H, Askari G. The effects of synbiotic supplementation on thyroid function and inflammation in hypothyroid patients: A randomized, double-blind, placebo-controlled trial. Complementary Therapies in Medicine. 2020;**48**:102234

[33] Spaggiari G, Brigante G, De Vincentis S, Cattini U, Roli L, De Santis MC, et al. Probiotics ingestion does not directly affect thyroid hormonal parameters in hypothyroid patients on levothyroxine treatment. Frontiers in Endocrinology (Lausanne). 2017;**8**:316

[34] Zawadzka K, Kałuzińska K, Świerz MJ, Sawiec Z, Antonowicz E, Leończyk-Spórna M, et al. Are probiotics, prebiotics, and synbiotics beneficial in primary thyroid diseases? A systematic review with meta-analysis. Annals of Agricultural and Environmental Medicine. 2023;**30**(2):217-223

Section 2

Diagnosis

Chapter 4

Intelligent Methods for Hypothyroidism Associations and Characterisation for Personalised Diagnosis and Treatment

Xinyu Zhang and Vincent C.S. Lee

Abstract

Hypothyroidism results from low levels of thyroid hormone produced and has varied aetiology and manifestations. It is potentially fatal in severe cases if it remains undetected and timely untreated. Accordingly, this research deploys intelligent machine learning-based methods to uncover its associations and facilitates accurate and efficient detection through case-based predictions. Specifically, data mining algorithms will be adopted to identify risk factors associated with hypothyroidism, including demographics and medical history. These identified associations can be applied to understand, screen, and predict hypothyroidism in individual patients. This intelligent approach enables proactive management of the disease in its early stages to mitigate the potential of developing subsequent diseases, such as heart disease, infertility, or thyroid tumours. The proposed intelligent methods not only advance our understanding of the disease pathogenesis but also achieve precise diagnosis, providing clinicians with valuable insights to support follow-up treatment decision-making.

Keywords: machine learning, association rule mining, hypothyroidism, disease associations, diagnosis and treatment

1. Introduction

Hypothyroidism occurs when the thyroid gland is under-active, failing to secrete sufficient hormones into one's bloodstream, thereby impeding the proper regulation of their metabolism [1]. Under this condition, hypothyroidism is associated with elevated morbidity and mortality rates related to subsequent thyroid disease [2], hypercholesterolemia [3], and cardiovascular disease [4]. Despite the critical consequences, the diagnosis and treatment of the disease appear to be overlooked by the public.

Hypothyroidism is known to be associated with various comorbidities, including infertility [5], reversible dementia [6], and Alzheimer's disease [7], to name a few. However, the identification of the aetiology has been somehow neglected in the existing literature body. A majority of those studies were derived from the clinical perspective, where the aetiology of hypothyroidism can be categorised into primary and secondary causes. The primary cause is a condition where the thyroid gland fails to produce sufficient levels of hormones, with the most common cause being the autoimmune condition known as Hashimoto's thyroiditis [8]. The secondary cause occurs when the pituitary gland fails to send thyroid-stimulating hormone (TSH) to the thyroid gland to maintain hormone balance. Despite conventional efforts to identify associations in the clinical domain, many of these associations remain controversial. This is due to variations in sample groups, scales, and diverse demographic features used in the analyses. Consequently, even though subsequent comorbidities associated with hypothyroidism have been extensively studied, the causes and associations related to its aetiology remain under-researched.

In addition to the overlooked etiological associations of hypothyroidism, its treatment has also received insufficient attention from the public. Chiovato et al. once suggested that 5% of the general population suffers from hypothyroidism, and an additional 5% of the population remains undiagnosed and untreated [4]. Statistics indicated that from 2012 to 2019, the potential instance rates of untreated hypothyroidism grew from 11.8 to 14.4% in the United States [9], and this number continues to increase steadily. The treatment of the disease necessitates constant medication intake, such as levothyroxine, to prevent potential symptoms like mental health issues, heart problems, and breathing issues from manifesting. However, an estimated 35–60% of hypothyroidism patients are either over-treated or under-treated [10]. This phenomenon should be seriously considered and addressed.

Derived from above, the hypothyroidism aetiology associations are pivotal for disease diagnosis and prevention, and its treatment is focal for promising prognosis. To reach personalised diagnosis and treatments, conventional clinical ways of identifying aetiology associations, diagnoses, and treatments should be more automated and intelligent to potentially accomplish precision medicine. Accordingly, this study endeavours to provide a computerised approach to streamline the process of understanding, diagnosing, and treating the disease through machine learning methods. Therefore, through data mining technique and tool, the disease aetiology can be thoroughly elucidated to clarify its intricate associations. Subsequently, these identified associations can be directly applied to screen and predict hypothyroidism in individual patients, thereby eliminating the need for all thyroid function blood examinations. Ultimately, individual patients with hypothyroidism will be suggested on medication intake choice. Such an intelligent approach contributes to advancing our understanding of the disease pathogenesis, enabling proactive management of the disease in its early stages, while offering "second opinions" for clinicians with valuable insights to support their decision-making.

2. Related works

To better capture the literature gaps, this section displays the findings of existing works regarding the pathogenesis associations, diagnosis, and treatments of hypothyroidism.

2.1 Associations

Existing studies identified several factors related to the pathogenesis of hypothyroidism within the clinical domain. For example, Ragusa et al. once proposed a comprehensive investigation on the epidemiology, pathogenesis, and therapy of Hashimoto's thyroiditis [8]. They have indicated that Hashimoto's thyroiditis is the leading cause of hypothyroidism when the iodine intake level is sufficient. In a study by Yaniv et al., they conducted questionnaires on 190 patients who had undergone thyroidectomy, revealing a significant relationship between thyroid surgeries and the development of hypothyroidism [11]. Choi et al. delved into the analysis of 4073 female patients who were treated with adjuvant radiation therapy, noting an apparent increase in the rate of hypothyroidism among this cohort [12]. Similarly, Milano et al. deployed a systematic review for investigating the association between radiation therapy and primary hypothyroidism in childhood cancer survivors. Their findings strongly support the association between radiation and hypothyroidism [13]. There are additional factors that contribute to the understanding of hypothyroidism, such as generic heredity [14, 15] and pregnancy [16, 17].

Nevertheless, existing studies often involve diverse sample groups with variations in size and demographics, leading to limited consensus on the investigated factors. Moreover, examining individual factors typically relies on long-established retrospective analyses in the clinical domain, often overlooking the intricate associations among these factors. Consequently, there is a pressing need for a more intelligent methodology to unveil the intricate associations among these factors for a comprehensive understanding of the underlying causes of hypothyroidism.

2.2 Diagnosis

In the clinical domain, the diagnosis of hypothyroidism typically relies on the thyroid function test, which applies blood examinations to assess the levels of TSH, thyroxine (T4), and free T4 (FT4). Broadly, if one has a high level of TSH yet a low level of T4, then they have an underactive thyroid [18].

However, the clinical diagnosis of hypothyroidism is a nuanced process. In practise, doctors always take other factors into consideration, such as the TSH reference range needs to be adjusted based on the individual's age, body weight, and comorbidities [19]. Therefore, an automated diagnosis needs to be achieved for individual patients by considering all the relevant facets. This approach holds the potential to significantly enhance diagnostic efficiency and accuracy in the assessment of hypothyroidism.

2.3 Treatments

The treatment process of hypothyroidism is pretty standardised, which requires the intake of medications to balance hormones. Levothyroxine, commonly referred to as "L-T4", is a form of the thyroid hormone thyroxine and also a critical medication usually used to treat patients with hypothyroidism or after surgeries [20]. Among the various brands of levothyroxine available globally, "Euthyrox" stands out as one of the most widely used. Over the last century, scholars have dedicated efforts to investigating the importance of taking L-T4 to replace hormones to get a promising prognosis of thyroid disease [21]. It should be well noticed that the dosage of L-T4 is highly dependent on several factors, including the patient's age, weight, body mass index (BMI), pregnancy status, and also medication doses for other diseases. Furthermore, the L-T4 dosage is not fixed for a patient at all times, and adjustments are often necessary with seasonal temperature changes or alterations in the patient's health status.

Therefore, to offer patients the most personalised recommendations for medication intake levels, this study aims to advocate considering individual's relevant features, such as demographics and aetiology associations. The proposed approach is designed to achieve precision diagnosis and treatments tailored to the specific characteristics of each patient.

3. Methodology

In order to achieve the objective of revealing hypothyroidism associations while diagnosing and treating the disease more effectively and accurately, this section exhibits the proposed intelligent approach.

3.1 Proposed Hypo-ADT framework

Figure 1 displays the proposed intelligent approach flowchart for hypothyroidism associations, diagnosis, and treatment, namely the Hypo-ADT framework. The framework consists of two main modules (i.e., the diagnostic module and the treatment module), tailored for personalised hypothyroidism diagnosis and treatments.

Within the diagnostic module, initially, integrated patient records are utilised for understanding the aetiology associations of hypothyroidism, including their demographics, medical history, comorbidity, and function tests. With the retrieved raw data, a series of pre-processing techniques are applied to standardise the data. More specifically, data wrangling methods are deployed to deal with duplicates and missing data [22, 23]. Moreover, all numerical values are formatted into categorical data for further association rule mining processing and analysis. Through mining from the process records, a set of critical features are extracted, which can be determined as aetiology associations of hypothyroidism, and they are also the most significant features to be employed for personalised diagnosis and treatments. When new cases occur, the individual patient can be diagnosed with the pre-identified significant features; if diagnosed as positive, a corresponding treatment protocol is eventually offered.

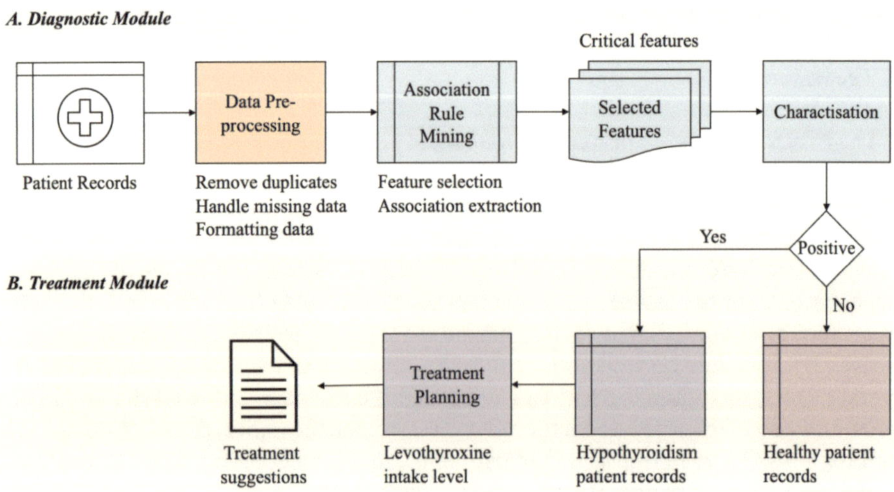

Figure 1.
Intelligent hypothyroidism associations, diagnosis, and treatment (Hypo-ADT) framework.

3.2 Association rule mining

Association rule mining (ARM) is a subset of data mining, which was introduced by Agrawal et al. [24] in the twentieth century. ARM has been applied in a wide range of domains as it is responsible for unravelling hidden patterns among complex data [25]. Thus, it has shown a promising capability of finding associations for specific diseases [26–29], yet the work on extracting associations of hypothyroidism is still absent. Therefore, this work deploys the most classic ARM Apriori algorithm for the aetiology association extraction of hypothyroidism.

The Apriori algorithm was introduced by Agrawal et al. [30], which aims to extract frequent patterns from unstructured datasets. Specifically, the algorithm generates rules that represent $X \Rightarrow Y$ where antecedents X are associated with consequence Y. The procedures are as follows:

- *Step 1*: Pre-define support and confidence thresholds for generated frequent itemsets and association rules.
- *Step 2*: Calculate the support values for all the individual items in the database, then prune the items which do not meet the threshold.
- *Step 3*: Loop through the entire database for each candidate item, pare up to form into an itemset until enumerating all items.
- *Step 4*: Calculate support values for all the candidate itemsets and prune the ones below the threshold.
- *Step 5*: Repeat steps 3 and 4, each time including one more item, until finishing listing all items in the database.
- *Step 6*: Final rules are the frequent itemsets that have support and confidence values above the thresholds.

Through the application of the Apriori algorithm, a set of association rules will be generated denoting the antecedents of hypothyroidism. In other words, these rules also represent the critical factors affecting the development of hypothyroidism and, thus, will be selected for further disease characterisation with individual patients.

3.3 Treatment planning

Within the treatment module, through the pre-defined characterisation classifier (i.e., random forest), the individual patient will be grouped into either positive (i.e., diagnosed with hypothyroidism) or negative (i.e., healthy patient). With the diagnosed positive patient, a treatment planning process is expected to provide corresponding treatment protocols for the individual patient based on their health conditions. More specifically, **Table 1** demonstrates the generally required daily L-T4 dosage under different age groups based on the averaged weights.

Such a treatment protocol regarding thyroxine intake dosage will be provided for patients with hypothyroidism while considering the patient's unique characteristics, including their age, gender, health conditions, thyroid function examination results, and medical history, to name a few.

Age group	Dosage
Neonates	10–15 *ug/kgBw*
Children aged between 8 and 12 months	8–10 *ug/kgBw*
Children aged between 2 and 10 years	4–6 *ug/kgBw*
Adolescents	2–3 *ug/kgBw*
Adults	2 *ug/kgBw*
Elderly	1–1.2 *ug/kgBw*
Pregnancy	1.8–2 *ug/kgBw*

Table 1.
The L-T4 intake dosage requirement (adapted from [31]).

4. Experimental setup

In order to validate the proposed Hypo-ADT framework, this section explains the deployed dataset and parameter settings for the experimental setup.

4.1 Dataset description

This study adopts an open-access dataset to conduct experiments in order to ensure reproducibility. The adopted dataset was contributed by Quinlan [32], which includes 3163 patient records with 25 attributes. After the data wrangling process (i.e., duplicates removal, dealing with missing variables), 2631 instances with 18 attributes were applied for further analysis. Dataset details can be viewed in **Table 2**.

4.2 Parameter setting

With the deployed open-access dataset, this study rigorously follows the Hypo-ADT framework to conduct experiments. More specifically, after pre-processing, for the association rule mining stage, the confidence thresholds were set to 0.9 to extract significant common and exception association rules (i.e., rules that are reliable and meaningful among the public).

With the selected features, the random forest classifier was applied to distinguish negative and positive cases. All the experiments were implemented on the Anaconda Python platform and trained/tested under the same computational environment. Through the 10-fold cross-validation, the classification performance was calculated through accuracy and standard deviation.

5. Results and discussion

This section exhibits the extracted hypothyroidism associations, diagnostic results, and case-based treatment protocols.

Attributes	Descriptions	Details
Age	Age group	18 and under, 18–30, 30–50, 50–70, 70+
Sex	M, F	M = Male, F = Female
On thyroxine	Take thyroxine	False or true
Query on thyroxine	Query thyroxine	False or true
On anti-thyroid med	Take anti-thyroid medication	False or true
Thyroid surgery	Had thyroid surgery	False or true
Query hypothyroid	Query hypothyroidism	False or true
Query hyperthyroid	Query hyperthyroidism	False or true
Pregnant	Current pregnant status	False or true
Sick	Current sick status	False or true
Tumour	Have or had tumour	False or true
Lithium	Have lithium	False or true
Goitre	Have or had goitre	False or true
TSH	TSH level	Normal (0.27–4.2) or abnormal
T3	T3 level	Normal (0.9–2.8) or abnormal
TT4	TT4 level	Normal (62–164) or abnormal
T4U	T4U level	Normal (0.7–1.8) or abnormal
FTI	FTI level	Normal (53–142) or abnormal
Class	Hypothyroidism	Negative or positive

Table 2.
Dataset descriptions.

5.1 Association results

With the Apriori algorithm, the top five association rules were identified and demonstrated in **Table 3**.

Based on the table, gender, age group, TSH, and FTI attributes showcase significant associations with the development of hypothyroidism. Specifically, the top rule is that if a patient has abnormal TSH and FTI function examinations, then he/she is very likely to be diagnosed with hypothyroidism. This rule has a 0.98 support value, indicating that 98% of the examined group diagnosed with the disease have the two attributes detected as abnormal. **Figure 2** exhibits the correlations of the incorporated functioning measurements. It suggests that TT4 and FTI have considerate associations, yet the correlation between TSH and FTI is not explicit. Therefore, the two factors are considered independent attributes associated with hypothyroidism.

Other than that, female patients tend to be diagnosed with hypothyroidism more often than male patients. When a female patient has an abnormal TSH level, then she will be likely to establish hypothyroidism, and this rule has a confidence of 1.0. Similarly, if a female patient has an abnormal FTI level, then she will also likely be diagnosed with hypothyroidism, with support and confidence of 0.74 and 1.0, respectively.

Moreover, two exception rules (i.e., low support and high confidence) were generated, indicating that the age group between 50 and 70 is likely to establish

Antecedence		Consequence	Support	Confidence
Abnormal_FTI, Abnormal_TSH	⇒	Hypothyroidism	0.98	1.00
Female, Abnormal_TSH	⇒	Hypothyroidism	0.75	1.00
Female, Abnormal_FTI	⇒	Hypothyroidism	0.74	1.00
Age group = 50–70	⇒	Hypothyroidism	0.37	1.00
Female, Age_group = 50–70	⇒	Hypothyroidism	0.26	1.00

Table 3.
Hypothyroidism associations.

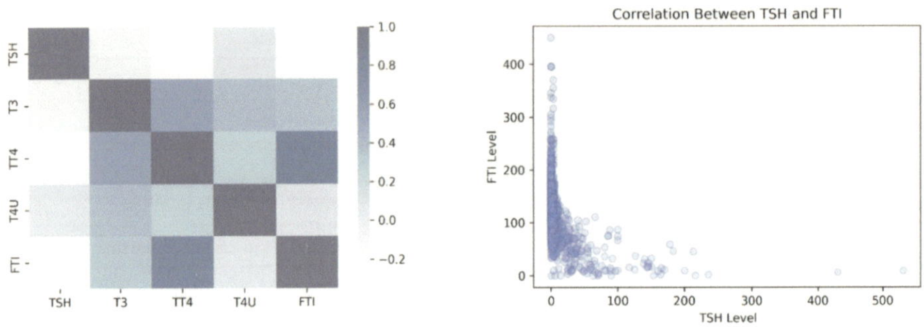

Figure 2.
Thyroid function examination associations. Left: Associations among the five blood measurements; Right: Associations between TSH and FTI.

hypothyroidism, with a support value of 0.37 and confidence of 1.0. When a female patient is within the age group, the rule stands still, also reaching a confidence of 1.0.

Gender disparity in thyroid disease is well established, where female patients are much more in quantity than male patients. Besides this, based on the results, FTI and TSH levels are proven to be two critical features affecting hypothyroidism, and this finding is in accordance with [33]. Liao et al. [33] deployed several machine learning models to confirm their associations, while our approach is much more efficient.

Besides, we found hypothyroidism is more common in the older population, and this finding is also consistent with [19, 34, 35]. Nevertheless, existing studies generally have a vague description of the ageing definition, which does not clearly determine the elderly age group interval. Yet, our finding indicates that patients aged from 50 to 70 have a more substantial probability of establishing hypothyroidism than those aged above 70, and this interesting finding will help formulate a more explicit guidance to monitor and surveillance the elderly's thyroid health. The specific associations are displayed in **Figure 3**.

5.2 Diagnosis results

In order to validate the extracted associations, this study involves three commonly used classifiers for classifying negative and positive classes, including random forest (RF), support vector machine (SVM), and multi-layer perceptron (MLP). The baseline experiments include all 18 features from the original database, and the feature

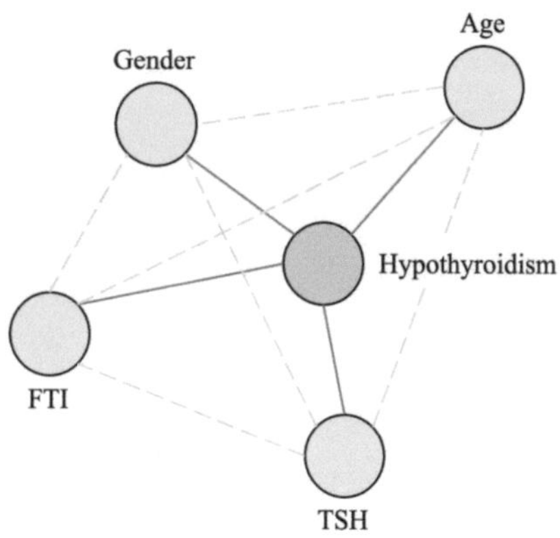

Figure 3.
Hypothyroidism associations. Solid lines represent determinate associations with hypothyroidism, and dashed lines represent hidden interconnected associations.

Type	Model	Accuracy
Baseline	Random forest	0.9821 ± 0.007
Feature selection		**0.9856 ± 0.007**
Baseline	Support vector machine	0.9821 ± 0.006
Feature selection		**0.9833 ± 0.007**
Baseline	Multi-layer perceptron	0.9806 ± 0.010
Feature selection		0.9806 ± 0.007

The bold entires in Table 4 highlight the better accuracies. This means increased performance when incorporating the feature selection approach.

Table 4.
Hypothyroidism diagnosis classification results.

selection experiments include the extracted four attributes (i.e., age, gender, FTI, and TSH). Details of the classification accuracy can be viewed in **Table 4** and **Figure 4**.

Based on the classification results, it is evident that random forest is the best-performing classifier for diagnosing hypothyroidism, reaching an accuracy of 0.9821 and 0.9856 rates for baseline and feature selection types. More importantly, the association rule mining-based feature selection approach demonstrates enhanced diagnostic accuracy using fewer attributes compared to incorporating all the features. Specifically, the random forest and support vector machines showcase enhanced diagnostic accuracy compared to baseline models (i.e., from 0.982 to 0.986 and from 0.982 to 0.983), and the multi-layer perceptron demonstrates the same accuracy rates (i.e., 0.981). Accordingly, the selected four features are determined as critical factors affecting hypothyroidism development and can be further used to monitor the disease more efficiently.

5.3 Treatment results

When an individual is diagnosed with hypothyroidism using the pre-defined classifier, he/she will be considered individually for personalised treatment protocol planning. Here, we use two case samples to demonstrate how the treatment suggestions are given.

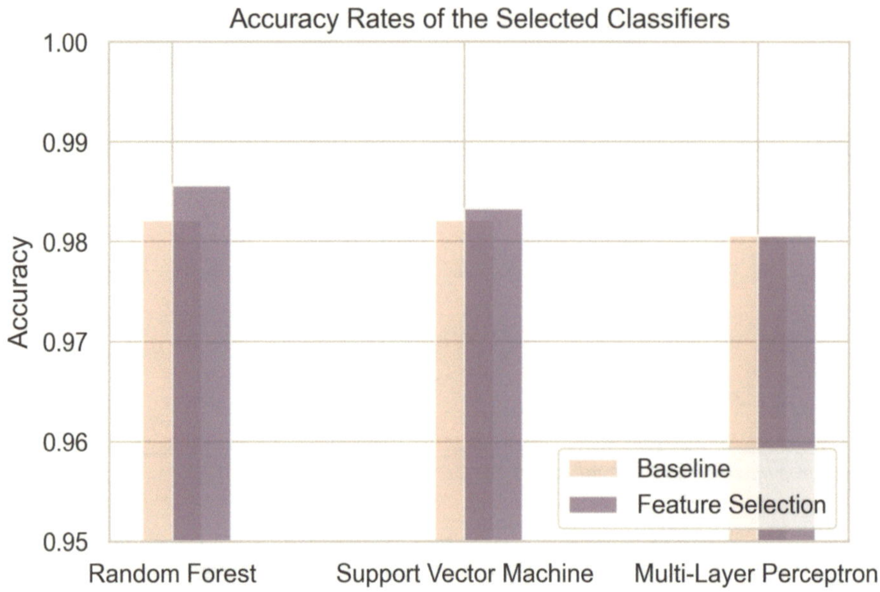

Figure 4.
Hypothyroidism diagnosis classification results.

5.3.1 Case #1

Consider a patient with the following characteristics: a female patient (indexed Case 7) aged 64, who had thyroid surgery in the past and is now with TSH measured of 7.7, T3 of 1.3, TT4 of 54, T4U of 0.86, and FTI of 63. Considering the normal range of the thyroid function test, it is evident that she has abnormal TSH and TT4 levels. Since she is not sick or has the pregnancy status, she is expected and required to have a daily L-T4 intake level of 1–1.2 *ug/kgBw* to make up for the thyroid hormones.

5.3.2 Case #2

Consider a patient with the following characteristics: a male patient (indexed Case 126) aged 35, who also experienced thyroid surgery in his medical history, and he now has TSH measured of 0.25, T3 of 0.4, TT4 of 38, T4U of 1.08, and FTI of 35. Based on the evaluation, he is experiencing abnormal TSH, T3, TT4, and FTI; thus, he is required to take a daily L-T4 of 2 *ug/kgBw*.

It should be noted that the suggestions provided in **Table 1** are based on normal averaged weight and BMI. Since the patient's weight, BMI, height, and seasonal information are all missing in our involved dataset, only such an approximate medication intake suggestion can be provided for individual patients. Therefore, to provide a more determinate suggestion, more information is required.

6. Conclusion

This study proposed an intelligent Hypo-ADT framework to reveal hypothyroidism associations, improve diagnostic accuracy and efficiency, and provide personalised treatment suggestions for individual patients. An open-access dataset is involved to evaluate the proposed framework, and satisfying performance was achieved. The proposed approach can also be adapted to other diseases, as it aims to help society understand the disease to a deeper extent, prevent it in an early stage, and support precision medicine.

There are some limitations embedded within this study, and the main one is with the deployed dataset. The sample size is a bit small, and the embedded attributes are limited in quantity and variety. Therefore, the findings of this study are not comprehensive enough. For future work, we will include more samples with more comprehensive factors to drive into a more solid and thorough analysis. Other than that, the dataset does not provide any related attributes or information on treatment protocols. Thus, future work will be designing and deploying a more robust model for intelligent treatment planning.

Abbreviations

ARM	association rule mining
BMI	body mass index
TSH	thyroid-stimulating hormone
T3	triiodothyronine
T4	thyroxine
FT4	free thyroxine
FTI	free thyroxine index
L-T4	levothyroxine
MLP	multi-layer perceptron
RF	random forest
SVM	support vector machine

Author details

Xinyu Zhang[1*] and Vincent C.S. Lee[2]

1 Northwestern Polytechnical University, Xi'an, China

2 Monash University, Melbourne, Australia

*Address all correspondence to: xinyu.zhang@nwpu.edu.cn

References

[1] Wilson SA, Stem LA, Bruehlman RD. Hypothyroidism: Diagnosis and treatment. American Family Physician. 2021;**103**(10):605-613

[2] Panfilova E, Kruk L, Isaeva M, Osmanova P, Bostanova F, Troshina E. The development of Graves' disease after long-term hypothyroidism due to Hashimoto's disease. Problemy Endokrinologii. 2020;**66**(5):24-30

[3] Bianco AC, Taylor P. Levothyroxine treatment and cholesterol in hypothyroidism. Nature Reviews Endocrinology. 2020;**16**(4): 193-194

[4] Chiovato L, Magri F, Carlé A. Hypothyroidism in context: Where we've been and where we're going. Advances in Therapy. 2019;**36**:47-58

[5] Koyyada A, Orsu P. Role of hypothyroidism and associated pathways in pregnancy and infertility: Clinical insights. Tzu-Chi Medical Journal. 2020;**32**(4):312

[6] Layal Chaker JJ, Bianco AC, Peeters RP. Hypothyroidism. The Lancet. 2017;**390**(10101):1550-1562

[7] AlAnazi FH, Al-Kuraishy HM, Alexiou A, Papadakis M, Ashour MHM, Alnaaim SA, et al. Primary hypothyroidism and Alzheimer's disease: A tale of two. Cellular and Molecular Neurobiology. 2023;**43**(7):3405-3416

[8] Ragusa F, Fallahi P, Elia G, Gonnella D, Paparo SR, Giusti C, et al. Hashimotos' thyroiditis: Epidemiology, pathogenesis, clinic and therapy. Best Practice & Research Clinical Endocrinology & Metabolism. 2019; **33**(6):101367. Autoimmune endocrine disorders: Part I

[9] Wyne KL, Nair L, Schneiderman CP, Pinsky B, Antunez Flores O, Guo D, et al. Hypothyroidism prevalence in the United States: A retrospective study combining national health and nutrition examination survey and claims data, 2009–2019. Journal of the Endocrine Society. 2023;7(1):bvac172

[10] Taylor PN, Iqbal A, Minassian C, Sayers A, Draman MS, Greenwood R, et al. Falling threshold for treatment of borderline elevated thyrotropin levels—Balancing benefits and risks: Evidence from a large community-based study. JAMA Internal Medicine. 2014;**174**(1): 32-39

[11] Yaniv D, Vainer I, Amir I, Robenshtok E, Hirsch D, Watt T, et al. Quality of life following lobectomy versus total thyroidectomy is significantly related to hypothyroidism. Journal of Surgical Oncology. 2022; **126**(4):640-648

[12] Choi SH, Chang JS, Byun HK, Son NH, Hong CS, Hong N, et al. Risk of hypothyroidism in women after radiation therapy for breast cancer. International Journal of Radiation Oncology* Biology* Physics. 2021; **110**(2):462-472

[13] Milano MT, Vargo JA, Yorke ED, Ronckers CM, Kremer LC, Chafe SM, et al. Primary hypothyroidism in childhood cancer survivors treated with radiation therapy: A PENTEC comprehensive review. International Journal of Radiation Oncology* Biology* Physics. 2021;**17**:S0360-3016(21) 00128-0

[14] Persani L, Rurale G, de Filippis T, Galazzi E, Muzza M, Fugazzola L. Genetics and management of congenital

hypothyroidism. Best Practice & Research Clinical Endocrinology & Metabolism. 2018;**32**(4): 387-396

[15] Kostopoulou E, Miliordos K, Spiliotis B. Genetics of primary congenital hypothyroidism—A review. Hormones. 2021;**20**:225-236

[16] Teng W, Shan Z, Patil-Sisodia K, Cooper DS. Hypothyroidism in pregnancy. The Lancet Diabetes & Endocrinology. 2013;**1**(3):228-237

[17] Li SW, Chan SY. Management of overt hypothyroidism during pregnancy. Best Practice & Research Clinical Endocrinology & Metabolism. 2020; **34**(4):101439

[18] Kalaria T, Sanders A, Fenn J, Ashby HL, Mohammed P, Buch HN, et al. The diagnosis and management of subclinical hypothyroidism is assay-dependent—Implications for clinical practice. Clinical Endocrinology. 2021; **94**(6):1012-1016

[19] Duntas LH, Yen PM. Diagnosis and treatment of hypothyroidism in the elderly. Endocrine. 2019;**66**:63-69

[20] Biondi B, Wartofsky L. Treatment with thyroid hormone. Endocrine Reviews. 2014;**35**(3):433-512

[21] Escobar-Morreale HF, Botella-Carretero JI, del Rey FE, de Escobar GM. Treatment of hypothyroidism with combinations of levothyroxine plus liothyronine. The Journal of Clinical Endocrinology & Metabolism. 2005; **90**(8):4946-4954

[22] Yu D, Wang X, Wu H. EHR data pre-processing and preparation. In: Statistics and Machine Learning Methods for EHR Data. New York: Chapman and Hall/ CRC; 2020. pp. 111-147

[23] Mazilu L, Konstantinou N, Paton NW, Fernandes AAA. Data wrangling for fair classification. In: Proceedings of the EDBT/ICDT 2021 Joint Conference (March 23–26, 2021, Nicosia, Cyprus). 2021. pp. 111-147. Available from: CEUR-WS.org

[24] Agrawal R, Imieliński T, Swami A. Mining association rules between sets of items in large databases. In: Proceedings of the 1993 ACM SIGMOD International Conference on Management of Data, Washington DC, 25-28 May 1993, Vol. 22 (2) of SIGMOD Records. 1993. pp. 207-216

[25] Telikani A, Gandomi AH, Shahbahrami A. A survey of evolutionary computation for association rule mining. Information Sciences. 2020; **524**:318-352

[26] Lakshmi K, Vadivu G. A novel approach for disease comorbidity prediction using weighted association rule mining. Journal of Ambient Intelligence and Humanized Computing. 2019:1-8

[27] Ren X, Shao XX, Li XX, Jia XH, Song T, Zhou WY, et al. Identifying potential treatments of COVID-19 from traditional Chinese medicine (TCM) by using a data-driven approach. Journal of Ethnopharmacology. 2020;**258**:112932

[28] Tandan M, Acharya Y, Pokharel S, Timilsina M. Discovering symptom patterns of COVID-19 patients using association rule mining. Computers in Biology and Medicine. 2021;**131**: 104249

[29] Alam TM, Shaukat K, Hameed IA, Khan WA, Sarwar MU, Iqbal F, et al. A novel framework for prognostic factors identification of malignant mesothelioma through association rule

mining. Biomedical Signal Processing and Control. 2021;**68**:102726

[30] Agrawal R, Srikant R. Fast algorithms for mining association rules. In: Laha AK, editor. Proceedings of the 20th International Conference on Very Large Data Bases. Vol. 1215. Santiago, Chile: VLDB; 1994. pp. 487-499

[31] Schäffler A. Hormone replacement after thyroid and parathyroid surgery. Deutsches Ärzteblatt International. 2010;**107**(47):827

[32] Quinlan R. Thyroid disease. UCI Machine Learning Repository. 1987. DOI: 10.24432/C5D010

[33] Liao B, Liang J, Guo B, Jia X, Lu J, Zhang T, et al. ILSHIP: An interpretable and predictive model for hypothyroidism. Computers in Biology and Medicine. 2023;**154**:106578

[34] Leng O, Razvi S. Hypothyroidism in the older population. Thyroid Research. 2019;**12**(1):1-10

[35] Biondi B, Cappola AR. Subclinical hypothyroidism in older individuals. The Lancet Diabetes & Endocrinology. 2022; **10**(2):129-141

Chapter 5

Optimizing TSH Testing: Minimizing Overdiagnosis and Unnecessary Interventions

Palacios-Bayona Karen Lorena

Abstract

In this chapter, the routine application of thyroid function tests for hypothyroidism detection is evaluated, with a focus on the problems of overdiagnosis and unnecessary treatment, especially in subclinical scenarios. It critically assesses the lack of solid evidence behind common interventions, like the widespread prescription of levothyroxine without definitive clinical need. Highlighting evidence-based guidelines for hypothyroidism screening, the chapter argues against indiscriminate thyroid testing. It advocates for a thoughtful approach to thyroid disorder management, urging cautious use of TSH tests to reduce needless medical actions and improve patient outcomes.

Keywords: thyroid screening, overdiagnosis, overtreatment, healthcare quality, evidence based practice

1. Introduction

The journey from clinical trial discoveries to their practical application in healthcare is remarkably slow, often taking up to 17 years. This slow process reveals a significant healthcare paradox: the hesitancy to adopt proven interventions while outdated or less effective practices continue, particularly in thyroid health management [1, 2]. This situation points to a significant gap between knowledge generation and its application, underscoring a critical area for improvement across all medical areas, including endocrinology [3]. The frequent use of Thyroid Stimulating Hormone (TSH) tests has come under scrutiny for contributing to the overdiagnosis and unnecessary treatment of conditions like subclinical hypothyroidism, which remains a contentious area in medical practice [4–6]. It advocates for a critical reassessment of TSH testing's role, aiming to align it more closely with the latest evidence and clinical guidelines without necessarily proposing new protocols but emphasizing the importance of evidence-based practice [7–9].

2. Challenges in hypothyroidism screening

In healthcare, screening is intended to detect diseases in apparently healthy individuals with risk factors, aiming to decrease morbidity and mortality through early

IntechOpen

intervention. In contrast, early diagnosis seeks to promptly identify diseases in individuals already exhibiting symptoms. The foundation for modern screening practices was established in 1968 by Wilson and Jungner in a seminal WHO publication, where they outlined key criteria [10]. Applying these principles to hypothyroidism screening reveals several challenges: limitations in the diagnostic accuracy of the TSH test, a weak association between symptoms and hypothyroidism diagnosis, and the inconsistent relationship between minor TSH elevations and adverse outcomes. Additionally, treatment with levothyroxine often lacks significant efficacy, leading to recommendations against treating most patients with subclinical hypothyroidism [5, 11]. These complexities are detailed in **Table 1**, which applies Wilson and Jungner's screening criteria to hypothyroidism, revealing the unique challenges in this field.

2.1 Limitations in TSH and symptom use for hypothyroidism diagnosis

TSH is critical for screening and early diagnosis of hypothyroidism. However, interpreting its levels is complex due to variations caused by circadian rhythms,

Principle	Assessment for hypothyroidism
1. The condition should be a significant health problem	Manifest hypothyroidism is significant due to its potential complications. However, the clinical relevance of subclinical hypothyroidism is debatable since its treatment has not shown to improve significant clinical outcomes in controlled trials.
2. There should be an accepted treatment for patients with recognized disease	Treatment with levothyroxine is common but does not necessarily improve clinical outcomes in subclinical hypothyroidism.
3. Facilities for diagnosis and treatment should be available	Broad access to TSH testing can promote its overuse, increasing the risk of unnecessary treatments that negatively impact patients and the healthcare system.
4. There should be a recognizable latent or early symptomatic stage	Early identification of hypothyroidism is complicated because general symptoms, such as fatigue and cold sensitivity, are not exclusive to this condition, making diagnosis based solely on clinical signs challenging.
5. There should be a suitable test or examination	TSH variability without proper age adjustments can lead to erroneous diagnoses and an increase in overdiagnosis, particularly in older populations.
6. The test should be acceptable to the population	The TSH test is a minimally invasive and low-risk procedure.
7. The natural history of the condition should be adequately understood	Uncertainty regarding the relationship between TSH levels and nonspecific symptoms, along with unclear therapeutic benefits, poses a challenge to understanding the natural course of subclinical hypothyroidism.
8. There should be an agreed policy on whom to treat as patients	There is widespread consensus against universal screening tests in the general population.
9. The cost of case finding should be economically balanced in relation to possible expenditure on medical care as a whole	Broad screening with TSH tests can lead to substantial expenses and the unjustified classification of patients, necessitating regular consultations, levothyroxine treatment, additional expenses, and more medical examinations.

Table 1.
Assessment of Wilson and Jungner's principles for population screening of hypothyroidism.

individual variability, and the effects of aging [12–14]. A longitudinal study observed individuals without thyroid conditions for 5 years, revealing that 62% of TSH levels initially ranging from 5.5 mIU/L to 10 mIU/L naturally returned to normal in later evaluations without any medical intervention [15]. This variability underscores the importance of confirming abnormal TSH levels with a subsequent measurement before initiating any treatment [4]. Adhering to the guidelines from the National Health and Nutrition Examination Survey (NHANES III), which recommend a TSH upper threshold of 7.5 mIU/L for individuals older than 80, is crucial. Ignoring the necessity for age-based threshold adjustments could inadvertently increase the likelihood of overdiagnosis and consequent unnecessary treatments, along with their potential adverse effects [3, 16].

Moreover, TSH diagnostic accuracy is influenced by pretest probability. It reliably indicates thyroid dysfunction in high-suspicion cases, such as patients with a history of thyroid surgery or using medications affecting the thyroid. However, its precision diminishes when solely assessing symptoms like fatigue, common in hypothyroidism [17–19]. Symptoms alone lack specificity, as population studies show no significant increase in mild thyroid dysfunction symptomatology compared to normal function [8]. Additionally, up to 25% of individuals without thyroid disorders may exhibit symptoms erroneously interpreted as hypothyroidism [20].

2.2 Adverse outcomes of subclinical hypothyroidism and effects of levothyroxine treatment

Observational studies suggest that TSH levels above 10 mIU/L are associated with an increased risk of cardiac events, such as heart failure and coronary artery disease [6]. However, for nonpregnant adults with subclinical hypothyroidism and TSH levels at or below 10 mIU/L, there is no consistent evidence linking these slight TSH elevations to an increased risk of mortality, cardiovascular events, cognitive impairment, frailty, decreased bone mineral density, worsened quality of life, or an increased occurrence of symptoms [4, 6, 21].

Moreover, substantial evidence supporting the effectiveness of levothyroxine treatment in these patients is lacking [22]. Results from various clinical trials, including the TRUST trial that enrolled 737 older patients with mild TSH elevations in a randomized, double-blind, placebo-controlled study, revealed no significant improvements in symptoms such as fatigue, quality of life, cognitive function, or cardiometabolic parameters after normalizing TSH levels with 12 months of levothyroxine use [23].

Despite these findings, the use of levothyroxine has significantly increased in many countries, with about 7% of the U.S. population now receiving this hormone therapy [24, 25]. Often, the indications for initiating thyroid hormone therapy include inappropriate criteria, such as patients with normal TSH levels, management of mild subclinical hypothyroidism, suppression of thyroid nodule growth, or addressing nonspecific symptoms like depression, weight loss, and fatigue [3, 26]. A study by Brito and colleagues examining levothyroxine use between 2008 and 2018 in 58,706 commercially insured adult patients and Medicare beneficiaries found that 30.5% began levothyroxine therapy despite having normal hormone levels, 61% for subclinical hypothyroidism, and 8.4% for overt hypothyroidism. Among those treated for subclinical hypothyroidism, the majority (57.9%) had TSH levels below 10 mIU/L, with primary care physicians initiating most prescriptions (47.5%) [26].

As previously discussed, the treatment for subclinical hypothyroidism, particularly with levothyroxine, does not clearly demonstrate benefits and is associated with significant adverse effects. The trend toward lowering the threshold for treating mild subclinical conditions has led to an increase in iatrogenic medical complications. Specifically, levothyroxine treatment resulting in suppressed TSH levels is linked to a heightened risk of arrhythmias and bone fractures, with hazard ratios of 1.60 (95% CI: 1.10–2.33) and 2.02 ([95% CI: 1.55–2.62]), respectively, compared to patients maintaining normal TSH levels [27]. Furthermore, research shows that 40–50% of patients over 65 on levothyroxine have TSH levels lower than 0.45 mIU/L, indicating widespread overtreatment [28]. This not only increases the burden of medication and its associated costs but also necessitates regular doctor visits, frequent blood tests, and lifestyle adjustments for taking medication on an empty stomach [29]. Importantly, once started, about 90% of patients with subclinical hypothyroidism are likely to require lifelong treatment, emphasizing the need for careful evaluation before initiating levothyroxine therapy [30].

2.3 Current guidelines for hypothyroidism screening

The perspectives of medical organizations on universal screening for hypothyroidism vary considerably. While the American Thyroid Association advocates for assessments every 5 years to identify thyroid dysfunction in asymptomatic individuals aged over 35, potentially impacting around 3.5 billion adults worldwide [28, 31], other medical organizations question this approach for nonpregnant adults [17, 32]. These guidelines, as outlined in **Table 2**, provide insights into the recommendations set forth by various medical bodies regarding hypothyroidism screening practices.

The United States Preventive Services Task Force (USPSTF), in its 2015 review, determined insufficient evidence to support mass thyroid screening in asymptomatic adults, citing a lack of conclusive data on its effect in preventing significant adverse outcomes such as cardiovascular diseases or improving cognitive function. Concerns about overdiagnosis and overtreatment were also emphasized [17].

Conversely, health authorities in the United Kingdom, including the Association for Clinical Biochemistry, British Thyroid Association, and British Thyroid Foundation, do not advocate for screening in the general healthy population. Instead, they promote an early diagnostic approach in high-risk individuals with indicative symptoms [33]. Despite these guidelines, up to 30% of individuals over 65 undergo thyroid evaluations annually [15, 34, 35]. An analysis of 2936 subjects in this age

Organization	Current guidelines
USPSTF (United States Preventive Services Task Force) [17]	Insufficient evidence to assess universal screening.
ATA (American Thyroid Association), AACE (American Association of Clinical Endocrinology) [27]	Identifying high-risk individuals and evaluating thyroid function every 5 years in asymptomatic individuals over 35.
Association for Clinical Biochemistry (ACB), the British Thyroid Association (BTA), and the British Thyroid Foundation (BTF) [30]	Do not endorse routine universal screening. Instead, they recommend identifying cases in women with nonspecific symptoms suggestive of an underlying thyroid disorder
Canadian Task Force on Preventive Health Care [29]	Do not perform screening tests for thyroid dysfunction in asymptomatic nonpregnant adults

Table 2.
Guidelines for hypothyroidism screening by medical organizations.

range, with normal or slightly altered thyroid results, revealed that less than 0.5% progressed to overt thyroid dysfunction within 5 years, raising questions about the necessity of screening in this age group [34]. This situation underscores the discrepancy between current medical practice and clinical consensus, highlighting the importance of reassessing screening practices to avoid unnecessary medical interventions [3].

3. Challenges and strategies for de-implementation

3.1 Barriers to de-implementation

De-implementation emerges as a critical strategy for reducing low-value care, such as the excessive use of TSH testing [36]. Its primary objectives are to minimize patient harm, optimize resource utilization, and enhance overall population health [37]. However, it encounters significant hurdles, including resistance and conflicting motivations from healthcare providers and patients, as well as external influences stemming from economic, political, cultural, and historical factors [38]. To tackle these barriers, a series of comprehensive approaches is outlined in **Table 3**. These strategies aim to navigate and overcome the obstacles to de-implementation, ultimately promoting the judicious use of the TSH test.

Norton and Chambers have underscored the multifaceted nature of the de-implementation process, where diverse factors exert influence across different levels [39]. Patient preferences significantly impact prescribing practices, posing challenges for physicians striving to adhere to evidence-based care [9]. Cognitive dissonance

Category	Strategy/insight	Implementation challenge	Example application
De-implementation challenges	Overcoming resistance from healthcare providers and patients; navigating economic, political, and cultural influences.	Resistance to change due to established practices and external pressures.	Implementing a multifaceted educational campaign to address misconceptions and emphasize the evidence-based approach to TSH testing.
Education and training	Updating healthcare professionals on current guidelines; emphasizing high-value care in medical training	Knowledge gaps; inertia in updating practices according to new evidence.	Hosting workshops and seminars to disseminate the latest research and guidelines on when TSH testing and treatment are warranted.
EHR-based tools	Utilizing CPOE and CDSS to guide clinical decisions and reduce inappropriate interventions.	Ensuring EHR tools are user-friendly and effectively integrated into clinical workflows.	Integrating alerts into EHRs that prompt for clinical justification when ordering TSH tests, especially for borderline cases.
Audit and feedback	Regular performance evaluations against standards to encourage adherence to evidence-based practices.	Establishing meaningful benchmarks and ensuring feedback is constructive and actionable.	Providing quarterly reports to clinicians comparing their TSH testing patterns with best practice guidelines, highlighting areas for improvement.

Category	Strategy/insight	Implementation challenge	Example application
Patient engagement	Involving patients in care decisions, particularly regarding the necessity and implications of TSH testing.	Balancing educational efforts to ensure patients have realistic expectations without undermining trust.	Developing patient education materials that detail the potential risks of overtreatment and the importance of evidence-based testing.
Institutional policy adjustments	Revising policies to limit TSH testing to clinically justified scenarios.	Aligning institutional policies with current evidence while managing stakeholder interests.	Instituting a review process for TSH test orders to ensure compliance with updated clinical guidelines.
Assessing sustainability	Evaluating long-term adherence to de-implementation strategies and maintaining practice change.	Addressing persistent or resurfacing inappropriate testing practices over time	Establishing an annual review process to assess the impact of de-implementation strategies on TSH testing rates and identify areas for ongoing improvement.
Cost-effectiveness and broader analysis	Considering the long-term financial impact of reducing unnecessary TSH tests.	Demonstrating the value of de-implementation beyond immediate cost savings.	Conducting a cost-benefit analysis to showcase the long-term savings from avoiding unnecessary treatments and complications.
Research and innovation	Encouraging research on TSH testing impacts and developing innovative approaches to reduce unnecessary testing.	Securing funding and interest for research focused on diagnostic stewardship.	Pilot studies assessing the impact of targeted educational programs on TSH testing rates.

Table 3.
Enhanced strategies for optimizing TSH testing.

arises when physicians recognize that certain interventions, such as thyroid screenings or treatments for subclinical hypothyroidism, may not benefit specific patients. However, addressing patient concerns, potential litigation, and the importance of maintaining the doctor-patient relationship complicate decision-making [40]. This internal conflict, compounded by external pressures such as malpractice concerns, fear of missing a diagnosis, and the need to meet patient expectations, is further influenced by habituation, extensive training, and years of practice [41].

Given these complexities, sociological theories, like Rogers' theory of the diffusion of innovations, suggest that the majority of physicians, around 84%, are often slow to adopt changes in their clinical practice [42]. Considering this delay in adopting new guidelines is crucial for developing effective communication strategies and ongoing training programs. These efforts should directly target perceived barriers and aim to expedite the adoption of evidence-based practices [43].

3.2 Strategies for de-implementation

The field of de-implementation is advancing with the emergence of more effective evidence-based strategies [44]. Addressing the identified challenges requires a comprehensive approach that involves the practices of healthcare professionals, incorporates the perspectives and needs of patients, and updates institutional policies [44, 45].

Several de-implementation strategies have been explored in the literature, which include support for clinical decision-making, education of both physicians and patients, and the implementation of multicomponent interventions, as reported in a systematic review that identified nine strategies for reducing low-value care. Additionally, other mentioned strategies include cost-sharing, which shifts the financial burden of low-value care onto patients; provider performance reports, providing patients with information about their healthcare provider's use of low-value care services; pay-for-performance, offering financial incentives to physicians; insurer restrictions that limit reimbursement for low-value care; risk-sharing; and provider feedback, also identified as effective interventions [46].

The majority of evidence suggests that multicomponent strategies are effective and could be applied in de-implementation programs targeting the indiscriminate use of TSH.

3.2.1 Education and training for healthcare professionals

The factors influencing healthcare professionals are closely tied to their beliefs, knowledge, and skills [47]. It is crucial to acknowledge that clinicians often encounter challenges in staying updated with scientific literature and may be influenced by habits acquired during their medical training, which typically prioritizes diagnosis over "do nothing" [48–50]. Therefore, resident training presents a critical opportunity to introduce the concept of high-value care, as behaviors learned during this period tend to persist throughout one's professional career [49].

Although some medical schools have integrated healthcare economics content into their curricula, many physicians still have significant knowledge gaps in these areas. Training programs frequently overlook resource management and cost-conscious practices, essential elements for promoting more efficient, evidence-based healthcare [50].

Recent reviews have indicated that the majority of de-implementation strategies focus on educational approaches aligned with the "Training and Education of Stakeholders" category of the ERIC (Expert Recommendations for Implementing Change) framework, emphasizing direct training and widespread dissemination of educational materials as key strategies [45]. To discourage the indiscriminate ordering of TSH tests, various educational strategies can be implemented, such as focused training sessions on updated guidelines, distribution of educational materials, and conducting periodic assessments. These initiatives should be complemented with specific, measurable, achievable, relevant, and time-bound (SMART) objectives [47]. For instance, evaluating the impact on reducing TSH tests by 15% among primary care physicians over the next 6 months would provide tangible and measurable results within a defined timeframe.

However, it is essential to recognize that education alone may not suffice to change deeply entrenched practices [1]. Research indicates that relying solely on education for de-implementation often yields limited effectiveness, emphasizing the need for a multifaceted, multi-level approach in current strategies, which has shown to yield more promising results [51]. Moreover, the implementation process tends to accelerate significantly when clear policies and effective communication channels are established among research, Pharmacy Benefit Management (PBM) Services, and clinical practice [1]. Therefore, it is critical to seamlessly integrate educational strategies into a comprehensive framework to ensure their effectiveness.

3.2.2 Use of EHR-based tools

The utilization of Electronic Health Record (EHR)-based tools, including Computerized Physician Order Entry (CPOE) and Clinical Decision Support Systems (CDSS), emerges as a powerful strategy to influence medical practice [45]. These tools rely on theories of individual and organizational learning, facilitating the implementation of effective strategies to replace inappropriate interventions with evidence-based ones [36]. However, it is paramount for these tools to remain intuitive and straightforward, incorporating contextual alerts that guide physicians in real-time and allowing for customization to meet patient needs. This ensures that the process does not deteriorate into a low-value management endeavor [52].

To illustrate, there are various approaches to reducing the number of requested TSH tests. For instance, implementing an alert within the CPOE system would trigger when a physician requests a TSH test without a clear indication or adherence to established clinical guidelines. This alert would prompt the physician to provide a specific justification for the TSH test order before proceeding. Additionally, regularly reviewing predefined order lists in the EHR system, which include the TSH test, proves effective [36, 44].

Clinical Decision Support Systems (CDSS) represent advanced tools for influencing behavior. They deliver real-time alerts on best practices, reminders, and evidence-based recommendations. For example, integrating alerts or reminders into CDSS prompts clinicians to reassess their decisions to request TSH tests without indication and opt for more appropriate interventions aligned with current best practices and guidelines, such as conducting TSH tests in populations truly at risk and benefiting from levothyroxine use [44]. In summary, effectively leveraging these EHR-based tools offers a potent avenue for enhancing clinical decision-making and optimizing patient care while also contributing to the de-implementation of indiscriminate TSH testing [36, 44].

3.2.3 Audit and feedback

Audit and feedback are essential tools in assessing professional performance, as they are evidence-based and designed to compare individual practice with established professional standards and objectives [53]. This evaluation process, known as "auditing" performance, is communicated both individually and collectively to motivate compliance with professional norms and standards, such as following recommendations to limit hypothyroidism screening or overuse of levothyroxine in various contexts [44, 53, 54].

Additionally, accessible dashboards can be utilized in this audit, allowing clinicians to compare their performance with others and pre-established benchmarks. These dashboards not only facilitate comparison but also provide an opportunity for clinicians to self-audit their performance and reflect on their own practices [44]. This, in turn, promotes continuous improvement in the quality of medical care provided [53].

3.2.4 Strengthening patient engagement in de-implementation processes

Engaging patients in the process of removing unnecessary medical practices through educational efforts and shared decision-making is key in medical settings, particularly when patients hold specific beliefs or expectations about certain treatments [44]. In scenarios like subclinical hypothyroidism, providing patients with thorough information about the risks, benefits, and alternatives to levothyroxine treatment helps to realign their expectations with evidence-based standards [45, 55]. Evidence from a systematic review and meta-analysis confirms that actively including patients and ensuring they have access to relevant information are effective strategies for phasing out unnecessary medical interventions [56]. These methods foster meaningful interactions between patients and healthcare providers, creating a culture of shared decision-making that effectively reduces the use of treatments that are not essential [56].

3.2.5 Institutional policy adjustment

To address the issue of excessive TSH screening and the overuse of LT4, it is crucial to implement changes in institutional policies. This could involve restricting access to these practices in cases where they are not supported by medical evidence. By establishing specific guidelines that limit the use of TSH testing and the prescription of LT4 to clinical scenarios where they are clearly indicated, we can promote a more evidence-based and patient-centered approach to medical care [36, 44].

4. Assessing long-term sustainability of de-implementation strategies

The evaluation of de-implementation and its long-term sustainability demands a comprehensive approach. While physicians and patients may acknowledge the risks associated with indiscriminate TSH testing, various psychological, cultural, and social factors may perpetuate its request, necessitating attention to overcome this barrier [36].

A thorough examination of cost-effectiveness is essential [9]. While the upfront expense of a TSH test is clear, it is imperative to consider broader implications for long-term savings. By forecasting outcomes for patients with undiagnosed subclinical hypothyroidism, potential cost savings become apparent. These savings stem from avoiding expenses associated with levothyroxine treatment, follow-up appointments, and complications arising from overdosing, such as hospitalizations for cardiac arrhythmias or costs related to bone fractures resulting from chronic levothyroxine overdose.

Furthermore, de-implementation represents an ongoing and dynamic process. Even if successful initially, it is crucial to assess its penetration, indicating the extent to which the practice discontinues across all levels of the healthcare system, and its sustainability, reflecting the ability to maintain the interruption of the practice over time [9].

An integral aspect of de-implementation science involves considering potential unintended consequences [36]. For instance, discontinuing a previously recommended intervention, such as including TSH testing in routine check-ups, may lead to patients losing confidence in the medical system. Additionally, clinicians may compensate for de-implementation by increasing the use of other medical interventions, such as conducting additional blood tests like free T4 or anti-TPO alongside TSH, or requesting thyroid ultrasounds in response to patient requests.

5. Conclusion

The significance of optimizing thyroid function tests to prevent unnecessary diagnoses and treatments, especially in cases of subclinical hypothyroidism, has been emphasized in this chapter. It is evident that adopting an individualized and risk-based approach to patient selection for thyroid function testing is crucial, given the variability of TSH levels and their limited correlation with symptoms. Despite the challenges in reducing the overuse of TSH testing, specific strategies, such as healthcare professional education, leveraging electronic health record-based tools, and enhancing patient engagement in the de-implementation process, have been identified as essential steps toward successfully de-implementing low-value medical practices.

Looking ahead, it is imperative to address the limitations present in current literature, including inconsistencies in terminology. Moreover, exploring variations in de-implementation strategies based on taxonomy, along with investigating combined de-implementation approaches and conducting further qualitative research to understand the preferences of physicians, payers, and patients, is crucial avenues for future exploration. By pursuing these paths, tailored interventions can be developed to effectively discourage the use of low-value medical practices across diverse geographical and economic contexts, thereby enhancing healthcare quality and promoting the efficient utilization of healthcare resources. Advancements in these proposed future directions hold the potential to optimize TSH testing, minimizing overdiagnosis and unnecessary interventions.

Acknowledgements

I express my heartfelt gratitude to my family members for their unwavering support and encouragement throughout the completion of this work.

Conflict of interest

The author declares no conflict of interest. This work is not funded.

Author details

Palacios-Bayona Karen Lorena[1,2]

1 Department of Endocrinology, Diabetes, and Metabolic Diseases, Clinica Diagnostica Especializada VID, Medellín, Colombia

2 Clinical Epidemiology, Academic Group of Clinical Epidemiology (GRAEPIC), University of Antioquia, Medellín, Colombia

*Address all correspondence to: lorena.palacios@udea.edu.co

References

[1] Campbell HM, Murata AE, Henrie AM, Conner TA. Combination therapy use and associated events in clinical practice following dissemination of trial findings: A de-implementation study using interrupted time series analysis. Clinical Therapeutics. 2024;**46**(1):40-49. DOI: 10.1016/j.clinthera.2023.10.009

[2] Hensher M, Tisdell J, Zimitat C. "Too much medicine": Insights and explanations from economic theory and research. Social Science & Medicine. 2017;**176**:77-84. DOI: 10.1016/j.socscimed.2017.01.020

[3] Perkins JM, Papaleontiou M. Towards de-implementation of low-value thyroid care in older adults. Current Opinion in Endocrinology, Diabetes, and Obesity. 2022;**29**(5):483-491. DOI: 10.1097/MED.0000000000000758

[4] Biondi B, Cappola AR, Cooper DS. Subclinical hypothyroidism: A review. Journal of the American Medical Association. 2019;**322**(2):153-160. DOI: 10.1001/jama.2019.9052

[5] Manolis AA, Manolis TA, Melita H, Manolis AS. Subclinical thyroid dysfunction and cardiovascular consequences: An alarming wake-up call? Trends in Cardiovascular Medicine. 2020;**30**(2):57-69. DOI: 10.1016/j.tcm.2019.02.011

[6] Rodondi N, den Elzen WP, Bauer DC, Cappola AR, Razvi S, Walsh JP, et al. Subclinical hypothyroidism and the risk of coronary heart disease and mortality. Journal of the American Medical Association. 2010;**304**(12):1365-1374. DOI: 10.1001/jama.2010.1361

[7] Barry MJ, Edgman-Levitan S. Shared decision making--pinnacle of patient-centered care. The New England Journal of Medicine. 2012;**366**(9):780-781. DOI: 10.1056/NEJMp1109283

[8] Cave E. Selecting treatment options and choosing between them: Delineating patient and professional autonomy in shared decision-making. Health Care Analysis. 2020;**28**(1):4-24. DOI: 10.1007/s10728-019-00384-8

[9] Prusaczyk B, Swindle T, Curran G. Defining and conceptualizing outcomes for de-implementation: Key distinctions from implementation outcomes. Implementation Science Communication. 2020;**1**:43. DOI: 10.1186/s43058-020-00035-3

[10] Wilson JMG, Jungner G, editors. Principles and Practice of Screening for Disease. Geneva, Switzerland: World Health Organization; 1968

[11] Jones CM, Boelaert K. The endocrinology of ageing: A mini-review. Gerontology. 2015;**61**(4):291-300. DOI: 10.1159/000367692

[12] Sviridonova MA, Fadeyev VV, Sych YP, Melnichenko GA. Clinical significance of TSH circadian variability in patients with hypothyroidism. Endocrine Research. 2013;**38**(1):24-31. DOI: 10.3109/07435800.2012.710696

[13] Andersen S, Pedersen KM, Bruun NH, Laurberg P. Narrow individual variations in serum T(4) and T(3) in normal subjects: A clue to the understanding of subclinical thyroid disease. The Journal of Clinical Endocrinology and Metabolism. 2002;**87**(3):1068-1072. DOI: 10.1210/jcem.87.3.8165

[14] Surks MI, Hollowell JG. Age-specific distribution of serum

thyrotropin and antithyroid antibodies in the US population: Implications for the prevalence of subclinical hypothyroidism. The Journal of Clinical Endocrinology and Metabolism. 2007;**92**(12):4575-4582. DOI: 10.1210/jc.2007-1499. Epub 2007 Oct 2

[15] Meyerovitch J, Rotman-Pikielny P, Sherf M, Battat E, Levy Y, Surks MI. Serum thyrotropin measurements in the community: Five-year follow-up in a large network of primary care physicians. Archives of Internal Medicine. 2007;**167**(14):1533-1538. DOI: 10.1001/archinte.167.14.1533

[16] Hollowell JG, Staehling NW, Flanders WD, Hannon WH, Gunter EW, Spencer CA, et al. Serum TSH, T(4), and thyroid antibodies in the United States population (1988 to 1994): National Health and Nutrition Examination Survey (NHANES III). The Journal of Clinical Endocrinology and Metabolism. 2002;**87**(2):489-499. DOI: 10.1210/jcem.87.2.8182

[17] LeFevre ML. U.S. Preventive Services Task Force. Screening for thyroid dysfunction: U.S. Preventive Services Task Force recommendation statement. Annals of Internal Medicine. 2015;**162**(9):641-650. DOI: 10.7326/M15 0183

[18] Carlé A, Karmisholt JS, Knudsen N, Perrild H, Thuesen BH, Ovesen L, et al. Does subclinical hypothyroidism add any symptoms? Evidence from a Danish population-based study. The American Journal of Medicine. 2021;**134**(9):1115-1126.e1. DOI: 10.1016/j.amjmed.2021.03.009

[19] Carlé A, Pedersen IB, Knudsen N, Perrild H, Ovesen L, Laurberg P. Hypothyroid symptoms and the likelihood of overt thyroid failure: A population-based case-control study. European Journal of Endocrinology. 2014;**171**(5):593-602. DOI: 10.1530/EJE-14-0481

[20] Canaris GJ, Manowitz NR, Mayor G, Ridgway EC. The Colorado thyroid disease prevalence study. Archives of Internal Medicine. 2000;**160**(4):526-534. DOI: 10.1001/archinte.160.4.526

[21] Gencer B, Collet TH, Virgini V, Bauer DC, Gussekloo J, Cappola AR, et al. Subclinical thyroid dysfunction and the risk of heart failure events: An individual participant data analysis from 6 prospective cohorts. Circulation. 2012;**126**(9):1040-1049. DOI: 10.1161/CIRCULATIONAHA.112.096024

[22] Feller M, Snel M, Moutzouri E, Bauer DC, de Montmollin M, Aujesky D, et al. Association of thyroid hormone therapy with quality of life and thyroid-related symptoms in patients with subclinical hypothyroidism: A systematic review and meta-analysis. Journal of the American Medical Association. 2018;**320**(13):1349-1359. DOI: 10.1001/jama.2018.13770

[23] Stott DJ, Rodondi N, Kearney PM, Ford I, Westendorp RGJ, Mooijaart SP, et al. Thyroid hormone therapy for older adults with subclinical hypothyroidism. The New England Journal of Medicine. 2017;**376**(26):2534-2544. DOI: 10.1056/NEJMoa1603825

[24] Kantor ED, Rehm CD, Haas JS, Chan AT, Giovannucci EL. Trends in prescription drug use among adults in the United States from 1999-2012. Journal of the American Medical Association. 2015;**314**(17):1818-1831. DOI: 10.1001/jama.2015.13766

[25] Ross JS, Rohde S, Sangaralingham L, Brito JP, Choi L, Dutcher SK, et al. Generic and brand-name thyroid hormone drug use among commercially insured and

medicare beneficiaries, 2007 through 2016. The Journal of Clinical Endocrinology and Metabolism. 2019;**104**(6):2305-2314. DOI: 10.1210/jc.2018-02197

[26] Brito JP, Ross JS, El Kawkgi OM, Maraka S, Deng Y, Shah ND, et al. Levothyroxine use in the United States, 2008-2018. JAMA Internal Medicine. 2021;**181**(10):1402-1405. DOI: 10.1001/jamainternmed.2021.2686

[27] Flynn RW, Bonellie SR, Jung RT, MacDonald TM, Morris AD, Leese GP. Serum thyroid-stimulating hormone concentration and morbidity from cardiovascular disease and fractures in patients on long-term thyroxine therapy. The Journal of Clinical Endocrinology and Metabolism. 2010;**95**(1):186-193. DOI: 10.1210/jc.2009-1625

[28] Somwaru LL, Arnold AM, Joshi N, Fried LP, Cappola AR. High frequency of and factors associated with thyroid hormone over-replacement and under-replacement in men and women aged 65 and over. The Journal of Clinical Endocrinology and Metabolism. 2009;**94**(4):1342-1345. DOI: 10.1210/jc.2008-1696

[29] Silverstein WK, Grady D. Overuse of levothyroxine in patients with subclinical hypothyroidism: Time to "Leve"-out-thyroxine. JAMA Internal Medicine. 2021;**181**(10):1286-1287. DOI: 10.1001/jamainternmed.2021.2690

[30] Taylor PN, Iqbal A, Minassian C, Sayers A, Draman MS, Greenwood R, et al. Falling threshold for treatment of borderline elevated thyrotropin levels-balancing benefits and risks: Evidence from a large community-based study. JAMA Internal Medicine. 2014;**174**(1):32-39. DOI: 10.1001/jamainternmed.2013.11312

[31] Garber JR, Cobin RH, Gharib H, Hennessey JV, Klein I, Mechanick JI, et al. Clinical practice guidelines for hypothyroidism in adults: Cosponsored by the American Association of Clinical Endocrinologists and the American Thyroid Association. Endocrine Practice. 2012;**18**(6):988-1028. DOI: 10.4158/EP12280.GL

[32] Birtwhistle R, Morissette K, Dickinson JA, Reynolds DL, Avey MT, Domingo FR, et al; Canadian Task Force on Preventive Health Care. Recommendation on screening adults for asymptomatic thyroid dysfunction in primary care. CMAJ 2019;**191**(46):E1274-E1280. DOI: 10.1503/cmaj.190395. PMID: 31740537; PMCID: PMC6861143

[33] Beastall G, Beckett G, Franklyn J, Fraser W, Hickey J, John R, et al. UK Guidelines for the Use of Thyroid Function Tests. London, UK: Association for Clinical Biochemistry, British Thyroid Association & British Thyroid Foundation; 2006. Available from: http://www.british-thyroid-association.org/sandbox/bta2016/uk_guidelines_for_the_use_of_ thyroid_function_tests.pdf

[34] Roberts L, McCahon D, Johnson O, Haque MS, Parle J, Hobbs FR. Stability of thyroid function in older adults: The Birmingham elderly thyroid study. The British Journal of General Practice. 2018;**68**(675):e718-e726. DOI: 10.3399/bjgp18X698861

[35] Kiel S, Ittermann T, Völzke H, Chenot JF, Angelow A. Frequency of thyroid function tests and examinations in participants of a population-based study. BMC Health Services Research. 2020;**20**(1):70. DOI: 10.1186/s12913-020-4910-7

[36] Ospina NS, Salloum RG, Maraka S, Brito JP. De-implementing low-value care in endocrinology. Endocrine. 2021;**73**(2):292-300. DOI: 10.1007/s12020-021-02732-y

[37] Marcotte LM, Zech JM, Liao JM. Key features underlying low-value care recommendations. American Journal of Medical Quality. 2021;**36**(2):99-102. DOI: 10.1177/1062860620930329

[38] van Bodegom-Vos L, Davidoff F, Marang-van de Mheen PJ. Implementation and de-implementation: Two sides of the same coin? BMJ Quality and Safety. 2017;**26**(6):495-501. DOI: 10.1136/bmjqs-2016-005473

[39] Norton WE, Chambers DA. Unpacking the complexities of de-implementing inappropriate health interventions. Implementation Science. 2020;**15**(1):2. DOI: 10.1186/s13012-019-0960-9

[40] Grimshaw JM, Patey AM, Kirkham KR, Hall A, Dowling SK, Rodondi N, et al. De-implementing wisely: Developing the evidence base to reduce low-value care. BMJ Quality and Safety. 2020;**29**(5):409-417. DOI: 10.1136/bmjqs-2019-010060

[41] Parker G, Kastner M, Born K, Shahid N, Berta W. Understanding low-value care and associated de-implementation processes: A qualitative study of choosing wisely interventions across Canadian hospitals. BMC Health Services Research. 2022;**22**(1):92. DOI: 10.1186/s12913-022-07485-6

[42] Rogers E. Diffusion of Innovations. 5th ed. New York City, USA: Simon & Schuster; 2003

[43] Penfield T, Baker MJ, Scoble R, Wykes MC. Assessment, evaluations, and definitions of research impact: A review. Research Evaluation. 2014;**23**(1):21-32. DOI: 10.1093/reseval/rvt021

[44] Kripalani S, Norton WE. Methodological progress note: De-implementation of low-value care. Journal of Hospital Medicine. 2024;**19**(1):57-61. DOI: 10.1002/jhm.13257

[45] Ingvarsson S, Hasson H, von Thiele SU, Nilsen P, Powell BJ, Lindberg C, et al. Strategies for de-implementation of low-value care-a scoping review. Implementation Science. 2022;**17**(1):73. DOI: 10.1186/s13012-022-01247-y

[46] Berger Z, Flickinger TE, Pfoh E, Martinez KA, Dy SM. Promoting engagement by patients and families to reduce adverse events in acute care settings: A systematic review. BMJ Quality and Safety. 2014;**23**(7):548-555. DOI: 10.1136/bmjqs-2012-001769

[47] van Dulmen SA, Naaktgeboren CA, Heus P, Verkerk EW, Weenink J, Kool RB, et al. Barriers and facilitators to reduce low-value care: A qualitative evidence synthesis. BMJ Open. 2020;**10**(10):e040025. DOI: 10.1136/bmjopen-2020-040025

[48] Kool RB, Verkerk EW, Winnemuller LJ, Wiersma T, Westert GP, Burgers JS, et al. Identifying and de-implementing low-value care in primary care: The GP's perspective-a cross-sectional survey. BMJ Open. 2020;**10**(6):e037019. DOI: 10.1136/bmjopen-2020-037019

[49] Asch DA, Nicholson S, Srinivas S, Herrin J, Epstein AJ. Evaluating obstetrical residency programs using patient outcomes. Journal of the American Medical Association. 2009;**302**(12):1277-1283. DOI: 10.1001/jama.2009.1356

[50] Vaassen S, Essers BAB, Stammen LA, Walsh K, Kerssens M, Evers SMAA, et al. Incorporating value-based healthcare projects in residency training: A mixed-methods study on the impact

of participation on understanding and competency development. BMJ Open. 2022;**12**(8):e060682. DOI: 10.1136/bmjopen-2021-060682

[51] Raudasoja AJ, Falkenbach P, Vernooij RWM, Mustonen JMJ, Agarwal A, et al. Randomized controlled trials in de-implementation research: A systematic scoping review. Implementation Science. 2022;**17**(1):65. DOI: 10.1186/s13012-022-01238-z

[52] Kerr EA, Friese CR, Conroy JM. Enhancing the value of clinical work-choosing wisely to preserve the clinician workforce. JAMA Health Forum. 2022;**3**(11):e224018. DOI: 10.1001/jamahealthforum.2022.4018

[53] Ivers N, Jamtvedt G, Flottorp S, Young JM, Odgaard-Jensen J, French SD, et al. Audit and feedback: Effects on professional practice and healthcare outcomes. Cochrane Database of Systematic Reviews. 2012;(6):CD000259. DOI: 10.1002/14651858.CD000259.pub3

[54] Esposito P, Dal Canton A. Clinical audit, a valuable tool to improve quality of care: General methodology and applications in nephrology. World Journal of Nephrology. 2014;**3**(4):249-255. DOI: 10.5527/wjn.v3.i4.249

[55] Jansen HI, Boelen A, Heijboer AC, Bruinstroop E, Fliers E. Hypothyroidism: The difficulty in attributing symptoms to their underlying cause. Frontiers in Endocrinology (Lausanne). 2023;**14**:1130661. DOI: 10.3389/fendo.2023.1130661

[56] Sypes EE, de Grood C, Whalen-Browne L, Clement FM, Parsons Leigh J, Niven DJ, et al. Engaging patients in de-implementation interventions to reduce low-value clinical care: A systematic review and meta-analysis. BMC Medicine. 2020;**18**(1):116. DOI: 10.1186/s12916-020-01567-0

Chapter 6

Thyroid Imaging Tests

Evangelia Zaromytidou and Athanasios Notopoulos

Abstract

Thyroid imaging tests provide more information about the thyroid gland's size, shape, and function. After the thyroid blood tests which are the gold standard for the assessment of conditions like hypothyroidism or hyperthyroidism, imaging tests are recommended to establish a diagnosis. Although the diagnosis of hypothyroidism in itself is not an indication of thyroid imaging, thyroid radionuclide scanning may be useful in elucidating several pathophysiological aspects of hyperthyroidism and in determining the cause of abnormal thyroid function. This may be especially crucial in deciding whether a person will take thyroxine replacement therapy. However, it is important to recognize whether the cause of hypothyroidism is transient or drug-induced because this may require no treatment or only short-term thyroxine supplementation.

Keywords: hypothyroidism, RAIU, RTCUT, imagine tests, thyroid scan

1. Introduction

Hypothyroidism is a clinical and biochemical disorder caused by a lack of thyroid hormones resulting in a slowing down of metabolic processes and potentially is fatal in severe cases if untreated. It may be due to a disease of either the thyroid gland (primary hypothyroidism), the pituitary gland (secondary), the hypothalamus (tertiary hypothyroidism) or rarely to a peripheral resistance to the actions of thyroid hormones [1].

The causes of hypothyroidism for primary hypothyroidism with goiter are hypertrophic form of Hashimoto's thyroiditis, thyroid hormone biosynthesis disorders and subacute thyroiditis. For primary hypothyroidism without goiter, is atrophic form of Hashimoto's thyroiditis, agenesis or hypoplasia of the thyroid, excessive iodine intake, inflammation, post thyroidectomy, post radioactive iodine therapy or post radiotherapy of the neck. It should be noted that TSH levels are high in these conditions. The causes of secondary hypothyroidism, in which TSH is invariably detected at low levels, are panhypopituitarism and isolated TSH deficiency. The causes of tertiary hypothyroidism are due to hypothalamic lesions where the TSH values are detected at low levels [1].

Nuclear medicine in the field of thyroid disorders provides important information for both diagnostic tests (in vitro and in vivo tests) and therapeutic interventions. A scintigraphic study is an in vivo imaging diagnostic study, performed after administration of a gamma photon- or positron- emitting radionuclide, which demonstrates in two or three dimensions the distribution of the radioactive tracer in the target organ of the human body. The uptake and distribution of radiopharmaceutical in the thyroid gland depends upon three factors, the metabolism, the physiology, and the pathophysiology of the gland [1, 2].

 IntechOpen

There are many radiopharmaceuticals available in the Nuclear Physician's quiver that provide them with the ability to study the biokinetic behavior of the non-radioactive tracer and to obtain functional quantitative and anatomical information about the thyroid gland. The most widely used radionuclides are 99 m-Technetium Pertechnetate, two isotopes of iodine I-123 and I-131, Thallium Chloride (201 T1) and Fluorine-18-fluorodeoxyglocose (FDG) [3].

2. Diagnostic applications of radiopharmaceuticals

2.1 99mTechnetium pertechnetate

Is widely used for imaging the thyroid gland. Technetium does not exist in nature but was first discovered in 1937 by Carlo Perrier and Emilio Segre at Palermo University. They managed to isolate technetium-97 from a sample of molybdenum irradiated with deuterons in the cyclotron [4]. It belongs to group VIIA of the Mendeleev Table of the Elements. The pertechnetate monovalent ion ([99mTc]-Tc04)- has similar chemical and physical characteristics to the iodide ion (i. e. ionic size and negative charge) and similar biological distribution, thus competing with it and its active uptake in the thyroid gland, salivary glands, choroidal plexuses and stomach [5, 6].

99mTechnetium Pertechnetate is trapped by the thyroid parenchyma after being mediated by the NIS (sodium/iodide symporter), a transmembrane glycoprotein located on the basolateral membrane of follicular cells. However, unlike iodine, pertechnetate ion does not undergo organification and is not incorporated into the thyroid hormones; therefore, it remains in the gland for a relative short period. It has replaced the 131I-sodium iodide in the imaging of the thyroid gland for five decades because:

- it has low cost
- is readily available from portable generators with molybdenum-99,
- the absorbed radiation dose to the thyroid gland is very low compared to 131I-sodium-iodine (it is about 2600 times lower per mCi),
- it provides good image quality of the gland
- it has short retention in the gland with short half-life (6 hours) and no β - radiation; therefore, imaging is performed about 20–30 min after the injection.

The administered dose for adults is 111–185 MBq (3–5 mCi) and for children is lower approximately 18,5–111 MBq (0.5–3 mCi) [6].

2.2 Radioiodine-123 and radioiodine-131

Radioiodine-123(Na[123I] I) due to its ideal characteristics, which are the short physical half-life (13 hours), the absence of β –emissions and the high ratio uptake in thyroid tissue compared to that in the surrounding tissues, is very suitable for scintigraphy. However, it has some disadvantages, being less readily available (produced by cyclotron) and more expensive than 99mTechnetium Pertechnetate. It has the same biokinetics as the stable iodine and is based on the basic principle of radiotracer and this fact allows the pathophysiological imaging and the quantitative study of (i) iodine behavior in the thyroid gland as well as in other organs related to the uptake, (ii) the organification of iodine into thyroid hormones, (iii) the metabolism and excretion of stable iodine. The administered dose is approximately 200–400 μCi (7.4–14.8 MBq). Radioiodine-123 has a preferable use for the detection of either ectopic thyroid tissue or lack of iodine organification.

Na[131I]I, is the first of all theragnostics radiopharmaceuticals used for to observe and quantify the iodine distribution and kinetics inside the thyroid gland, whereas β-particles emission was used to obtain the therapeutic effect. Based on its physical characteristics, the long half-life (8.02 days), the high absorbed radiation dose, the β-electrons emission and the emitting of an electromagnetic photon with a principal gamma-ray of 364 keV, it is no longer used for routine diagnostic scintigraphy. However, it is still usable for evaluating mediastinal masses and detecting of recurrences in differentiated thyroid cancer and metastases. The administered diagnostic dose is approximately 2–5 mCi (74–185 MBq).

Regarding its therapeutic properties, Na[131I]I is the preferable agent for the treatment of hyperthyroidism and thyroid cancer, due to the high activity of β- particles which drastically destroy thyroid tissue. The administered therapeutic dose is based on the uptake measurement, on the radioactivity (MBq) we want to be delivered per gram of tissue and the mass of the gland [6].

2.3 Thallium chloride (201 T1)

Its use is limited only in the imaging and confirmation of metastases from adenocarcinomas of the thyroid gland in some patients with total thyroidectomy without interrupting the replacement therapy, as it is required when using Na[131I]I in follicular carcinomas in order to increase TSH. It has a high importance of monitoring thyroidectomized patients having negative whole-body scintigraphy with iodine-131 and elevated thyroglobulin values which indicate the presence of metastases of differentiated cancer. It is disadvantaged in that its uptake is nonspecific and may be observed in benign as well as malignant conditions [6].

2.4 Fluorine-18-fluorodeoxyglocose (FDG)

It is only used in evaluating a variety of neoplasms including differentiated thyroid cancer, not visualized at radioiodine imaging, and to assess prognosis. It also has the advantage to detect the nonfunctioning as well as functioning thyroid cancers and to distinguish benign thyroid nodudes from cancer, based on the higher FDG metabolism seen in tumors [6].

3. The in vivo tests of thyroid function

The purpose of the in vivo diagnostic tests for thyroid gland is:

i. to measure thyroid function with uptake tests with and

ii. to obtain an image of the location, size, morphology and the evaluation of the functionality of the thyroid gland by scintigraphy using either 99mTechnetium

Pertechnetate or Radioiodine-123, if the evaluation of the patient's history, vitro tests and other diagnostic tests have been carried out previously [7].

i. *Uptake Test:* The uptake test refers to the percentage uptake of a radiopharmaceutical by the thyroid gland in relation to the administered dose at specified intervals. Several methods of functional assessment have been used in the past, which have gradually been limited and nowadays mainly the Radioiodine Uptake (RAIU) and the 99mTechnetium Pertechnetate Thyroid Uptake (RTCUT) have remained in use.

Radioiodine Uptake (RAIU) illustrates the functional state of thyroid gland and helps to determine the dose of 131-I in a post-operative therapy (ablation). The main indications for its performances are the confirmation of hyperthyroidism, the estimation of the therapeutic dose of 131-I, the determination of the thyroid tissue autonomy, and the clarification of the cause of thyrotoxicosis.

The RAIU test can also be performed with 123-I in conjunction with scintigraphy.

The factors affecting thyroid uptake of iodine are dietary restrictions, impaired kidney function, radiological studies with iodine-contrast, antithyroid medications, amiodarone and thyroid hormones. In addition, there are pathological disorders that either increase or decrease the RAIU (**Table 1**).

The normal range for RAIU in thyroid gland is from 10 to 30%.

99mTechnetium Pertechnetate Thyroid Uptake (RTCUT), as a substitute for iodine indicates the temporary trapping that iodine would have had, not its organification. For this reason, RTCUTs values are indicative and not as precise as those of RAIU. It is performed in conjunction with scintigraphy within 20 minutes after the intravenous administration. The main indications for its performance are Grave's disease, subacute thyroiditis, drug-induced thyrotoxicosis, evaluation and monitoring of hyperthyroidism, evaluation of hypothyroidism caused by an impairment of the organification, evaluation of treatment or withdrawal of treatment in persons receiving either methimazole, either propylthiouracil.

The normal values of RTCUT at 20 minutes range from 0,24 to 3,34% [7].

ii. *Thyroid scan* is a simple, non-invasive, cost effective tool for assessment of most thyroid disorders. The advantage of scintigraphy is that it can provide an immediate assessment of the morphological and functional status of the

Increase RAIU	Decrease RAIU
Hyperthyroidism	Blocked Trapping
Rebound effect from abrupt withdrawal of antithyroid drugs	Acute Subacute and Chronic lymphocytic thyroiditis
Enzyme disorders	Blocked Organification
Long-term antithyroid therapy (↑TSH ↓ T4)	Exogenous intake of thyroid hormones
Lithium	Ablation
Thyroiditis onset	Struma Ovari
Rebound effect from post thyroiditis	Antithyroid drugs

Table 1.
Thyroid disorders which increase or decrease the RAIU.

thyroid gland. Thyroid scan plays a complementary role in diagnosis of hypothyroidism in infancy to confirm the underlying etiology. It detects patients who should be given lifelong replacement therapy (hypo-plastic ectopic thyroid) and identifies patients who need reevaluation (non-visualization or dyshormonogenesis).

The clinical indications for thyroid scintigraphy are:

- the evaluation of thyroid size, shape, position and function
- further evaluation and identification of findings on physical examination
- determination of functional status of thyroid nodules
- follow up of radioiodine therapy for thyroid cancer
- diagnosis and monitoring of thyroiditis
- diagnosis, treatment, follow-up, and prognosis of the goiter
- assessment of extrathyroidal tissue and mediastinal masses
- screening after head and neck irradiation

99mTechnetium Pertechnetate imaging: An intravenous injection of 1–5 mCi (37 185 MBq) is administered and images are obtained 20 minutes p.i. in the anterior and the 45° right anterior oblique and 45° left anterior oblique views. The 99mTc Pertechnetate is actively transported and trapped into the follicular cells but it is not bound to tyrosine. Therefore, the study reflects the measurement of trapping.

Radioiodine 123 imaging: the tracer is administered orally in capsule form of 100–400 μCi (3,7–15 MBq) and images are obtained at 6 and 24 hours in the anterior and the 45° right anterior oblique and 45° left anterior oblique views. This isotope of iodine is handled by the body exactly like ^{127}I (a nonradioactive iodine) and after administration it is absorbed by the intestine into the extrathyroidal iodide pool. Extrathyroidal iodine is actively transported across the membrane of the follicular cell where it binds to tyrosine, through interaction with thyroid peroxidase, it is organized and incorporated into thyroid hormone. Therefore, the study reflects the distribution of tissue that possesses the functions of trapping and organifying [7–9].

4. Hypothyroidism nuclear medicine imaging

Introduction: Primary hypothyroidism is associated with insufficient production of thyroid hormones by the thyroid gland, while secondary hypothyroidism is related to impaired signaling to a normal thyroid gland by an abnormal pituitary gland or hypothalamus.

Iodine deficiency is the most common cause of hypothyroidism worldwide, while Hashimoto thyroiditis is the prevailing cause of hypothyroidism in developed countries (**Table 2**).

Primary Hypothyroidism	Secondary Hypothyroidism
• autoimmune thyroid diseases • iodine deficiency • thyroiditis (postpartum, silent, subacute, Riedel, Van Wyk-Grumbach syndrome) • post-radiation, –surgery, –radioiodine therapy • infiltrative disease (lymphoma, amyloidosis, sarcoidosis, tuberculosis) • congenital hypothyroidism • antithyroid drugs	• pituitary lesions (adenoma, panhypopituitarism, infiltrative disease, post-radiation) • central congenital hypothyroidism • drug-induced • amiodarone

Table 2.
Causes of primary and secondary hypothyroidism.

In the following paragraphs the imaging features of some of the above disorders and conditions will be dealt.

4.1 Autoimmune thyroid diseases (AITDs)

AITDs are increasingly seen due to:

- the widespread use of (i) anti-tumor targeted therapies such as tyrosine kinase inhibitors (TKIs) and (ii) immunotherapies with checkpoint inhibitors (CPIs)
- SARS-CoV-2 infection

Lymphocytic infiltration of the thyroid gland is the hallmark of AITD.

NM techniques, such as radioiodine upta.ke (RAIU) and thyroid scintigraphy, using 99mTc-pertechnetate (Na[99mTc]TcO4) or 123-Iodine (Na[123I]I), play a clear role in the differential diagnosis [10].

4.1.1 Hashimoto thyroiditis (HT)

Being a subtype of autoimmune thyroiditis, it is also known as lymphocytic thyroiditis or chronic autoimmune thyroiditis. It typically affects middle-aged females (30–50-year age group with an F:M ratio of 10–15:1).

In developed countries, it is the most common cause of hypothyroidism. The inflammation enhanced by the lymphocytic infiltration of the gland induces (i) follicular cell destruction, necrosis, and apoptosis, (ii) fibrosis, (iii) a humoral antibody (Ab)-mediated response directed against TPO or/and Tg, (iv) hypothyroidism [11].

Imaging is usually not necessary to diagnose HT. In selected cases, it helps to estimate the size and composition of the gland, as well as to detect any co-existing nodules.

- *US*

In the initial phase the gland is usually depicted enlarged and heterogeneous, while in chronic cases it may be atrophic. Diffuse hypoechoicity and development of micro-pseudonodules with surrounding echogenic septations (pseudolobulated changes) are frequently observed [12, 13]. The degree of echogenicity shows a satisfactory negative correlation with the degree of lymphocytic infiltration [14], but not with the biochemical indices of thyroid function [15]. Color Doppler usually shows normal or decreased flow, but occasionally it might appear hypervascular similar to a thyroid inferno; in HT hypervascularity does not reflect thyrotoxicosis. It is difficult to reliably sonographically differentiate HT from other thyroid pathology.

Annual ultrasound screening is recommended for early detection of nodules [16]. Nodular HT is associated with the presence of large nodules. Sometimes prominent reactive cervical nodes with normal morphologic features may be observed. The presence of any calcifications may either reflect the presence or indicate an increased risk of papillary thyroid carcinoma [17].

- *Thyroid scan*

The pertechnetate thyroid scintigraphy illustrates the functional state of the thyroid gland. In the initial phase of the disease, a diffusely increased concentration of the radiopharmaceutical is observed in the thyroid, a finding that reflects the stimulation of the gland by TSH, produced by the pituitary gland and compensating for the early reduction of thyroid hormones. The image should be differentiated from Graves' disease and color flow Doppler may contribute to the differential diagnosis [18]. As the disease progresses, the thyroid parenchyma is replaced by lymphocytes and fibrous tissue and the gland becomes unable to respond to stimulation by elevated TSH levels. In such cases, the common findings on pertechnetate thyroid scintigraphy include symmetrical enlargement of the gland's borders, slightly inhomogeneous distribution of the radiopharmaceutical in the thyroid parenchyma, without the existence of defined focal findings [19]. This relative heterogeneity is attributed to the variable response of the follicles to their stimulation by TSH. In children and adolescents with HT, the distribution of the radiopharmaceutical is more homogeneous compared to the adult picture [20].

Iodine-123 thyroid scintigraphy is rarely needed in the investigation of HT [21].

FDG-PET scan shows a diffusely increased uptake and may reveal autoimmune thyroiditis as a consequence of cancer immunotherapy, especially when using CPIs.

4.2 Thyroiditis

4.2.1 Post-partum thyroiditis

It is a transient disorder, which occurs in women who have a high titer of antibodies against TPO, which are involved in enhancing the rebound stimulation of the immune mechanisms, after the period of relative immune-suppression, which is constituted by pregnancy [22]. It affects approximately 6–10% of births [23, 24]. 33–50% of pregnant women with elevated Ab-TPO in early pregnancy will develop transient, postpartum thyroiditis [25]. Ab-TPO and Ab-Tg cross the placenta, but do not appear to exert any adverse effect on the fetus [26]. Women with HLA haplotype DR-3, DR-4 or DR-5 are at increased risk of postpartum thyroiditis. In women with type 1 diabetes mellitus, the incidence of postpartum thyroiditis is three times that of the general population [27].

Ultrasound is the imaging test of choice; the gland often appears hypoechoic, but variable findings may be noted. Scintigraphically, a reduced uptake of the radiopharmaceutical by the thyroid parenchyma is observed [28]. The immunohistochemical pattern of the thyroid in postpartum thyroiditis resembles that of Hashimoto's thyroiditis, except that Hurthle cells are not often seen.

About 20–25% of women with postpartum thyroiditis will develop hypothyroidism a few years later. A positive correlation has been observed between the probability of permanent hypothyroidism and the values of TSH and Ab-TPO. Also, subsequent pregnancy can cause recurrence of the disease in up to 70% of cases. Of the group of women with elevated Ab-TPO without postpartum thyroiditis in the initial pregnancy, 25% will develop the disease in a subsequent pregnancy [29].

4.2.2 Silent thyroiditis

It is a form of subacute thyroiditis associated with HLA-DR-3 and elevated levels of Ab-TPO and Ab-Tg. It is usually characterized by the recent onset of symptoms and the lack of thyroidal pain or tenderness. An initial transient hyperthyroid period is followed by hypothyroidism and finally the euthyroid state is attained.

Scintigraphically the thyroid parenchyma typically shows markedly reduced radiotracer uptake, while the gland may have normal to moderately enlarged size.

4.2.3 Riedel thyroiditis (RT)

It is a rare disease tending to affect middle-aged persons (30–60 years old with an F:M ratio of 3:1). Its etiology being rather obscure, RT seems to be characterized by a fibroinflammatory process derived from autoimmune signaling [30].

- US

The thyroid gland appears diffusely hypoechoic and ischaemic due to extensive fibrosis; hyperechoic bands correspond to the fibrosis [31]. US elastography may reveal significant stiffness of the gland.

- CT

Within the thyroid parenchyma, hypodense areas are observed, which remain unaltered after administration of a contrast agent [32]. CT imaging of the chest or abdomen may show more systemic involvement.

- MRI

The main findings are: (i) hypointense images in T1- and T2-sequences, (ii) uniform enhancement of variable intensity can be observed following IV Gd administration.

- Pertechnate Thyroid Scan

No radiotracer is detected within the affected tissue, which appears as a photopenic area.

- FDG-PET Scan

Intense uptake is observed corresponding to the areas of inflammation–fibrosis in RT [33, 34].

4.2.4 Subacute thyroiditis (DE QUERVAIN)

It is a self-limited thyroiditis usually preceded by an upper respiratory tract viral infection. In the initial phase, patients present with a painful neck along with thyrotoxicosis, followed by a period of hypothyroidism. In most cases a euthyroid state is finally achieved without requiring a specific treatment.

- US

The affected areas appear as irregularly confined lesions of decreased echogenicity and vascularity. They can be bilateral or unilateral. The gland size is usually normal but can occasionally be enlarged or smaller. After the resolution of the disease, the sonographic pattern and enlargement of the thyroid resolve with some strands of fbrosis refecting the residual thyroid damage.

- Thyroid scan

In patients with the appropriate clinical setting and ultrasound findings, low or absent uptake of the radiotracer is observed, rendering difficult the clear delineation of the gland from the surrounding tissues.

4.2.5 Van Wyk-Grumbach syndrome

This syndrome is characterized by chronic hypothyroid autoimmune thyroiditis, delayed bone age and precocious puberty (usually early menarche and breast development, without pubic and axillary hair growth) due to the stimulation of ovarian FSH receptors by the excess of TSH.

Plain radiographs wrist and hand are used to detect delayed bone age.

4.3 Infiltrative thyroid disease

The imaging features of these entities are nonspecific and may pose diagnostic challenges being difficult to differentiate from primary thyroid malignancies, HT and other forms of thyroiditis [35].

4.3.1 Thyroid lymphoma

It is a rare disease (1–2 patients per 1,000,000 people) mainly affecting 50–70 year old females (F:M = 3). It commonly presents as a rapidly enlarging goiter with accompanying compressive symptoms and cervical lymphadenopathy. Hashimoto thyroiditis has been associated with an increased risk for thyroid lymphoma.

- US

It may appear as nodular (hypoechoic mass) or diffuse (mixed echotexture) or mixed [36], while calcifications are uncommon 4.

- CT

Its usual appearance is a goiter, hypodense compared to the adjacent muscles, which may show heterogeneous enhancement but still less than adjacent muscle [37].

- MRI

The gland may appear iso- to hyper-intense on T1/T2 sequences. A pseudocapsule may be detected.

4.3.2 Thyroid amyloidosis

It is due to the deposition of amyloid protein and fat within the thyroid gland.

- US

An enlarged gland showing complex or hypoechoic areas maybe extending to the mediastinum.

- CT

A diffuse or/and multinodular thyroid enlargement at varying extents depending on the amount of fat and amyloid deposited within the thyroid parenchyma [38].

- MRI

Proteinaceous substances within the nodules result in high intensity T1 images, fibrillar amyloid structures in increased signal on T2 images and fatty infiltration in increased T1 and T2 signals [39]. Cases with diffuse fatty infiltration can be difficult to differentiate from thyrolipomatosis.

4.3.3 Thyroid sarcoidosis

Involvement of the thyroid gland by sarcoidosis is very rare, affecting 4.5% of patients with sarcoidosis. It may present as (i) a gradual enlargement of the gland, eventually causing compressive symptoms, (ii) a multinodular goiter, (iii) cold solitary thyroid nodules, with or without cervical lymphadenopathy [40]. Its diagnosis may be elusive given the imaging similarities with other thyroid diseases and the limitations of FNA due to either the scattered pattern of granulomatous infiltration or the formation of hyperplastic papillary structures [41].

4.3.4 Thyroid tuberculosis

It is extremely unusual and the diagnosis can be easily disregarded as the clinical and imagological findings are usually non-specific. The gland may appear either diffusely enlarged or with a heterogeneous (micro)-nodular composition [42]. Cervical lymphadenopathy may also be present.

4.4 Congenital hypothyroidism

4.4.1 Introduction

The most common causes of congenital hypothyroidism [43, 44] are presented in **Table 3**. In developing countries, the main cause is the endemic lack of iodine in mother and fetus.

• *Thyroid dysgenesis* (most common cause: 80–85% of cases, 1:4500 births)
• agenesis • hypoplasia • ectopy (67% of cases): usually found at the base of the tongue, but also anywhere along the thyroglossal duct. Despite the existence of functional thyroid parenchyma, the production of thyroid hormones is usually insufficient to ensure normal development
• *Dyshormogenesis* (10–15% of congenital hypothyroidism cases, 1:30000 births)
• decreased response to TSH: it affects 1% of cases; it is due to a mutation of the TSH receptor gene and more rarely to a mutation of the Gs_{α}-gene (pseudohyperparathyroidism type 1a or Albright's hereditary osteodystrophy) • disorder in iodine trapping (dysfunction of the sodium-iodine cotransporter) • problematic organification of iodine (disorders either of the TPO enzyme or of H_2O_2 production, Pendred syndrome) • disorders of the enzyme iodotyrosine dehalogenase • disorders of synthesis, iodination and transport of thyroglobulin • presence of abnormal iodoproteins (iodotyrosine deiodinase disorders)
• *Central congenital hypothyroidism* (5% of cases, 1:50000–100,000 births)
• isolated hypothalamic lesion (insufficient TRH secretion or resistance to its action) • hypothalamic lesion combined with midline abnormalities and brain malformations • structural abnormalities of TSH molecule • pituitary hypoplasia / ectopy

Table 3.
The most common causes of congenital hypothyroidism.

4.4.2 Imaging investigation in neonates with congenital hypothyroidism

After performing the screening test, as long as TSH < 10mIU/L, no further action is needed. Newborns with a moderate increase in TSH (10mIU/L < TSH < 20mIU/L) are invited for a confirmatory test of TSH and measurement of T4 and FT4 (blood collection by venipuncture); if hypothyroid hormone levels are confirmed, they are referred to a pediatric endocrinologist and treatment begins. Neonates with TSH > 20mIU/L are referred directly to a pediatric endocrinologist for further testing and treatment.

In cases of single measurement of TSH or total T4 (TT4), the following observations have emerged from their application in clinical practice: The measurement of TT4 is advantageous in the detection of cases with central hypothyroidism and is accompanied by fewer false positive results (TT4 does not change during the first 24–48 hours of life, as it has been observed with TSH). It is difficult to define a cutoff (threshold) low enough to avoid false-positive results and high enough to detect cases with an ectopic thyroid gland, resulting in about 7% false-negative results. The measurement of TSH has the advantage of having fewer false negative results and is furthermore highly recommended in the detection of congenital hypothyroidism due to iodine deficiency, as well as in cases with mild hypothyroidism [45].

- Radiographs

The knee joints may be X-rayed to determine the bone age (bone epiphyses study).

- US

It can provide additional information about (i) the anatomy of the gland, (ii) the presence of cysts or thymic tissue in the thyroid region in patients with thyroid dysgenesis, and (iii) allow the gland to be detected in some cases in the absence of radiopharmaceutical uptake during scintigraphic testing [46, 47]. In the latter cases, there arises a suspicion of some form of dyshormonogenesis (specifically that due to a reduced response to TSH) or of the transplacental passage of antibodies against TSH receptors. Antibodies against TSH receptors completely inhibit TSH-induced uptake of the radiopharmaceutical by the thyroid parenchyma [48]. The measurement of thyroglobulin can help detect residual functional thyroid tissue.

- Thyroid scan

It is particularly useful in ruling out any dysgenesis and is much more sensitive than ultrasound in revealing ectopic thyroid tissue [49]. It is performed with either radioactive technetium (1–5 MBq/kg 99mTc-pertechnenate) or radioactive iodine-123 (0.1–0.3 MBq/kg 123I). 123I is the radionuclide of choice when ectopic or dystopic thyroid tissue is suspected, due to its superior properties such as higher gamma energy (159 keV) compared to 99mTechnetium (140 keV), thus allowing for better penetration of osseous structures and detection of retrosternal, intrathoracic and abdominal thyrogenous masses. Sensitivity and specifcity of scintigraphy gets further increased if SPECT/CT hybrid imaging is available for anatomic correlation and attenuation correction.

It appears that thyroid dysgenesis is a multigene (disruption of several genes is required to manifest the specific phenotype) and multifactorial (synergy of genetic and environmental factors is required) disease [50]. In 40–60% of cases there is residual thyroid tissue, but thyroid scintigraphy (even with 123I) has relatively limited sensitivity for its detection.

Except in the case of decreased response to TSH, in congenital hypothyroidism due to dyshormonogenesis, the thyroid gland is visualized in situ (and is often enlarged and/or shows increased radiopharmaceutical uptake).

In dyshormonogenesis due to iodine trapping disorder, hypothyroidism is accompanied by goiter and a low uptake of the radiopharmaceutical is observed in the thyroid parenchyma. As hypothyroidism is usually detected late, mental retardation coexists. Potassium iodide 1–5 mg is given and then thyroxine.

In the case of decreased response to TSH, the thyroid gland is not visualized on scintigraphy (same picture as that of agenesis), while the thyroid tissue is revealed on ultrasound examination and serum thyroglobulin is measured in approximately normal ranges [51]. The dissociation between the gland size and thyroglobulin concentration is partly explained by the fact that the regulation of thyroglobulin secretion is not solely dependent on TSH.

The use of recombinant TSH is a satisfactory alternative to scintigraphic study and potassium perchlorate discharge test, avoiding discontinuation of replacement therapy [52].

In conclusion, the combination of scintigraphy and thyroid ultrasound is the best imaging approach for congenital hypothyroidism [53].

DOI: http://dx.doi.org/10.5772/intechopen.1004702

Author details

Evangelia Zaromytidou* and Athanasios Notopoulos
Nuclear Medicine Department, Hippokration General Hospital, Thessaloniki, Greece

*Address all correspondence to: evazarom4@gmail.com; enmf23@gmail.com

References

[1] Mariani G, Tonacchera M, Grosso M, et al. The role of nuclear medicine in the clinical management of benign thyroid disorders, part 2: Nodular goiter, hypothyroidism, and subacute thyroiditis. Journal of Nuclear Medicine. 2021;**62**:88

[2] Atkins HL. Technetium-99m pertechnetate uptake and scanning in the evaluation of thyroid function. Seminars in Nuclear Medicine. 1971;**1**(3):345-55.6-895

[3] Chaudhary V, Bano S. Imaging of the thyroid: Recent advances. Indian Journal of Endocrinology and Metabolism. 2012;**16**(3):371-376

[4] De Jonge FA, Pauwels EK. Technetium, the missing element. European Journal of Nuclear Medicine. 1996;**23**(3):336-344. DOI: 10.1007/bf00837634

[5] Lakshmanan M, Schaffer A, Robbins J, Reynolds J, Norton J. A simplified low iodine diet in I-131 scanning and therapy of thyroid cancer. Clinical Nuclear Medicine. 1988;**13**(12):866-868

[6] Intenzo CM, Dam HQ, Manzone TA, Kim SM. Imaging of the thyroid in benign and malignant disease. Seminars in Nuclear Medicine. 2012;**42**(1):49-61

[7] Giovanella L, Avram AM, Iakovu I. EANM practice guideline/SNMMI procedure standard for RAIU and thyroid scintigraphy. European Journal of Nuclear Medicine and Molecular Imaging. 2019;**46**:2514-2525

[8] Qiao T, Liu S, Cui Z, et al. Deep learning for intelligent diagnosis in thyroid scintigraphy. The Journal of International Medical Research. 2021;**49**(1):300060520982842. DOI: 10.1177/0300060520982842

[9] Smith JR, Oates E. Radionuclide imaging of the thyroid gland: Patterns, pearls, and pitfalls. Clinical Nuclear Medicine. 2004;**29**:181-193

[10] Petranović Ovčariček P, Görges R, Giovanella L. Autoimmune thyroid diseases. Seminars in Nuclear Medicine. 2023;**S0001-2998**(23):00090-00099

[11] Vargas-Uricoechea H. Molecular mechanisms in autoimmune thyroid disease. Cells. 2023;**12**:918

[12] Aydin O, Apaydin FD, Bozdogan R, Pata C, Yalcinoglu O, Kanik A. Cytological correlation in patients who have a pre-diagnosis of thyroiditis ultrasonographically. Endocrine Research. 2003;**29**:97-106

[13] Yeh HC, Futterweit W, Gilbert P. Micronodulation: Ultrasonographic sign of Hashimoto thyroiditis. Journal of Ultrasound in Medicine. 1996;**15**:813-819

[14] Yoshida A, Adachi T, Noguchi T, Urabe K, Onoyama S, Okamura Y, et al. Echographic findings and histological feature of the thyroid: A reverse relationship between the level of echo-amplitude and lymphocytic infiltration. Endocrinologia Japonica. 1985;**32**:681-690

[15] Set PA, Oleszczuk-Raschke K, von Lengerke JH, Bramswig J. Sonographic features of Hashimoto thyroiditis in childhood. Clinical Radiology. 1996;**51**:167-169

[16] Pedersen OM, Aardal NP, Larssen TB, Varhaug JE, Myking O,

Vik-Mo H. The value of ultrasonography in predicting autoimmune thyroid disease. Thyroid. 2000;**10**:251-259

[17] Ohmori N, Miyakawa M, Ohmori K, Takano K. Ultrasonographic findings of papillary thyroid carcinoma with Hashimoto's thyroiditis. Internal Medicine. 2007;**46**:547-550

[18] Erdogan MF, Anil C, Cesur M, Baskal N, Erdogan G. Color flow Doppler sonography for the etiologic diagnosis of hyperthyroidism. Thyroid. 2007;**17**:223-228

[19] Intenzo CM, Capuzzi DM, Jabbour S, Kim SM, dePapp AE. Scintigraphic features of autoimmune thyroiditis. Radiographics. 2001;**21**:957-964

[20] Alos N, Huot C, Lambert R, Van Vliet G. Thyroid scintigraphy in children and adolescents with Hashimoto disease. The Journal of Pediatrics. 1995;**127**:951-953

[21] Paltiel HJ, Summerville DA, Treves ST. Iodine-123 scintigraphy in the evaluation of pediatric thyroid disorders: A ten year experience. Pediatric Radiology. 1992;**22**:251-256

[22] Muller AF, Drexhage HA, Berghout A. Postpartum thyroiditis and autoimmune thyroiditis in women of childbearing age: Recent insights and consequences for antenatal and postnatal care. Endocrine Reviews. 2001;**22**:605-630

[23] Lervang HH, Pryds O, Kristensen HP. Thyroid dysfunction after delivery: Incidence and clinical course. Acta Medica Scandinavica. 1987;**222**:369-374

[24] Lucas A, Pizarro E, Granada ML, Salinas I, Foz M, Sanmarti A. Postpartum thyroiditis: Epidemiology and clinical evolution in a nonselected population. Thyroid. 2000;**10**:71-77

[25] Freeman R, Rosen H, Thysen B. Incidence of thyroid dysfunction in an unselected postpartum population. Archives of Internal Medicine. 1986;**146**:1361-1364

[26] Amino N, Tada H, Hidaka Y. Postpartum autoimmune thyroid syndrome: A model of aggravation of auto-immune disease. Thyroid. 1999;**9**:705-713

[27] Alvarez-Marfany M, Roman SH, DrexlerAJ,RobertsonC,Stagnaro-GreenAS. Long-term prospective study of postpartum thyroid dysfunction in women with insulin dependent diabetes mellitus. The Journal of Clinical Endocrinology and Metabolism. 1994;**79**:10-16

[28] Parkes AB, Othman S, Hall R, John R, Richards CJ, Lazarus JH. The role of complement in the pathogenesis of postpartum thyroiditis. The Journal of Clinical Endocrinology and Metabolism. 1994;**79**:395-400

[29] Lazarus JH, Ammari F, Oretti R, Parkes AB, Richards CJ, Harris B. Clinical aspects of recurrent postpartum thyroiditis. The British Journal of General Practice. 1997;**47**:305-308

[30] Czarnywojtek A, Pietrończyk K, Thompson LDR, Triantafyllou A, Florek E, Sawicka-Gutaj N, et al. IgG4-related sclerosing thyroiditis (Riedel-Struma): A review of clinicopathological features and management. Virchows Archiv. 2023;**483**:133-144

[31] Lu L, Gu F, Dai WX, Li WY, Chen J, Xiao Y, et al. Clinical and pathological features of Riedel's thyroiditis. Chinese Medical Sciences Journal. 2010;**25**(3):129-134

[32] Ozgen A, Cila A. Riedel's thyroiditis in multifocal fibrosclerosis: CT and MR imaging findings. AJNR. American Journal of Neuroradiology. 2000;**21**:320-321

[33] Slman R, Monpeyssen H, Desarnaud S, Haroche J, Fediaevsky Ldu P, Fabrice M, et al. Ultrasound, elastography, and fluorodeoxyglucose positron emission tomography/computed tomography imaging in Riedel's thyroiditis: Report of two cases. Thyroid. 2011;**21**:799-804

[34] Kotilainen P, Airas L, Kojo T, Kurki T, Kataja K, Minn H, et al. Positron emission tomography as an aid in the diagnosis and follow-up of Riedel's thyroiditis. European Journal of Internal Medicine. 2004;**15**:186-189

[35] Lee YJ, Jung SJ, Kim DW, Cho HJ, Ahn KJ. Amyloid goiter mimicking subacute thyroiditis on clinical and imaging findings: A case report. Journal of Clinical Ultrasound. 2018;**46**:497-500

[36] Walsh S, Lowery AJ, Evoy D, et al. Thyroid lymphoma: Recent advances in diagnosis and optimal management strategies. The Oncologist. 2013;**18**:994-1003

[37] Wang JH, Chen L, Ren K. Identification of primary thyroid lymphoma with medical imaging: A case report and review of the literature. Oncology Letters. 2014;**8**:2505-2508

[38] Bakan S, Kandemirli SG, Akbas S, Cingoz M, Ozcan Guzelbey B, Kantarci F, et al. Amyloid Goiter: A diagnosis to consider in diffuse fatty infiltration of the thyroid. Journal of Ultrasound in Medicine. 2017;**36**:1045-1049

[39] Aksu AO, Ozmen MN, Oguz KK, Akinci D, Yasavun U, Firat P. Diffuse fatty infiltration of the thyroid gland in amyloidosis: Sonographic, computed tomographic, and magnetic resonance imaging findings. Journal of Ultrasound in Medicine. 2010;**29**:1251-1255

[40] Manchanda A, Patel S, Jiang JJ, Babu AR. Thyroid: An unusual hideout for sarcoidosis. Endocrine Practice. 2013;**19**:e40-e43

[41] Katsamakas M, Tzitzili E, Boudina M, Kiziridou A, Valeri R, Zafeiriou G, et al. Thyroid sarcoidosis: A rare entity in the differential diagnosis of thyroid cancer. Endocrinology, Diabetes & Metabolism Case Reports. 2021;**2021**:21-0095

[42] Araújo AN, Matos T, Boavida J, Bugalho MJGM. Thyroid tuberculosis: An unexpected diagnosis. BML Case Reports. 2021;**14**:e238795

[43] Avramidis A. Endocrinology. In: Thyroid. Vol. 1. Thessaloniki: University Studio Press; 2000

[44] De Vijlder JJ. Primary congenital hypothyroidism: Defects in iodine pathways. European Journal of Endocrinology. 2003;**149**:247-256

[45] Buyukgebiz A. Newborn screening for congenital hypothyroidism. Journal of Pediatric Endocrinology & Metabolism. 2006;**19**:1291-1298

[46] Bubuteishvili L, Garel C, Czernichow P, Leger J. Thyroid abnormalities by ultrasonography in neonates with congenital hypothyroidism. The Journal of Pediatrics. 2003;**143**:759-764

[47] Kreisner E, Camargo-Neto E, Maia CR, Gross JL. Accuracy of ultrasonography to establish the diagnosis and aetiology of permanent primary congenital hypothyroidism.

Clinical Endocrinology. 2003;**59**:361-365

[48] Garel C, Leger J. Thyroid imaging in children. Endocrine Development. 2007;**10**:43-61

[49] Iranpour R, Hashemipour M, Amini M, Talaei SM, Kelishadi R, Hovsepian S, et al. [Tc]-99m thyroid scintigraphy in congenital hypothyroidism screening program. Journal of Tropical Pediatrics. 2006;**52**:411-415

[50] Abramowicz MJ, Vassart G, Refetoff S. Probing the cause of thyroid dysgenesis. Thyroid. 1997;7:325-326

[51] Gagne N, Parma J, Deal C, Vassart G, Van Vliet G. Apparent congenital athyreosis contrasting with normal plasma thyroglobulin levels and associated with inactivating mutations in the thyrotropin receptor gene: Are athyreosis and ectopic thyroid distinct entities? The Journal of Clinical Endocrinology and Metabolism. 1998;**83**:1771-1775

[52] Fugazzola L, Persani L, Vannucchi G, Carletto M, Mannavola D, Vigone MC, et al. Thyroid scintigraphy and perchlorate test after recombinant human TSH: A new tool for the differential diagnosis of congenital hypothyroidism during infancy. European Journal of Nuclear Medicine and Molecular Imaging. 2007;**34**:1498-1503

[53] Perry RJ, Maroo S, Maclennan AC, Jones JH, Donaldson MD. Combined ultrasound and isotope scanning is more informative in the diagnosis of congenital hypothyroidism than single scanning. Archives of Disease in Childhood. 2006;**91**:972-976

Section 3

Causes of Hypothyroidism

Chapter 7

Hashimoto's Thyroiditis

Sedat Carkit

Abstract

Hashimoto's thyroiditis is the most common type of thyroiditis, an inflammatory disease of the thyroid gland. Antibodies that the body normally produces against substances foreign to the body, together with the immune system, attack the thyroid cells and cause inflammation and damage to the thyroid gland. Thus, the thyroid gland cannot fulfill its function, and the level of hormones it secretes decreases over time. It is familial and is mostly seen in women between the ages of 30–50. Hashimoto's thyroid is one of the causes of "hypothyroidism", a condition in which the thyroid gland is underactive. The thyroid hormone, which regulates the body's metabolic rate and thus affects all tissues, decreases over time in these patients, and the risk of hypothyroidism increases with age. Another problem that Hashimoto's thyroid can cause in the thyroid gland is nodule formation. In general, enlargement of the thyroid gland is common, especially in the beginning, and this may be accompanied by nodule formation in the process. Hashimoto's thyroid should be detected early, and thyroid hormone levels should be monitored at regular intervals and replaced with medication if necessary. With close follow-up and treatment, patients do not experience adverse effects related to Hashimoto's thyroid.

Keywords: Hashimoto's thyroiditis, hypothyroidism, thyroid antibodies, thyroid peroxidase, chronic autoimmune thyroiditis

1. Introduction

In areas with adequate iodine, Hashimoto's thyroiditis is the primary reason for hypothyroidism. Hashimoto initially described this condition in 1912, and it primarily affects women, impacting approximately 10% of the population. As individuals age, the prevalence of this disease rises [1]. We now acknowledge Hashimoto's thyroiditis as an autoimmune thyroid disorder with a rising incidence [2].

Presently, Hashimoto's thyroiditis is the primary cause of hypothyroidism [3], and patients with this condition face an elevated risk of cardiovascular diseases and malignancies [4]. The disease's progression involves lymphocytic infiltration and autoimmune damage to the thyroid gland. Nearly all patients with this disease exhibit elevated serum antibody levels against thyroid antigens, along with extensive lymphocytic infiltration primarily involving thyroid-specific B and T cells.

The disease typically involves follicular destruction, which results from a combination of genetic predisposition and environmental factors. Despite their distinct clinical presentations, the familial link between Graves' disease and the occasional transition from Graves' disease to Hashimoto's thyroiditis suggests a related pathophysiological connection between these two disorders [5].

Here, we discuss the etiological factors and pathophysiological changes that contribute to the development of the disease. Diagnostic methods, various treatment strategies, and important considerations in patient management are also discussed.

2. Epidemiology

Over the last three decades, there has been a significant rise in the occurrence of Hashimoto's thyroiditis [6]. Presently, Hashimoto's thyroiditis ranks among the most prevalent thyroid disorders, affecting 0.3–1.5 cases per 1000 people [7]. Over 10% of women test positive for antibodies related to Hashimoto's thyroiditis, and around 2% experience clinical symptoms.

Although Hashimoto's thyroiditis is less common among Pacific Islanders, individuals of white ethnicity have a higher incidence compared to those of black ethnicity [8].

The prevalence of the disease increases with age. The exact reasons behind the elevated prevalence of Hashimoto's thyroiditis in women remain unclear. However, potential factors include similarities to animal models of other autoimmune diseases and the influence of X chromosome inactivation and fetal microchimerism due to female sex hormone exposure [9].

Hashimoto's thyroiditis can present itself in three ways: on its own, in conjunction with other autoimmune diseases like type 1 diabetes mellitus and Sjögren syndrome, or paired with other thyroid conditions. It is worth noting that within this last category, the incidence of papillary thyroid cancer can vary between 0.5% and 30%.

The development of Hashimoto's thyroiditis has been linked to climatic factors. For instance, Siberian women exhibit a greater density of thyroid peroxidase (TPO) antibodies compared to the overall population [10]. Additionally, Hashimoto's thyroiditis may be more prevalent in specific conditions, including myasthenia gravis (MG) and systemic sclerosis.

Hashimoto's thyroiditis serves as a typical illustration of organ-specific autoimmune conditions and frequently coexists with other autoimmune diseases within the same patient or family, implying a shared genetic foundation [11]. Notably, Hashimoto's thyroiditis and systemic lupus erythematosus were the initial diseases where a genetic underpinning for autoimmunity, specifically associated with MHC class II genes, was established during the early 1970s.

Despite extensive research spanning four decades, only a handful of susceptibility genes have been pinpointed for Hashimoto's thyroiditis, each exerting a modest influence on the disease phenotype via mechanisms that remain unclear [12].

3. Etiology

There are primary and secondary causes.

3.1 Primary Hashimoto's disease

The most prevalent type of Hashimoto's thyroiditis is the primary form, which includes cases where no specific causes can be identified. This form encompasses a clinical and pathological spectrum comprising six main variants: the classical form, fibrous variant, IgG4-related variant, juvenile form, Hashitoxicosis, and painless (or silent) thyroiditis [13].

The latter variant may occur sporadically or postpartum. The typical clinical presentation involves enlargement of the thyroid gland (goiter), with or without hypothyroidism. Pathologically, all these variants share a common feature: pronounced lymphocytic infiltration within the thyroid gland.

3.2 Secondary Hashimoto's disease

These forms involve identifiable etiological agents. More frequently, it results from medical intervention and the use of immunomodulatory medications. A case in point is interferon-alpha, which, when used to treat hepatitis C viral infection, can trigger or worsen thyroiditis [14].

Recent progress in cancer immunotherapy has revealed various immune-related adverse events, including thyroiditis, associated with the use of monoclonal antibodies that block CTLA-4 or cancer vaccines.

4. Pathogenesis

The development of Hashimoto's thyroiditis involves a complex, multistep process influenced by genetic, environmental, and immunological factors. In essence, the breakdown of immune tolerance toward normal thyroid cells results in the production of antibodies targeting thyroid tissue, leading to thyroid gland destruction. The initial inflammatory changes occur when genetically susceptible individuals encounter the aforementioned environmental factors.

Following this, cells expressing major histocompatibility complex (MHC) class 2 antigens, including dendritic cells and macrophages, infiltrate the thyroid gland. These cells present the thyroid's autoantigens to the immune system for recognition and processing. Among the various potential auto-antigens, thyroglobulin, the primary protein produced in thyroid tissue, plays a central role in the disease's pathogenesis [15]. Notably, thyroglobulin protein encompasses approximately 40 distinct epitope types critical to the disease process [16].

In the disease's pathogenesis, thyroid peroxidase an enzyme responsible for iodine oxidation serves as a crucial autoantigen. Moreover, 180 different types of thyroid peroxidase antibodies have been identified to date. Studies have confirmed that antibodies against the thyrotropin receptor and the sodium iodide symporter, which have been detected in patients with autoimmune thyroid disease, do not play a significant role in the pathogenesis of this condition.

Initially, a functional alteration occurs in B cells, leading to the production of autoantibodies in the disease process. Furthermore, T cell dysfunction contributes to the disturbance of immune balance targeting thyroid tissue [17]. Hence, we can infer that both cellular and humoral immunity play a role in the development of Hashimoto's thyroiditis. Cellular immunity has been found in Hashimoto's patients with CD8+ T cells against thyroglobulin and TPO [18].

Nevertheless, only a small proportion (approximately 2–3%) of CD8+ cells specifically target TG/TPO, indicating that the majority are not thyroid antigen-specific. Furthermore, recent studies have revealed that cell death in autoimmune thyroiditis is not only dependent on cytotoxicity but also on apoptotic processes. "Suppressor T cells", a specialized population of CD8+ cells, are thought to be able to inhibit harmful immune responses. It is hypothesized that Hashimoto's thyroiditis involves altered function of T cell suppressors targeting specific thyroid antigens. Certain functions attributed to T suppressor cells are also carried out by T regulatory cells [19].

A key hallmark of Hashimoto's thyroiditis is the generation of specific antibodies targeting thyroid tissue [20]. In most cases, Hashimoto's patients produce autoantibodies against thyroglobulin (TG) and thyroid peroxidase (TPO). Furthermore, analyzing anti-TPO antibodies proves valuable in predicting the development of hypothyroidism. A recent description of Hashimoto's includes a variant known as IgG4 thyroiditis, characterized by the presence of IgG4-positive cells within the context of a systemic autoimmune disorder [21].

Several studies have reported elevated serum levels of Th1 cells, as well as IL-17 and IL-22 cytokines, in individuals with Hashimoto's thyroiditis [22]. Evidence indicates that IL-12 cytokine levels are elevated in 56% of Hashimoto's patients [23]. A recent study proposed that circulating exosomes actively contribute to the pathogenesis of Hashimoto's thyroiditis (HT) [24]. Exosomes possess the ability to transport bioactive molecules to other cells, impacting biological processes. They participate in diverse cellular functions, including antigen presentation, inflammatory activation, autoimmune conditions, and tumor metastasis. Hashimoto-specific exosomes can present antigens to dendritic cells (DCs), triggering DC activation through the NFκB signaling pathway by binding to TLR2/3. This process may disrupt CD4+ T lymphocyte differentiation and potentially contribute to the development of Hashimoto's thyroiditis.

A similar process has been observed in systemic lupus erythematosus; however, further studies are necessary to validate this hypothesis in Hashimoto's patients. Hashimoto's thyroiditis (HT) frequently coexists with other autoimmune disorders, suggesting a potential shared poly-autoimmune origin. In a large prospective study involving 3209 patients with Graves' disease, Ferrari and colleagues investigated the association of this thyroid disorder with other autoimmune conditions.

A significant proportion of Graves' patients (16.7%) presented with additional autoimmune diseases, including vitiligo, autoimmune gastritis, rheumatoid arthritis, polymyalgia rheumatica, multiple sclerosis, and celiac disease. Notably, some patients were diagnosed with three or more associated autoimmune disorders [25].

5. Symptoms and diagnosis

The current diagnostic criteria for Hashimoto's thyroiditis involve evaluating clinical features, detecting serum antibodies against thyroid antigens (primarily thyroperoxidase and thyroglobulin), and assessing the thyroid sonogram. Radioactive iodine uptake and cytological examination of thyroid aspirate are infrequently employed in the diagnostic process.

5.1 Clinical features

Hashimoto's thyroiditis (HT) manifests with both local and systemic symptoms, as well as features specific to different forms of the disease. Local symptoms arise due to pressure on cervical structures near the thyroid gland. These include dysphonia (caused by involvement of the recurrent laryngeal nerve), dyspnea (due to tracheal constriction), and dysphagia (resulting from pressure on the esophagus).

DOI: http://dx.doi.org/10.5772/intechopen.1005431

Systemic symptoms emerge from thyroid gland dysfunction, leading to primary hypothyroidism. Given the far-reaching impact of thyroid hormones on various organs and tissues, the signs and symptoms of hypothyroidism are diverse and variable.

5.1.1 Gastrointestinal system

Hypothyroid patients frequently report constipation as their primary complaint. Reduced peristalsis can occasionally result in pseudo-obstruction or ileus. Additionally, gallbladder hypotonia and alterations in bile composition may contribute to an increased risk of bile duct stone formation.

5.1.2 Skin involvement

Hypothyroid patients commonly exhibit skin alterations, including dryness, coldness, yellowness, and thickening. These changes arise from the accumulation of hydrophilic mucoproteins, such as hyaluronic acid, in the skin, leading to myxedema. Additionally, sweat gland atrophy contributes to these manifestations. Hair becomes coarse and prone to falling out, while nails become thin and brittle.

5.1.3 Cardiovascular system

Hypothyroidism is characterized by classic signs, including bradycardia and reduced amplitude of cardiac waves on electrocardiogram. These manifestations result from decreased ventricular contractility, increased peripheral resistance, and their combined impact on cardiac output. Cardiomegaly may be present, often accompanied by pericardial effusion. Additionally, hypothyroid patients frequently experience coronary artery disease, likely influenced by the effects of thyroid hormones on lipid metabolism. Notably, hypothyroidism leads to reduced levels of cholesterol and LDL cholesterol, both recognized as atherogenic factors.

5.1.4 Skeletal muscles

The muscles appear hypertrophic due to the myxedematous infiltration of the connective tissue. The contraction and relaxation times are delayed and may cause pain and cramps.

5.1.5 Pulmonary system

Common respiratory abnormalities are bradypnea and hypoxia. These are caused by obstruction of the upper airways by enlarged soft tissues, weakness of the respiratory muscles, decreased chest wall and lung compliance, increased capillary permeability, and pleural effusion. Respiratory failure may occur in patients with myxedematous coma.

5.1.6 Hematopoietic system

Anemia is common in hypothyroidism. It can be normocytic (due to decreased renal secretion of erythropoietin), hypochromic, and microcytic (due to impaired iron absorption) or megaloblastic (due to gastric atrophy with B12 vitamin malabsorption).

5.1.7 Reproductive system

Oligomenorrhea and/or menometrorrhagia are common. Menstrual cycles are often anovulatory due to impaired conversion of estrogen precursors. Hypothyroidism during pregnancy has been associated with an increased rate of miscarriage.

5.1.8 Urinary system

Fluid retention caused by decreased glomerular filtration has been described.

5.1.9 Neuro-psychiatric system

Patients with Hashimoto's thyroiditis (HT) often experience difficulty concentrating, memory loss, and depression. A more contentious issue is Hashimoto's encephalopathy, which was first reported in 1966 [26]. It manifests insidiously, resembling truncal ataxia associated with spino-cerebellar degeneration. Additionally, paroxysmal dyskinesia has been documented [27]. Over time, patients develop cognitive impairments affecting episodic memory, attention, executive function, and visual–spatial abilities, while retaining naming ability. Diagnostic criteria remain unclear, necessitating a diagnosis based on excluding other potential causes of encephalopathy in patients with HT.

5.2 Clinical variants

Hashimoto's thyroiditis (HT) typically presents in the fifth decade of life and is more prevalent in women. The thyroid gland exhibits enlargement and firmness. Approximately 75% of patients are euthyroid at the time of diagnosis, while the remaining minority display a spectrum of dysfunction ranging from subclinical hypothyroidism (characterized by elevated TSH levels but thyroid hormones within the normal range) to overt hypothyroidism. The fibrous variant of HT, also more common in women but occurring at older ages, often presents with symptomatic goiter. The thyroid's lobulated appearance can resemble benign nodules.

Most patients with HT experience hypothyroidism and require prompt thyroid hormone replacement. In advanced age, this fibrous variant progresses to a severe form of thyroid atrophy, clinically manifesting as idiopathic myxedema. Although the thyroid gland is non-palpable, patients exhibit hypothyroid symptoms that may be challenging to distinguish from age-related signs.

The IgG4-associated variant of HT, akin to the classic form, typically emerges in the fifth decade of life but at a younger age [28]. Unlike the disproportionately high female-to-male ratio of the classic form, this variant affects both sexes equally. Despite synthetic thyroid hormone administration, the IgG4-associated variant often follows a more aggressive course, leading to persistent subclinical hypothyroidism in many patients.

The juvenile form of Hashimoto's thyroiditis (HT) typically appears before the age of 18, with the average age at referral being 11 [29]. While it is more prevalent in females, the ratio of females to males is lower. A majority of children show signs of goiter, but they usually do not exhibit any symptoms.

At the point of diagnosis, 43% of children have normal thyroid function (euthyroid), 24% have mild (subclinical) hypothyroidism, 21% have severe (overt) hypothyroidism, 9% have severe (overt) hyperthyroidism, and 3% have mild (subclinical) hyperthyroidism [30]. The disease progression can vary, including periods of remission, relapse, and eventual progression to permanent hypothyroidism.

The Hashitoxicosis variant, initially described by Fatourechi in 1971 [31], combines the clinical features of Graves' hyperthyroidism with the pathological appearance of HT. The initial hyperthyroid phase closely resembles Graves' disease, characterized by high thyroid uptake of radioactive iodine and the presence of thyroid-stimulating immunoglobulins. However, hyperthyroidism is transient, eventually transitioning to permanent hypothyroidism within a period of 3 to 24 months.

Silent thyroiditis, also known as painless thyroiditis, refers to a lymphocytic inflammation affecting the thyroid gland. It may manifest sporadically or more frequently within a year after childbirth. These two forms share indistinguishable characteristics, with the second form, associated with pregnancy, being termed postpartum thyroiditis. In regions with higher dietary iodine intake [32], painless thyroiditis tends to be more prevalent.

Scientifically, it is described as exhibiting a triphasic model, involving an initial phase of thyrotoxicosis, followed by hypothyroidism, and ultimately leading to recovery. Postpartum thyroiditis occurs in approximately 8% of all pregnancies [13], although estimates may vary based on the studied population and the frequency of follow-up.

Thyrotoxicosis, which typically occurs two to five months after delivery, has a duration of approximately one month. It is generally mild and seldom necessitates treatment, although beta-blockers can be employed. The underlying mechanism for the elevation in serum thyroid hormone levels is not excessive production by the thyroid gland (hyperthyroidism). Instead, it results from the release of previously synthesized hormones from thyroid follicles, triggered by destructive inflammation. Consequently, antithyroid drugs are not recommended during this phase.

Following thyrotoxicosis, a hypothyroid phase ensues, lasting approximately two to six months. During this period, symptoms are mild, and patients may be mistakenly attributed to postpartum depression. Fortunately, most women (80%) eventually recover normal thyroid function within a year after delivery. However, permanent hypothyroidism is more likely in women with multiple pregnancies and a history of postpartum thyroiditis.

5.3 Thyroperoxidase antibodies

Thyroid peroxidase antibodies serve as the optimal serological marker for diagnosing Hashimoto's thyroiditis (HT). These antibodies are present in approximately 95% of HT patients, whereas they are rare in healthy individuals. In the context of postpartum thyroiditis, thyroid peroxidase antibodies also play a unique role by increasing the risk of hypothyroidism and long-term thyroid dysfunction in pregnant women who have them at the beginning of pregnancy.

The correlation between thyroid peroxidase antibody levels and the number of autoreactive lymphocytes infiltrating the thyroid is evident. Additionally, it relates to the degree of sonographic hypoechogenicity. On the other hand, thyroglobulin antibodies, which constitute the most abundant protein in the thyroid gland, are less sensitive than thyroid peroxidase antibodies (positive in only 60–80% of HT patients) and less specific (positive in a higher proportion of healthy controls).

Despite this, they serve their own purposes. In clinical practice, both antibodies are simultaneously assessed and fluctuate together following treatment interventions.

Interestingly, thyroid antibodies exhibit poor correlation with each other. The interplay between thyroglobulin and thyroid peroxidase antibodies represents distinct facets of the autoimmune response against the thyroid gland.

Thyroglobulin antibodies might signify an initial, more innate immune response, whereas thyroid peroxidase antibodies could represent a subsequent adaptive immune response, a type of immune intensification. In line with this theory, thyroglobulin antibodies are anticipated to be present at the beginning of a disease that is inherently associated with thyroiditis.

Indeed, in mouse models of spontaneous autoimmune thyroiditis, thyroglobulin antibodies emerge before thyroid peroxidase antibodies. The commencement of disease is seldom seen in human autoimmune diseases. For instance, in the case of HT, the majority of patients have been living with the disease for a minimum of 7 years before they are clinically diagnosed. Hence, in humans, thyroid peroxidase antibodies are predicted to be more prevalent and elevated compared to thyroglobulin antibodies.

5.4 Ultrasonography

Among patients with thyroid conditions, neck ultrasound has become the most commonly employed imaging technique [33]. In Hashimoto's thyroiditis (HT), there is a characteristic reduction in echogenicity, distinguishing it on ultrasound. The normal thyroid gland, composed of varying-sized thyroid follicles, scatters ultrasound, causing the lobes to appear bright.

Conversely, in HT, the destruction of thyroid follicles by small lymphocytes results in a significant decrease in echogenicity, making the thyroid parenchyma similar to the adjacent strap muscles.

Different forms of HT exhibit distinct characteristics; for example, the IgG4-associated variant [34] displays more pronounced hypoechogenicity, while the fibrous variant shows irregularity and nodularity due to collagen fiber accumulation. Thyroid ultrasound also allows for the measurement of the thyroid gland's volume. The field of thyroid ultrasound is rapidly advancing, with ongoing efforts to improve visual impressions, facilitate point-of-use applications for endocrinologists and surgeons, and integrate with Doppler or elastography for additional information.

Lastly, ultrasound is commonly used in various centers to guide needle placement during fine needle aspiration, enhancing precision in targeting thyroid nodules.

5.5 Thyroid function tests, radioiodine uptake, and fine needle aspiration

The assessment of thyroid function in patients with HT is conducted by measuring the levels of serum thyrotropin (TSH) and free thyroxine (FT4). TSH serves as the most crucial indicator for monitoring thyroid function as its levels precisely adjust to the slightest changes in circulating thyroid hormones. Due to the variability in results, the 24-hour thyroid radioactive iodine uptake is seldom employed for diagnosing HT.

However, it proves beneficial in painless thyroiditis. During the hyperthyroid phase of this HT variant, contrary to what is expected in hyperthyroidism, the radioiodine uptake is reduced rather than increased. This is because the rise in circulating thyroid hormones is attributed to the destruction of thyroid follicles and the release of preformed thyroid hormones (thyrotoxicosis), not due to the enhanced function of the thyroid gland (hyperthyroidism).

Fine needle aspiration is commonly performed when a thyroid nodule is present in the patient. The majority of thyroid nodules are genuine neoplastic nodules, and most of them are benign tumors. However, in the fibrous variant of HT, considering that the dense keloid-like fibrosis disrupts the thyroid structure and gives the gland a lobular appearance, "pseudo-nodules" may be present. When thyroid antibodies and a nodule are present, it becomes challenging to determine whether the patient has two coexisting thyroid diseases or only the fibrous variant of HT.

Hence, fine needle aspiration is carried out, and the interpretation of the cytological results can be challenging. HT cytology typically presents a polymorphic lymphoid cell population (small mature lymphocytes, larger active lymphocytes, and occasionally plasma cells) along with Hurtle cells. Lymphocytes frequently interact with thyroid cell groups; this characteristic is believed to be beneficial in differentiating HT from thyroid neoplasms [35].

However, in some aspirates, there are no lymphoid cells, and they are composed almost entirely of Hurtle cells, which complicates the determination of whether these cells are Hurtle cells found in HT or those found in other oncocytic lesions of the thyroid, such as oncocytic adenomatoid nodule, Hurtle cell adenoma, or Hurtle cell carcinoma [36].

For these aspirates that are primarily composed of Hurtle cells, the cytopathologist employs the term "atypia of undetermined significance" [37] to denote the features that are neither benign nor malignant. Despite the Bethesda system's recommendation for this category being conservative treatment and the fact that most of these Hurtle cell lesions are benign [38], numerous patients are referred to a surgeon, and thyroidectomy is frequently performed.

6. Treatment

The primary objective of HT treatment is to manage hypothyroidism, which involves the oral intake of a synthetic hormone, Levo-Thyroxine 4 (L-T4), at a dosage of 1.6–1.8 micrograms per kilogram of body weight. Lifelong substitution therapy is necessary to achieve normal levels of circulating thyrotropin (TSH).

In certain cases, L-T4 therapy might not be needed, and mere clinical observation could suffice. The use of glucocorticoids has been debated as they can control thyroiditis and rapidly enhance thyroid function, but the risks linked with high dosage and prolonged treatment are believed to surpass the benefit [39].

However, the short-term usage of prednisolone may offer a longer-term advan tage in the IgG4 disease subgroup [40]. In recent times, the supplementary role of a specific diet in managing HT has been scrutinized. Overconsumption of iodine has been proposed to trigger thyroid autoimmunity in genetically susceptible individuals by amplifying the immunogenicity of thyroglobulin [41].

Therefore, even though a supplement suitable for a total intake of 250 g/day during pregnancy is advised, high iodine supplementation in HT should likely be avoided as it could pose a risk.

Selenium, which is involved in various selenoproteins, plays a crucial role in the homeostasis of human thyroid hormones, but the effectiveness of selenium supplementation in HT patients is a matter of debate [42].

The oral intake of selenium in the form of seleno-methionine could be advantageous for HT patients with a selenium deficiency and is expected to shield the thyroid gland from autoimmune damage. Numerous studies have demonstrated an association between Vitamin D deficiency and the pathogenesis and hypofunction of the thyroid in HT [43].

Given the affordability and minimal side effects of oral vitamin D supplementation, it may be advisable to screen and supplement HT patients for vitamin D deficiency, with clinical necessity dictating monthly monitoring of calcium and 25[OH]D levels [42].

The scope of HT surgery is restricted in the presence of a nodule with cervical anatomical structures or features of malignant transformation [44]. However, thyroidectomies performed on HT patients tend to have more complications than other thyroid disorders [45]. Looking ahead, the transplantation of the thyroid gland has been proposed as a solution to hypothyroidism, but further studies are required for confirmation [46].

7. Conclusions

In this section, we delved into the epidemiology, assumed pathogenesis, diagnosis, and treatment of Hashimoto's thyroiditis. We also explored other autoimmune diseases and potential complications. Hashimoto's thyroiditis often serves as a model for autoimmune disease in many respects. We also highlighted how environmental exposure can alter genetic susceptibility. As is the case with many subjects, increased knowledge often leads to more questions about what we understand. Consequently, HT remains a disease with an unknown pathogenesis, intricate and continually evolving, awaiting prevention strategies or novel treatment methods.

Conflict of interest

There are no conflicts of interest.

Financial support and sponsorship

The author reports no funding sources for this article.

Author details

Sedat Carkit
Erciyes University Faculty of Medicine, General Surgery Department, Kayseri, Turkey

*Address all correspondence to: opdrsedatcarkit@gmail.com

References

[1] Hollowell JG, Staehling NW, Flanders WD, Hannon WH, Gunter EW, Spencer CA, et al. Serum TSH, T4, and thyroid antibodies in the United States population (1988 to 1994): National Health and nutrition examination survey (NHANES III). The Journal of Clinical Endocrinology and Metabolism. 2002;**87**(2):489-499

[2] Antonelli A, Ferrari SM, Corrado A, Di Domenicantonio A, Fallahi P. Autoimmune thyroid disorders. Autoimmunity Reviews. 2015;**14**(2):174-180

[3] McLeod DS, Cooper DS. The incidence and prevalence of thyroid autoimmunity. Endocrine. 2012;**42**:252-265

[4] Chen W-H, Chen Y-K, Lin C-L, Yeh J-H, Kao C-H. Hashimoto's thyroiditis, risk of coronary heart disease, and L-thyroxine treatment: A nationwide cohort study. The Journal of Clinical Endocrinology and Metabolism. 2015;**100**(1):109-114

[5] Kralem Z, Baron E, Kahana L, Sadeh O, Shelnfeld M. Changes in stimulating and blocking TSH receptor antibodies in a patient undergoing three cycles of transition from hypo to hyper-thyroidism and back to hypothyroidism. Clinical Endocrinology. 1992;**36**(2):211-214

[6] Ott J, Meusel M, Schultheis A, Promberger R, Pallikunnel SJ, Neuhold N, et al. The incidence of lymphocytic thyroid infiltration and Hashimoto's thyroiditis increased in patients operated for benign goiter over a 31-year period. Virchows Archiv: An International Journal of Pathology. 2011;**459**(3):277-281

[7] Caturegli P, De Remigis A, Chuang K, Dembele M, Iwama A, Iwama S. Hashimoto's thyroiditis: Celebrating the centennial through the lens of the Johns Hopkins hospital surgical pathology records. Thyroid. 2013;**23**(2):142-150

[8] McLeod DS, Caturegli P, Cooper DS, Matos PG, Hutfless S. Variation in rates of autoimmune thyroid disease by race/ethnicity in US military personnel. Journal of the American Medical Association. 2014;**311**(15):1563-1565

[9] Brix TH, Hansen PS, Kyvik KO, Hegedus L. Aggregation of thyroid autoantibodies in twins from opposite-sex pairs suggests that microchimerism may play a role in the early stages of thyroid autoimmunity. The Journal of Clinical Endocrinology and Metabolism. 2009;**94**(11):4439-4443

[10] Weetman AP. The immunopathogenesis of chronic autoimmune thyroiditis one century after Hashimoto. European Thyroid Journal. 2013;**1**(4):243-250

[11] Cárdenas-Roldán J, Rojas-Villarraga A, Anaya J-M. How do autoimmune diseases cluster in families? A systematic review and meta-analysis. BMC Medicine. 2013;**11**:1-22

[12] Simmonds MJ, Gough SC. The search for the genetic contribution to autoimmune thyroid disease: The never ending story? Briefings in Functional Genomics. 2011;**10**(2):77-90

[13] Stagnaro-Green A. Approach to the patient with postpartum thyroiditis. The Journal of Clinical Endocrinology & Metabolism. 2012;**97**(2):334-342

[14] Mandac JC, Chaudhry S, Sherman KE, Tomer Y. The clinical and physiological spectrum of

interferon-alpha induced thyroiditis: Toward a new classification. Hepatology. 2006;**43**(4):661-672

[15] Champion BR, Page KR, Parish N, Rayner DC, Dawe K, Biswas-Hughes G, et al. Identification of a thyroxine-containing self-epitope of thyroglobulin which triggers thyroid autoreactive T cells. The Journal of experimental medicine. 1991;**174**(2):363-370

[16] Male D, Champion B, Pryce G, Matthews H, Shepherd P. Antigenic determinants of human thyroglobulin differentiated using antigen fragments. Immunology. 1985;**54**(3):419

[17] McLachlan SM, Rapoport B. Breaking tolerance to thyroid antigens: Changing concepts in thyroid autoimmunity. Endocrine Reviews. 2014;**35**(1):59-105

[18] Ehlers M, Thiel A, Bernecker C, Porwol D, Papewalis C, Willenberg HS, et al. Evidence of a combined cytotoxic thyroglobulin and thyroperoxidase epitope-specific cellular immunity in Hashimoto's thyroiditis. The Journal of Clinical Endocrinology and Metabolism. 2012;**97**(4):1347-1354

[19] MacDonald T. Suppressor T cells, rebranded as regulatory T cells, emerge from the wilderness bearing surface markers. Gut. 2002;**51**(3):311-312

[20] Weetman A. Cellular immune responses in autoimmune thyroid disease. Clinical Endocrinology. 2004;**61**(4):405-413

[21] Hamano H, Kawa S, Horiuchi A, Unno H, Furuya N, Akamatsu T, et al. High serum IgG4 concentrations in patients with sclerosing pancreatitis. New England Journal of Medicine. 2001;**344**(10):732-738

[22] Figueroa-Vega N, Alfonso-Perez M, Benedicto I, Sanchez-Madrid F, Gonzalez-Amaro R, Marazuela M. Increased circulating pro-inflammatory cytokines and Th17 lymphocytes in Hashimoto's thyroiditis. The Journal of Clinical Endocrinology and Metabolism. 2010;**95**(2):953-962

[23] Ruggeri RM, Saitta S, Cristani M, Giovinazzo S, Tigano V, Trimarchi F, et al. Serum interleukin-23 (IL-23) is increased in Hashimoto's thyroiditis. Endocrine Journal. 2014;**61**(4):359-363

[24] Cui X, Liu Y, Wang S, Zhao N, Qin J, Li Y, et al. Circulating exosomes activate dendritic cells and induce unbalanced CD4+ T cell differentiation in Hashimoto thyroiditis. The Journal of Clinical Endocrinology and Metabolism. 2019;**104**(10):4607-4618

[25] Ferrari SM, Fallahi P, Ruffilli I, Elia G, Ragusa F, Benvenga S, et al. The association of other autoimmune diseases in patients with Graves' disease (with or without ophthalmopathy): Review of the literature and report of a large series. Autoimmunity Reviews. 2019;**18**(3):287-292

[26] Jellinek E, Ball K. Hashimoto's disease and encephalopathy. The Lancet. 1966;**288**(7462):512-514

[27] Liu MY, Zhang SQ, Hao Y, Zheng HM. Paroxysmal kinesigenic dyskinesia as the initial symptom of Hashimoto encephalopathy. CNS Neuroscience and Therapeutics. 2012;**18**(3):271

[28] Li Y, Zhou G, Ozaki T, Nishihara E, Matsuzuka F, Bai Y, et al. Distinct histopathological features of Hashimoto's thyroiditis with respect to IgG4-related disease. Modern Pathology. 2012;**25**(8):1086-1097

[29] Demirbilek H, Kandemir N, Gonc E, Ozon A, Alikasifoglu A, Yordam N.

Hashimoto's thyroiditis in children and adolescents: A retrospective study on clinical, epidemiological and laboratory properties of the disease. Journal of Pediatric Endocrinology and Metabolism. 2007;**20**(11):1199-1206

[30] Wasniewska M, Corrias A, Salerno M, Mussa A, Capalbo D, Messina MF, et al. Thyroid function patterns at Hashimoto's thyroiditis presentation in childhood and adolescence are mainly conditioned by patients' age. Hormone Research in Paediatrics. 2012;**78**(4):232-236

[31] Fatourechi V, McConahey W, Woolner L, editors. Hyperthyroidism associated with histologic Hashimoto's thyroiditis. In: Mayo Clinic Proceedings. Vol. 46, Issue no 10; 1971. pp. 682-689

[32] Nishimaki M, Isozaki O, Yoshihara A, Okubo Y, Takano K. Clinical characteristics of frequently recurring painless thyroiditis: Contributions of higher thyroid hormone levels, younger onset, male gender, presence of thyroid autoantibody and absence of goiter to repeated recurrence. Endocrine Journal. 2009;**56**(3):391-397

[33] Lee JH, Anzai Y, editors. Imaging of thyroid and parathyroid glands. In: Seminars in roentgenology. Vol. 48, Issue no. 1; 2013. pp. 87-104

[34] Li Y, Nishihara E, Hirokawa M, Taniguchi E, Miyauchi A, Kakudo K. Distinct clinical, serological, and sonographic characteristics of Hashimoto's thyroiditis based with and without IgG4-positive plasma cells. The Journal of Clinical Endocrinology and Metabolism. 2010;**95**(3):1309-1317

[35] Harvey AM, Truong LD, Mody DR. Diagnostic pitfalls of Hashimoto's/lymphocytic thyroiditis on fine-needle aspirations and strategies to avoid overdiagnosis. Acta Cytologica. 2012;**56**(4):352-360

[36] Yang G, Schreiner A, Sun W. Can abundant colloid exclude oncocytic (Hürthle cell) carcinoma in thyroid fine needle aspiration? Cytohistological correlation of 127 oncocytic (Hürthle cell) lesions. Cytopathology. 2013;**24**(3):185-193

[37] Cibas ES, Ali SZ. The Bethesda system for reporting thyroid cytopathology. Thyroid. 2009;**19**(11):1159-1165

[38] Rossi ED, Martini M, Straccia P, Raffaelli M, Pennacchia I, Marrucci E, et al. The cytologic category of oncocytic (Hurthle) cell neoplasm mostly includes low-risk lesions at histology: An institutional experience. European Journal of Endocrinology. 2013;**169**(5):649-655

[39] Topliss DJ. Clinical update in aspects of the management of autoimmune thyroid diseases. Endocrinology and Metabolism. 2016;**31**(4):493-499

[40] Watanabe T, Maruyama M, Ito T, Fujinaga Y, Ozaki Y, Maruyama M, et al. Clinical features of a new disease concept, IgG4-related thyroiditis. Scandinavian Journal of Rheumatology. 2013;**42**(4):325-330

[41] Carayanniotis G. Recognition of thyroglobulin by T cells: The role of iodine. Thyroid. 2007;**17**(10):963-973

[42] Liontiris MI, Mazokopakis EE. A concise review of Hashimoto thyroiditis (HT) and the importance of iodine, selenium, vitamin D and gluten on the autoimmunity and dietary management of HT patients. Points that need more investigation. Hellenic Journal of Nuclear Medicine. 2017;**20**(1):51-56

[43] Bruscolini A, Sacchetti M, La Cava M, Nebbioso M, Iannitelli A, Quartini A, et al. Quality of life and neuropsychiatric disorders in patients with Graves' orbitopathy: Current concepts. Autoimmunity Reviews. 2018;**17**(7):639-643

[44] Gan T, Randle RW. The role of surgery in autoimmune conditions of the thyroid. Surgical Clinics. 2019;**99**(4):633-648

[45] McManus C, Luo J, Sippel R, Chen H. Is thyroidectomy in patients with Hashimoto thyroiditis more risky? Journal of Surgical Research. 2012;**178**(2):529-532

[46] Davies TF. Is Thyroid Transplantation on the Distant Horizon? 140 Huguenot Street, 3rd Floor New Rochelle, NY 10801 USA: Mary Ann Liebert, Inc; 2013. pp. 139-141

Chapter 8

Central Hypothyroidism

Huiwen Tan, Yuke Liu and Sumita Cholekho

Abstract

Central hypothyroidism is a state of thyroid hormone deficiency due to disorders of the pituitary gland, hypothalamus, or hypothalamic–pituitary portal circulation, often due to low thyrotropin-releasing hormone (TRH), insufficient stimulation of normal thyroid-stimulating hormone (TSH), or both. Over the recent decades, a number of advances have been made in the etiology and clinical management of central hypothyroidism, and our knowledge about central hypothyroidism has accumulated at a rapid pace. The recent publication of expert guidelines for the diagnosis and management of central hypothyroidism will be helped to improve understanding and standardize the management of this endocrine disorder.

Keywords: central hypothyroidism, hypopituitarism, hypothalamic-pituitary-thyorid axis, diagnosis, treatment

1. Introduction

Hypothyroidism is an endocrine disorder caused by a decrease in the synthesis and secretion of thyroid hormones, or insufficient thyroid hormone physiologic effects, or thyroid hormone resistance with a range of etiologic factors [1]. It is characterized by the accumulation of mucopolysaccharides in tissues and skin, which presents as systemic hypo-metabolic syndrome and mucous edema [2]. Hypothyroidism, according to the etiology, is classified as primary hypothyroidism, central hypothyroidism (secondary hypothyroidism), or peripheral hypothyroidism (thyroid hormone resistance syndrome) based on pathology in the thyroid, the hypothalamus or pituitary, or peripheral tissue, respectively [1–3].

Central hypothyroidism(CH) results from decreased production and secretion of thyrotropin-releasing hormone (TRH) or thyroid-stimulating hormone (TSH) caused by lesions of the hypothalamus or pituitary gland [4]. Central hypothyroidism is a rare form of heterogeneous hypothyroidism caused by inadequate stimulation of the otherwise normal thyroid gland by a lack of thyrotropin or TRH [1]. The negative feedback regulation of the hypothalamic-pituitary-thyroid axis is shown in the **Figure 1**. This loss of central thyroid stimulation may be caused by a functional or anatomical disorder of the pituitary and/or hypothalamus, resulting in inadequate TRH or TSH secretion and consequently inadequate thyroid hormone levels [5]. Central hypothyroidism could be isolated or combined with other pituitary-related hormone deficiencies, which are mostly acquired and are rarely congenital [6, 7].

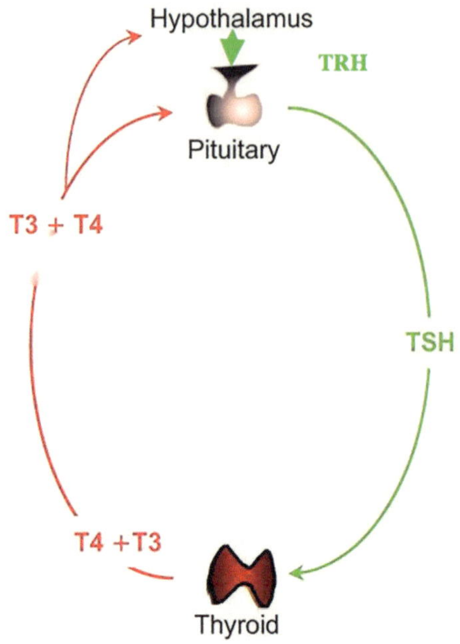

Figure 1.
Negative feedback regulation of the hypothalamic-pituitary-thyroid axis.

2. Epidemiology of central hypothyroidism

Worldwide, central hypothyroidism can affect patients of all ages; however, this hypothalamus–pituitary–thyroid (HPT) condition is commonly overlooked [8]. Central hypothyroidism is a rare cause of hypothyroidism, and there is no female predominance which is unlike what is observed in primary hypothyroidism [1, 9]. Globally, the estimated prevalence of central hypothyroidism in the general population ranging from approximately 1:20,000 to 1:100,000 [10]. The incidence of congenital central hypothyroidism (CCH) in neonates is usually quoted as having an incidence of around 1/60,000 live births, with regional and ethnic variations [11]. This variation is also associated with differences in the sensitivity of diagnostic strategies [12].

A recent retrospective investigation identified 42,861 cases of primary congenital hypothyroidism out of 91,921,334 newborns examined in China between 2013 and 2018. In the general population, the frequency of congenital hypothyroidism is 4.66 per 10,000 people (95% confidence interval [CI]: 4.62–4.71) [13]. In Japan, a case of congenital hypothyroidism of central origin was identified in 1:160,000 live newborns using neonatal screening programs for hypothyroidism based on a cohort of babies with TSH or T4 readings falling in the hypothyroid range [13, 14].

3. Pathogenesis of central hypothyroidism

The pathogenesis of central hypothyroidism remains undetermined, although they involve both hypothalamic and pituitary cells [15, 16]. They can be congenital or acquired [17, 18]. Central hypothyroidism is mainly caused by a decrease in the level of TSH secreted by the pituitary gland due to a variety of factors such as genetics or development, trauma, surgery, and radiation damage, which in turn leads to insufficient levels of thyroid hormone synthesized and secreted by the thyroid gland, the target gland of HPT [17–21].

The thyroid gland mainly synthesizes and secretes two biologically active thyroid hormones, one is tetraiodothyronine, thyroxine (T4); the other is triiodothyronine (T3) [22]. Thyroid hormones have a wide range of physiological effects in the body, the most important of which are to promote the oxidation and the production of heat, and to regulate or promote the growth and maturation of the human body, the functional state of the nervous system and the cardiovascular system, as well as the metabolism of certain substances [23]. Under physiological circumstances, the vast majority of T3 and T4 are bound to plasma proteins, and only a very small portion of them exists freely, which is called free thyroid hormone (i.e., fT3 and fT4). Although fT3 and fT4 are small in amount, they can exert biological effects in target tissue cells through cell membranes, and they are

Head trauma
Traumatic delivery
Medical causes
Medications (e.g. toxoids or mitotane)
Skull surgery
Irradiation
Pituitary macroadenoma
Craniopharyngioma
Meningiomas and gliomas
Rathke's cystic fissure
Metastatic seeding
Carotid aneurysm
Vascular accident
Heenan syndrome
Inferior iliac hemorrhage
Autoimmune inflammation
Postpartum
Infiltrative lesions Iron overload
Nodular disease
Histiocytosis X
Immune-checkpoint inhibitors therapy
Infectious diseases
Mycobacteria
Tuberculosis
Syphilis

Table 1.
Causes of acquired central hypothyroidism (ACH).

the most sensitive indexes to directly respond to the function of the thyroid gland [22, 24, 25].

Congenital central hypothyroidism (CCH) is a congenital disorder caused by insufficient production of thyroid hormones or defects in their receptors [26, 27]. CCH is one of the most common causes of mental retardation and poor physical development in children; fortunately, the condition can be treated with hormone replacement therapy [28]. CCH usually manifests in infancy, but sometimes there is a delayed onset in childhood or adulthood [29, 30]. Pediatric patients (younger than 14 years of age) with central hypothyroidism accompanied by other pituitary hormone deficiencies might have a congenital form of the disease, and clinicians should screen patients for gene mutations of several pituitary transcription factors [31].

The genes for central hypothyroidism can be categorized as those that lead to isolated forms or forms that combine with MPHD [32]. Central hypothyroidism often involves mechanisms including (1) hypothalamic factors or modifications to thyroid hormone feedback set points that impair thyroid stimulation (e.g., TRH resistance or mutations in IGSF1 or TBL1X or IRS4 or hypothalamic lesions), (2) decreased pituitary TSH reserve (e.g., TSHβ mutations or insufficient thyrocyte numbers or pituitary pathology resulting loss of thyrotrophin, and (3) impaired intrinsic biological activity of secreted TSH molecules [33–36]).

Acquired central hypothyroidism is primarily associated with expansive lesions of the hypothalamic/pituitary region. However, it can also be caused by head trauma, vascular accidents, autoimmunity, hemochromatosis or iron overload, and several medical causes of central hypothyroidism [37–42].

Acquired central hypothyroidism (ACH) is certainly more common in adulthood, and the condition is primarily caused by pituitary macroadenomas and their surgical or radiation treatment [43–45]. Recent evidence suggests that immunotherapy may also cause ACH [46]. Craniopharyngioma is the most common expansive lesion associated with central hypothyroidism in pediatric patients [47]. The increased use of immune checkpoint inhibitors (ICIs) in oncologic therapy over the past decade has led to an upsurge in central hypothyroidism associated with pituitary inflammation, although the exact mechanisms remain poorly understood [48]. The causes of acquired central hypothyroidism are shown in **Table 1**.

4. Clinical symptoms of central hypothyroidism

The clinical symptoms of central hypothyroidism are the same as those of primary hypothyroidism. The main clinical manifestations are fatigue, fear of cold, weight gain, memory loss, slow reaction, drowsiness, depression, etc. [16, 49, 50]. These symptoms are accompanied by muscle weakness, temporary muscle stiffness, and other muscle and joint reactions. The involvement of the cardiovascular system is often manifested in myocardial mucous edema leading to decreased myocardial contractility, bradycardia, decreased cardiac output, etc. Additionally, anorexia, abdominal distension, constipation, and other digestive reactions often appear [51–53]. Furthermore, coma with mucus edema often occurs in patients with severe disease [54].

Of note, most patients with central hypothyroidism rarely present at birth with the typical manifestations of severe congenital hypothyroidism. This is due to the efficient stimulation of the fetal thyroid gland by chorionic gonadotropin, which contrasts with primary thyroid defects. Additionally, thyroid function is not completely defective, especially when hypothalamic stimulation is predominantly affected [55].

Mental retardation may be particularly severe if there is a delay in the diagnosis of isolated congenital central hypothyroidism associated with a double allelic TSHβ mutation because of false-negative results of primary thyroid defects on neonatal TSH screening [56]. Genetic central hypothyroidism may be associated with growth retardation, delayed pubertal development, and/or variable neurologic deficits. Some patients with congenital central hypothyroidism have specific genetic defects, such as macrobiosis in IGSF1 or hearing defects in TBL1X [57–59].

Acquired forms of central hypothyroidism are usually disseminated and in most cases are due to the presence of saddle-occupying pituitary macroadenomas, craniopharyngiomas, and other tumors, head trauma, vascular accidents, or intracranial radiation therapy [60].

The size tumor may result in defective neuropituitary function causing uropygia and/or compression of the optic nerve block, which directly affects the quality of the visual field [60]. In addition, these lesions typically affect pituitary and hypothalamic function, resulting in clinical manifestations of MPHDs and hyperprolactinemia secondary to pituitary stalk removal or compression [61]. Consequently, the signs and symptoms resulting from this MHPD disorder, such as alopecia, diarrhea, pallor, headaches, menstrual disorders, decreased libido, visual deficits, and lipid metabolism disorder, may overlap and encompass specific manifestations resulting from hypothyroidism [62]. All of these problems can seriously impair the health and quality of life of patients [63].

5. Screening and diagnosis of central hypothyroidism

Diagnosing central hypothyroidism often requires a combination of clinical presentation, hormone level analysis, imaging studies, and genetic tests [12]. The clinical presentation of hypothyroidism is highly variable and often nonspecific. Therefore, the diagnosis of central hypothyroidism is predominantly based on biochemical and hormone evaluation [64, 65].

5.1 Clinical manifestations (symptoms of hypothyroidism)

A typical example is congenital central hypothyroidism in infants presenting with jaundice and poor growth associated with muscle dystonia [66]. Patients with signs and symptoms of hypothyroidism, recurrent headaches, or visual field defects should be investigated for central hypothyroidism [67].

5.2 Biochemical hormone and imaging findings

Diagnosis is usually made biochemically with low circulating fT4 concentrations associated with low/normal serum TSH levels. Subjects with a low serum concentration of FT4 should be considered for a diagnosis of abnormal CH, and further measurement of TSH by a reliable method is required to contribute to a correct diagnosis [68]. Serum TSH concentrations are also slightly elevated in some patients with CH who have predominantly hypothalamic defects. In this subgroup of patients,

TSH levels can be superimposed on those found in subclinical or mild primary hypothyroidism, although the molecule lacks full biological activity and fT4 is already in the hypothyroid range [68, 69]. If serum TSH is elevated and fT4 is decreased, diagnose primary congenital hypothyroidism [69]. If serum fT4 is decreased and TSH is decreased, normal, or slightly elevated, central congenital hypothyroidism should be considered [70]. If serum TSH is increased and fT4 is in the normal range, the diagnosis is hyperthyrotropinemia [71, 72]. FT4 and TSH levels of different diseases are shown in **Figure 2** and **Table 2**.

Serum TSH concentrations in patients with central hypothyroidism are usually within the reference range. However, the secreted TSH isoforms, while immunoreactive, have severely impaired biological activity [72]. Thus, the combination of inappropriately normal serum TSH and low circulating fT4 levels is common in patients with central hypothyroidism. In addition, transient or reversible forms of this

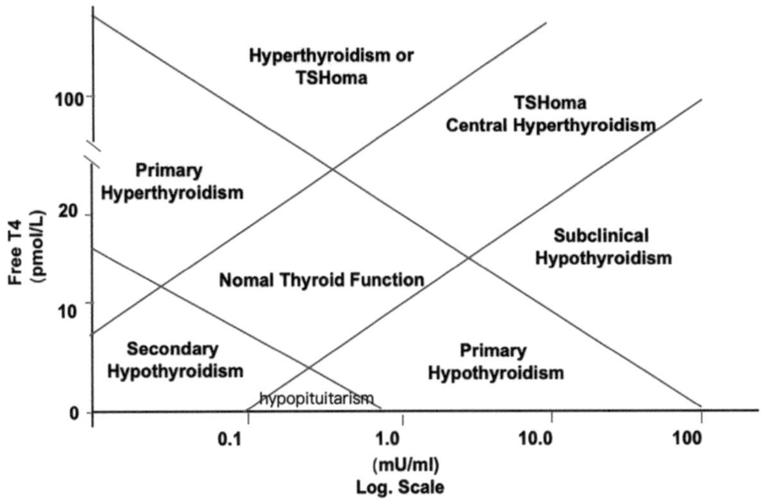

Figure 2.
Serum levels of FT4 and immunoreactive TSH in patients with CH and other conditions.

	TSH	T4/fT4	True status
Congenital central hypothyroidism	low/normal	reduced	Hypothyroid
Hypopituitarism (central hypothyroidism)	Normal (but patient not euthyroid)	Low	Hypothyroid
TSH-secreting pituitary tumor	High	High	Hyperthyroid
Thyroid hormone resistance	Normal	High	Variable usually euthyroid
Laboratory error	Normal	High or low	Hypothyroid or hyperthyroid
Abnormal protein	Normal	High	Euthyroid

Table 2.
Biochemical findings in patients with central hypothyroidism and other different thyroid conditions.

disorder may occur in patients with chronic thyrotoxicosis, in neonates of hyperthyroid mothers, and patients treated with growth hormone inhibitors, glucocorticoids, antineoplastic agents, or dopaminergic compounds [5, 73].

In patients with central congenital hypothyroidism, further testing of adrenal function and other functions of the anterior pituitary gland is recommended [74]. In all children with congenital hypothyroidism, vigilance should be exercised for the presence of heteromorphic features of congenital hypothyroidism syndrome and congenital malformations (especially of the heart) [26]. The most common presentation of congenital central hypothyroidism is characterized by reduced fT4 levels and inappropriately low or normal TSH levels. This condition may be identified at birth through a positive newborn screen or during biochemical testing in patients with known lesions in the hypothalamic–pituitary region, either during initial evaluation or follow-up. With central hypothyroidism, hormone test results are often present with lowered TSH and fT4 or markedly lowered fT4 without an elevation in TSH suggestive of pituitary or hypothalamic insufficiency. Clinically hypopituitary hypothyroidism is often associated with deficient levels of other pituitary-target gland hormones as well [75].

Thyroid imaging should be performed in patients with confirmed central hypothyroidism. Thyroid radioisotope scanning and/or perchlorate discharge test or ultrasonography are recommended [76]. Children and adolescents with primary congenital hypothyroidism due to hypoplasia of the thyroid gland may present with goiter and thyroid nodules. Therefore, regular thyroid ultrasonography is recommended to assess and monitor thyroid morphology (volume changes) [76, 77]. If ultrasound reveals suspicious nodules, fine needle aspiration cytological biopsy is recommended. Bone age or wrist or knee X-rays are recommended to assess the severity of intrauterine hypothyroidism [78].

Genetic testing: The experience of patients with congenital central hypothyroidism diagnosed by genetic testing has taught us that genetic defects may be a possible cause of mild idiopathic central hypothyroidism detected in puberty or adulthood after the incidental finding of low fT4 [79]. Genetic testing can help in the diagnosis, treatment, and prognosis of congenital hypothyroidism [79, 80]. Patients with a confirmed diagnosis of primary hypothyroidism may undergo genetic testing if conditions permit. Genetic testing is recommended for familial hypothyroidism, central hypothyroidism, and congenital hypothyroidism associated with any syndrome [80]. It is recommended that genetic analysis should be completed in cases of familial, congenital, or syndromic central hypothyroidism [70]. The identification of a pathogenic variant in a candidate gene can reveal possible carriers, enable early diagnosis in affected families, and support the diagnosis of central hypothyroidism in uncertain cases. This includes those with delayed evidence or the presence of biochemical abnormalities without an obvious cause. Genetic analyses can be performed by automated direct sequencing of specific genes, following a phenotype-driven approach, or by using targeted next-generation sequencing technologies that allow multiple candidate gene clusters to be run simultaneously [34]. Genetic testing should be performed using newer technologies such as array comparative genomic hybridization (aCGH), targeted sequencing in next-generation DNA sequencing (NGS), or whole exome sequencing (WES) [81]. It is important to note that genetic testing is not perfect, and the child's guardian should be informed of the limitations of genetic testing before proceeding with the test [82].

5.3 Differential diagnosis

Central hypothyroidism needs to be differentiated from the following conditions:

1. Drug-related pseudohypothyroidism

Drugs that inhibit TSH secretion include metformin, dopamine, glucocorticoids, cocaine, and antiepileptic and antipsychotic drugs [5, 37]. Other therapies that may cause central hypothyroidism include mitotane, as well as toxoid toxins that directly inhibit TSHβ expression (e.g., bexarotene) and newer biologic agents that induce pituitary inflammation, such as ipilimumab or other immune checkpoint inhibitors [83]. It is therefore recommended that TSH and fT4 should be checked repeatedly before and during the use of these therapeutic agents. Dopamine agonists and growth inhibitor analogs may produce a more mild and transient suppression of thyroid hormones [84].

2. Severe forms of non-thyroidal disease or euthyroid sick syndrome (ESS)

Non-thyroidal disease or ESS is most common in hospitalized patients with severe underlying disease or the elderly. It is marked by a prevalent and usually isolated decrease in T3 or fT3 levels and concomitant severe or chronic disease states (previously named low T3 syndromes) [85].

3. Thyrotoxicity-related conditions

Levothyroxine withdrawal syndrome, long-term TSH suppression after recovery from thyrotoxicosis [86]. Pharmacological treatments capable of suppressing TSH secretion or recovery from a state of thyrotoxicosis may sometimes be confused with CCH.

4. Pregnancy-related conditions

(a) Isolated maternal hypothyroxinemia (interpreted in the context of pregnancy-specific FT4 reference ranges in pregnant women) [87]. (b) Preterm labor (delayed rise in TSH in hypothyroid infants) [88]. Hypothyroxinemia in pregnancy can be diagnosed in the differential by CH, but this risk may be greatly reduced by defining a trimester-specific FT4 reference level. The delayed rise in TSH in preterm infants may be associated with transient CH, which is usually of short duration and in most cases does not require treatment [88].

Genetic factors: (a) Alan Herndon Dudley syndrome (a pathogenic allelic variant of the MCT8 gene); (b) RTHα due to heterozygous mutations in THRA; (c) TSHβ allelic variant with conserved bioactivity but loss of immune reactivity to circulating TSH [89–91].

A thorough personal history, repeat biochemical tests, and exclusion of underlying primary thyroid disease are recommended in the differential diagnosis. A careful and meticulous differential is key to detecting this possibility [92]. In addition, patients with rare genetic defects in thyroid hormone action may have low FT4 and normal or slightly elevated TSH [33]. However, patients affected by mutations in MCT8 or THRA that result in Alan Herndon Dudley syndrome or resistance to thyroid hormone alpha (RTHα) have distinctive and typical clinical features, with T3 levels at the upper end of the normal range [33, 89–91].

DOI: http://dx.doi.org/10.5772/intechopen.1005432

6. Treatment of central hypothyroidism

The first-line treatment for central hypothyroidism remains levothyroxine (L-T4) replacement therapy. Once concomitant cortisol deficiency has been ruled out, treatment is recommended for all patients who receive the diagnosis. In those who present with adrenal insufficiency or whose presence cannot be ruled out, supplemental L-T4 should be adequately treated with glucocorticoids to prevent induction of adrenal crisis [93].

6.1 Treatment of central hypothyroidism in adults

For adult patients with central disease, replacement L-T4 therapy is recommended to be tailored to each patient's weight and age (35) [12]. For patients over 65 years of age and those with cardiovascular comorbidities, the starting dose should be between 1.0 and 1.2 mcg/kg/day. In addition, treatment of milder forms of CH (fT4 values within the lower limit of the normal range) may be avoided in subjects over 75 years of age, as studies have shown that mild or subclinical primary hypothyroidism is protective against the risk of cardiovascular mortality in the elderly [94]. In addition, in elderly patients and patients with long-term illness and high cardiovascular risk, the ETA Task Force recommends starting with L-T4 therapy with a lower dose and then gradually increasing the dose over the next few weeks or months. It is important to assess the adequacy of the replacement after 6–8 weeks of measuring fT4 and targeting this parameter above the median value of the reference range [39].

Once treatment has been judged adequate, it should be reassessed annually with measurement of serum fT4. Measurement of TSH and T3 may be useful only to exclude suspects of under and over-treatment, respectively. Inadequate replacement therapy should be suspected whenever FT4 concentrations are found to be below or at the lower end of the normal range, especially when manifestations of hypothyroidism are present or when TSH remains within the normal range. In contrast, excessive intake of LT4 should be considered whenever fT4 concentrations are above or at the upper limit of the normal range, especially when clinical manifestations of thyrotoxicosis and/or high FT3 levels are present [12, 39, 94].

6.2 Treatment of congenital central hypothyroidism

Treatment of congenital central hypothyroidism should be initiated as soon as possible and no later than 2 weeks after birth [95]. Neonates with a positive confirmatory test should be started immediately. Treatment is preferred to LT4, which is given orally once daily at the same time. To enhance compliance in neonates and infants, LT4 may be taken with food. However, coadministration with foods or medications that may reduce LT4 absorption, such as soy protein, plant fibers, iron, and calcium, should be avoided [96]. Immediate initiation of LT4 therapy is recommended for young children and adolescent patients with reduced serum fT4 and significantly increased TSH. Due to higher thyroid hormone levels in childhood, children require higher doses of LT4 [97].

In children with congenital central hypothyroidism, it is recommended that LT4 therapy be initiated with normal adrenal function in order to prevent the development of adrenal crisis. If the presence of central adrenal insufficiency cannot be excluded, glucocorticosteroid therapy is mandatory before LT4 therapy.

In children with severe primary congenital hypothyroidism, i.e., FT4 < 5 pmol/L or very low TT4 concentrations with elevated TSH (based on the day and gestational age above the normal range), a starting dose of 10–15 μg/(kg-d) of LT4 is recommended.

For children with mild primary congenital hypothyroidism (FT4 > 10 pmol/L and elevated TSH), the initial LT4 dose is 10 μg/(kg-d); for children whose FT4 is within the age-specific reference range, the starting LT4 dose is 5 to 10 μg/(kg-d).

For children with severe central congenital hypothyroidism (FT4 < 5 pmol/L), the recommended starting dose of LT4 is 10 ~ 15 μg/(kg-d); and for children with milder central congenital hypothyroidism (fT4 5 ~ 15 pmol/L), the recommended starting dose of LT4 is 5 ~ 10 μg/(kg-d) [98].

6.3 Treatment of central hypothyroidism in pregnant women

During pregnancy, it is recommended to increase hormone supplementation by 20–50% of the initial dose and to maintain fT4 levels in the upper quartile of the reference range to compensate for the expanding extracellular T4 pool and to avoid fetal hypothyroidism [11].

7. Efficacy observation and follow-up of central hypothyroidism

Once replacement therapy is initiated, pediatric patients should be monitored to maintain FT4 levels within the reference range for age, and their follow-up should be similar to that of primary hypothyroidism [99]. In children with central hypothyroidism, LT4 treatment is accompanied by an accelerated growth rate so that target heights can be achieved. During follow-up, the frequency of assessment should be increased if fT4 or TSH abnormalities occur if patient compliance is questioned [100]. Additional assessments should be performed 4–6 weeks after changing the LT4 dose or dosage form. If an increase in LT4 dose is unexpectedly required, consideration should be given to the presence of other medical conditions (e.g., gastrointestinal disorders), foods, or medications that cause decreased absorption or increased metabolism of LT4. Poor compliance is also a common cause in adolescents and pubertal children. Malabsorption should be suspected when there is an insufficient increment of serum FT4 or its decrease during treatment with a given dose of L-T4 [101].

Unlike the treatment of primary hypothyroidism, where TSH is an excellent marker of adequate replacement, the management of central hypothyroidism is more complex. Even low doses of L-T4 are capable of suppressing TSH secretion [102]. In a comparison between adequately treated patients with primary thyroid disease and other patients presenting with hypothalamic–pituitary lesions [103]. If fT4 levels were significantly lower in central hypothyroidism, Koulouri et al. suggested the presence of inadequate replacement therapy in most cases [104]. Indeed, in acquired forms of central hypothyroidism such as surgery or radiotherapy for pituitary lesions or after initiation of treatments with an inherent risk of central hypothyroidism, it may be useful to assess fT4 concentrations before interventions and LT4 replacements can eventually achieve previous fT4 levels [104]. It may sometimes be useful to assess biochemical indicators of thyroid hormone metabolism and tissue action, such as sex hormone-binding globulin (SHBG), bone gamma-carboxyglutamic acidprotein (BGLAP) for thyrotoxicosis, or under-treated cholesterol [105].

8. Prognosis of central hypothyroidism

Most patients with CH can recover normal thyroid function after active and appropriate treatment [106]. Most children and adolescents with congenital hypothyroidism have normal neuro-development and schooling levels after early diagnosis and appropriate treatment [107]. However, children with severe hypothyroidism may have mild cognitive and motor deficits and lower educational attainment [108]. These deficits may be associated with prenatal brain damage caused by intrauterine thyroxine insufficiency. Children with central hypothyroidism may have reduced hippocampal volume and thinning or thickening of the cerebral cortex, which may lead to deficits in memory, language, sensorimotor, and visuospatial functions [109, 110]. Recent prospective studies have suggested a negative metabolic impact of under-treatment of central hypothyroidism as assessed by dual-energy x-ray (DXA) scanning for lipid distribution and body fat mass [111]. These data, in addition to supporting the need for appropriate treatment to maintain fT4 values at the upper limit of normality, suggest negative effects even in the usually undiagnosed form of occult central hypothyroidism.

Infants with congenital hypothyroid syndrome may also exhibit other neurological deficits not directly related to hypothyroidism [112]. Appropriately treated children with central hypothyroidism have an age of onset of puberty, age of first female menstruation, and menstrual cycles similar to those of the normal population [113]. In adults, fertility does not differ from normal [114].

Women with hypothyroidism are at increased risk for adverse pregnancy outcomes. Appropriately treated children have a better prognosis for physical development and also have normal skeletal, metabolic, and cardiovascular health [115]. Long-term studies of patients with hypothyroidism have shown that patients who begin appropriate treatment early have normal bone density, normal growth patterns, and height in adulthood. Children and adults with hypothyroidism have a body mass index comparable to that of the normal population [116]. Young patients have normal blood pressure, glucose, and lipid metabolism, as well as normal carotid intima-media thickness [117]. However, there is an increased risk of minor cardiovascular dysfunction in the presence of repeated undertreatment [118]. Examples include reduced exercise capacity, impaired diastolic function, increased carotid intima-media thickness, and mild endothelial dysfunction. Whether these minor abnormalities result in impaired quality of life or lead to an increased risk of cardiovascular disease requires further study [119].

Most children with congenital central hypothyroidism have a good prognosis after early diagnosis and appropriate treatment [120]. Therefore, it is recommended that enhanced patient education starts with the diagnosis of the disease, which could improve patients' and families' understanding of congenital hypothyroidism, promote self-management, and help improve the clinical prognosis and quality of life in patients with central hypothyroidism.

Acknowledgements

We thank Prof. Yerong Yu and Jianwei Li of the Department of Endocrinology and Metabolism, West China Hospital, Sichuan University, and Professor Hoffman R. Andrew Department of Endocrinology, Gerontology, & Metabolism, Stanford University School of Medicine.

Conflict of interest

The authors declare no conflict of interest.

Author details

Huiwen Tan*, Yuke Liu and Sumita Cholekho
Department of Endocrinology and Metabolism, West China Hospital of Sichuan University, Chengdu, China

*Address all correspondence to: huiwent2016@scu.edu.cn

References

[1] Chaker L et al. Hypothyroidism. Lancet. 2017;**390**(10101):1550-1562

[2] Persani L. Clinical review: Central hypothyroidism—Pathogenic, diagnostic, and therapeutic challenges. The Journal of Clinical Endocrinology and Metabolism. 2012;**97**(9):3068-3078

[3] Chaker L et al. Hypothyroidism. Nature Reviews. Disease Primers. 2022;**8**(1):30

[4] Devdhar M, Ousman YH, Burman KD. Hypothyroidism. Endocrinology and Metabolism Clinics of North America. 2007;**36**(3):595-615, v

[5] Rizzo LFL, Mana DL, Serra HA. Drug-induced hypothyroidism. Medicina (B Aires). 2017;**77**(5):394-404

[6] Feldt-Rasmussen U, Effraimidis G, Klose M. The hypothalamus-pituitary-thyroid (HPT)-axis and its role in physiology and pathophysiology of other hypothalamus-pituitary functions. Molecular and Cellular Endocrinology. 2021;**525**:111173

[7] Wilson SA, Stem LA, Bruehlman RD. Hypothyroidism: Diagnosis and treatment. American Family Physician. 2021;**103**(10):605-613

[8] Chiovato L, Magri F, Carlé A. Hypothyroidism in context: Where we've been and where We're going. Advances in Therapy. 2019;**36**(Suppl. 2):47-58

[9] Beck-Peccoz P et al. Central hypothyroidism—A neglected thyroid disorder. Nature Reviews. Endocrinology. 2017;**13**(10):588-598

[10] Benvenga S et al. Less known aspects of central hypothyroidism: Part 1—Acquired etiologies. Journal of Clinical & Translational Endocrinology. 2018;**14**:25-33

[11] van Trotsenburg P et al. Congenital hypothyroidism: A 2020-2021 consensus guidelines update-an ENDO-European reference network initiative endorsed by the European Society for Pediatric Endocrinology and the European Society for Endocrinology. Thyroid. 2021;**31**(3):387-419

[12] Lauffer P et al. Diagnosis and Management of Central Congenital Hypothyroidism. Frontiers in Endocrinology (Lausanne). 2021;**12**:686317

[13] Liu L et al. Global prevalence of congenital hypothyroidism among neonates from 1969 to 2020: A systematic review and meta-analysis. European Journal of Pediatrics. 2023;**182**(7):2957-2965

[14] Asakura Y et al. Hypothalamo-pituitary hypothyroidism detected by neonatal screening for congenital hypothyroidism using measurement of thyroid-stimulating hormone and thyroxine. Acta Paediatrica. 2002;**91**(2):172-177

[15] Hughes K, Eastman C. Thyroid disease: Long-term management of hyperthyroidism and hypothyroidism. Australian Journal of General Practice. 2021;**50**(1-2):36-42

[16] Jansen HI et al. Hypothyroidism: The difficulty in attributing symptoms to their underlying cause. Frontiers in Endocrinology (Lausanne). 2023;**14**:1130661

[17] Cherella CE, Wassner AJ. Update on congenital hypothyroidism. Current

Opinion in Endocrinology, Diabetes, and Obesity. 2020;**27**(1):63-69

[18] Lauridsen MB, Nærå RW, Leunbach TL. Acquired hypothyroidism in children and adolescents. Ugeskrift for Laeger. 2023;**185**(22):V10220628

[19] Zwaveling-Soonawala N, van Trotsenburg P. Genetics of primary congenital hypothyroidism. Pediatric Endocrinology Reviews. 2018;**15**(3):200-215

[20] Ahmad T, Muhammad ZA, Nadeem S. Is hypothyroidism associated with outcomes in fracture patients? Data from a trauma registry. The Journal of Surgical Research. 2021;**268**:527-531

[21] Takamizawa T et al. Central hypothyroidism related to pituitary adenomas: Low incidence of central hypothyroidism in patients with acromegaly. The Journal of Clinical Endocrinology and Metabolism. 2019;**104**(10):4879-4888

[22] Huang W et al. Identification of thyroid hormones and functional characterization of thyroid hormone receptor in the pacific oyster crassostrea gigas provide insight into evolution of the thyroid hormone system. PLoS One. 2015;**10**(12):e0144991

[23] Moran C et al. Genetic disorders of thyroid development, hormone biosynthesis and signalling. Clinical Endocrinology. 2022;**97**(4):502-514

[24] Iwen KA, Oelkrug R, Brabant G. Effects of thyroid hormones on thermogenesis and energy partitioning. Journal of Molecular Endocrinology. 2018;**60**(3):R157-r170

[25] Bassett JH, Williams GR. Role of thyroid hormones in skeletal development and bone maintenance. Endocrine Reviews. 2016;**37**(2):135-187

[26] Schoenmakers N et al. Recent advances in central congenital hypothyroidism. The Journal of Endocrinology. 2015;**227**(3):R51-R71

[27] Peters C, van Trotsenburg ASP, Schoenmakers N. Diagnosis of Endocrine disease: Congenital hypothyroidism—Update and perspectives. European Journal of Endocrinology. 2018;**179**(6):R297-r317

[28] Bauer AJ, Wassner AJ. Thyroid hormone therapy in congenital hypothyroidism and pediatric hypothyroidism. Endocrine. 2019;**66**(1):51-62

[29] Diaz A, Lipman Diaz EG. Hypothyroidism. Pediatrics in Review. 2014;**35**(8):336-347. quiz 348-9

[30] Sugisawa C et al. Adult thyroid outcomes of congenital hypothyroidism. Thyroid. 2023;**33**(5):556-565

[31] Rey RA et al. Diagnosing and treating anterior pituitary hormone deficiency in pediatric patients. Reviews in Endocrine & Metabolic Disorders. 2024;**25**(3):555-573

[32] Naafs JC et al. Cognitive and motor outcome in patients with early-detected central congenital hypothyroidism compared with siblings. The Journal of Clinical Endocrinology and Metabolism. 2021;**106**(3):e1231-e1239

[33] Beck-Peccoz P et al. Syndromes of hormone resistance in the hypothalamic-pituitary-thyroid axis. Best Practice & Research. Clinical Endocrinology & Metabolism. 2006;**20**(4):529-546

[34] Boelen A, van Trotsenburg ASP, Fliers E. Congenital isolated central

hypothyroidism: Novel mutations and their functional implications. Handbook of Clinical Neurology. 2021;**180**:161-169

[35] McDermott MT. Hypothyroidism. Annals of Internal Medicine. 2020;**173**(1):Itc1-itc16

[36] Qian F et al. Novel non-synonymous mutations of PAX8 in a cohort of Chinese with congenital hypothyroidism. Chinese Medical Journal. 2019;**132**(11):1322-1327

[37] Wu J, Huang H. Acquired hypothyroidism in patients with metastatic renal cell carcinoma treated with tyrosine kinase inhibitors. Drug Design, Development and Therapy. 2020;**14**:3977-3982

[38] Comité Nacional de Endocrinología de la Sociedad Argentina de Pediatría. Alteraciones tiroideas en la infancia y en la adolescencia. Parte 2: hipotiroidismo [Thyroid disorders in childhood and adolescence. Part 2: Hypothyroidism]. Archivos Argentinos de Pediatría. 2021;**119**(1):s8-s16

[39] Persani L, Cangiano B, Bonomi M. The diagnosis and management of central hypothyroidism in 2018. Endocrine Connections. 2019;**8**(2):R44-r54

[40] Persani L, Bonomi M. The multiple genetic causes of central hypothyroidism. Best Practice & Research. Clinical Endocrinology & Metabolism. 2017;**31**(2):255-263

[41] Heinen CA et al. Mutations in IRS4 are associated with central hypothyroidism. Journal of Medical Genetics. 2018;**55**(10):693-700

[42] Reiners C, Drozd V, Yamashita S. Hypothyroidism after radiation exposure: Brief narrative review. Journal of Neural Transmission (Vienna). 2020;**127**(11):1455-1466

[43] FitzGerald TJ et al. Treatment toxicity: Radiation. Hematology/Oncology Clinics of North America. 2019;**33**(6):1027-1039

[44] Lohiya S et al. Pituitary macroadenoma secondary to congenital hypothyroidism with growth failure and developmental delay: A rare presentation. Cureus. 2023;**15**(5):e39655

[45] Benea SN et al. Central hypothyroidism in severe sepsis. Acta Endocrinology (Buchar). 2019;**15**(3):372-377

[46] Kassi E et al. Endocrine-related adverse events associated with immune-checkpoint inhibitors in patients with melanoma. Cancer Medicine. 2019;**8**(15):6585-6594

[47] Sadashivam S et al. Adult craniopharyngioma: The role of extent of resection in tumor recurrence and long-term functional outcome. Clinical Neurology and Neurosurgery. 2020;**192**:105711

[48] Johnson DB et al. Immune-checkpoint inhibitors: Long-term implications of toxicity. Nature Reviews. Clinical Oncology. 2022;**19**(4):254-267

[49] Mavromati M, Jornayvaz FR. Hypothyroidism-associated dyslipidemia: Potential molecular mechanisms leading to NAFLD. International Journal of Molecular Sciences. 2021;**22**(23):12797

[50] Rose SR et al. Congenital hypothyroidism: Screening and management. Pediatrics. 2023;**151**:1

[51] Tysoe O. Skeletal muscle weakness in hypothyroidism. Nature Reviews. Endocrinology. 2021;**17**(8):447

[52] Paschou SA et al. Thyroid disorders and cardiovascular manifestations: An update. Endocrine. 2022;**75**(3):672-683

[53] Herrmann B et al. Central hypothyroidism impairs heart rate stability and prevents thyroid hormone-induced cardiac hypertrophy and pyrexia. Thyroid. 2020;**30**(8):1205-1216

[54] Kaur K et al. Central hypothyroidism with myxoedema: A less known but clinically challenging presentation. BMJ Case Reports. 13 Sep 2022;**15**(9):e250282

[55] Nicholas AK et al. Molecular spectrum of TSHβ subunit gene defects in central hypothyroidism in the UK and Ireland. Clinical Endocrinology. 2017;**86**(3):410-418

[56] Karguppikar MB et al. Rare case of central congenital hypothyroidism due to a TSHβ mutation presenting with macro-orchidism. BMJ Case Reports. 14 Nov 2023;**16**(11):e252796

[57] Costas Eimil J, Sánchez-Sobrino P. IGSF1 mutation as a cause of isolated central hypothyroidism. Endocrinología, Diabetes and Nutrición (English ed.). 2022;**69**(10):913-914

[58] Nikolaou M et al. Hepatomegaly and fatty liver disease secondary to central hypothyroidism in combination with macrosomia as initial presentation of IGSF1 deficiency syndrome. Hormones (Athens, Greece). 2023;**22**(3):515-520

[59] García M et al. Central hypothyroidism and novel clinical phenotypes in Hemizygous truncation of TBL1X. Journal of the Endocrine Society. 2019;**3**(1):119-128

[60] Galal A, Ahmed OEF. Determinants of visual and endocrinological outcome after early endoscopic endonasal surgery for pituitary apoplexy. Surgical Neurology International. 2022;**13**:433

[61] Poppe K. Management of endocrine disease: Thyroid and female infertility—More questions than answers?! European Journal of Endocrinology. 2021;**184**(4):R123-r135

[62] Alexander EK et al. 2017 guidelines of the American thyroid association for the diagnosis and management of thyroid disease during pregnancy and the postpartum. Thyroid. 2017;**27**(3):315-389

[63] Ellegård L et al. Health-related quality of life in hypothyroidism-a population-based study, the WHO MONICA project. Clinical Endocrinology. 2021;**95**(1):197-208

[64] Gottwald-Hostalek U, Schulte B. Low awareness and under-diagnosis of hypothyroidism. Current Medical Research and Opinion. 2022;**38**(1):59-64

[65] Davis MG, Phillippi JC. Hypothyroidism: Diagnosis and evidence-based treatment. Journal of Midwifery & Women's Health. 2022;**67**(3):394-397

[66] Mantri R, Bavdekar SB, Save SU. Congenital hypothyroidism: An unusual combination of biochemical abnormalities. Case Reports in Pediatrics. 2016;**2016**:2678578

[67] Nakhleh A et al. Outcomes of pituitary apoplexy: A comparison of microadenomas and macroadenomas. Pituitary. 2021;**24**(4):492-498

[68] Chen J et al. Epidemiologic characteristics and risk factors for congenital hypothyroidism from 2009 to 2018 in Xiamen, China. Endocrine Practice. 2020;**26**(6):585-594

[69] Boelen A et al. Neonatal screening for primary and central congenital hypothyroidism: Is it time to go Dutch? European Thyroid Journal. 27 Jul 2023;**12**(4):e230041

[70] Klosinska M, Kaczynska A, Ben-Skowronek I. Congenital hypothyroidism in preterm newborns—The challenges of diagnostics and treatment: A review. Frontiers in Endocrinology (Lausanne). 2022;**13**:860862

[71] Croce L et al. Unexplained Hyperthyrotropinemia: A biochemical and clinical challenge. Journal of Clinical Medicine. 18 Apr 2023;**12**(8):2934

[72] Agretti P et al. A fast method to detect cell surface expression of thyrotropin receptor (TSHr): The microchip flow cytometry analysis. Thyroid. 2007;**17**(9):861-868

[73] Hoang TD et al. Over-the-counter-drug-induced thyroid disorders. Endocrine Practice. 2013;**19**(2):268-274

[74] Silva JE. Pituitary-thyroid relationships in hypothyroidism. Baillière's Clinical Endocrinology and Metabolism. 1988;**2**(3):541-565

[75] Fliers E, Boelen A, van Trotsenburg AS. Central regulation of the hypothalamo-pituitary-thyroid (HPT) axis: Focus on clinical aspects. Handbook of Clinical Neurology. 2014;**124**:127-138

[76] Graber E et al. The role of ^{123}I imaging in the evaluation of infants with mild congenital hypothyroidism. Hormone Research in Pædiatrics. 2015;**83**(2):94-101

[77] Borges MF et al. Timing of thyroid ultrasonography in the etiological investigation of congenital hypothyroidism. Archives of Endocrinology and Metabolism. 2017;**61**(5):432-437

[78] Esposito A et al. Effect of initial levothyroxine dose on neurodevelopmental and growth outcomes in children with congenital hypothyroidism. Frontiers in Endocrinology (Lausanne). 2022;**13**:923448

[79] Kara C et al. Genetic testing can change diagnosis and treatment in children with congenital hypothyroidism. European Thyroid Journal. 13 Apr 2023;**12**(3):e220212

[80] Naafs JC et al. Clinical and genetic characteristics of Dutch children with central congenital hypothyroidism, early detected by neonatal screening. European Journal of Endocrinology. 2020;**183**(6):627-636

[81] Strom CM. Changing trends in laboratory testing in the United States: A personal, historical perspective. Clinics in Laboratory Medicine. 2012;**32**(4):651-664

[82] Majumder MA, Guerrini CJ, McGuire AL. Direct-to-consumer genetic testing: Value and risk. Annual Review of Medicine. 2021;**72**:151-166

[83] Wright JJ, Powers AC, Johnson DB. Endocrine toxicities of immune checkpoint inhibitors. Nature Reviews. Endocrinology. 2021;**17**(7):389-399

[84] Bowden SA, Goldis M. Congenital hypothyroidism. 5 Jun 2023. In: StatPearls [Internet]. Treasure Island, Tampa, Florida, United States: StatPearls Publishing; Jan 2025

[85] Fliers E, Boelen A. An update on non-thyroidal illness syndrome. Journal

of Endocrinological Investigation. 2021;**44**(8):1597-1607

[86] van Veelen NM et al. Compartment syndrome of the leg after thyroid hormone withdrawal; two cases and a systematic review of the literature. BMC Endocrine Disorders. 2020;**20**(1):80

[87] Chen L et al. Association between third trimester maternal isolated hypothyroxinemia and adverse pregnancy outcomes. Endocrine Journal. 2023;**70**(6):611-618

[88] Derakhshan A et al. Association of maternal thyroid function with birthweight: A systematic review and individual-participant data meta-analysis. The Lancet Diabetes and Endocrinology. 2020;**8**(6):501-510

[89] Groeneweg S et al. Disease characteristics of MCT8 deficiency: An international, retrospective, multicentre cohort study. The Lancet Diabetes and Endocrinology. 2020;**8**(7):594-605

[90] Ortiga-Carvalho TM, Sidhaye AR, Wondisford FE. Thyroid hormone receptors and resistance to thyroid hormone disorders. Nature Reviews. Endocrinology. 2014;**10**(10):582-591

[91] Sasaki S et al. The mechanism of negative transcriptional regulation by thyroid hormone: Lessons from the thyrotropin β subunit gene. Vitamins and Hormones. 2018;**106**:97-127

[92] Campi I et al. Unusual causes of hyperthyrotropinemia and differential diagnosis of primary hypothyroidism: A revised diagnostic flowchart. European Thyroid Journal. 9 Jun 2023;**12**(4):e230012

[93] Hahner S et al. Epidemiology of adrenal crisis in chronic adrenal insufficiency: The need for new prevention strategies. European Journal of Endocrinology. 2010;**162**(3):597-602

[94] Dore R et al. Resistance to thyroid hormone induced tachycardia in RTHα syndrome. Nature Communications. 2023;**14**(1):3312

[95] Jonklaas J. Optimal thyroid hormone replacement. Endocrine Reviews. 2022;**43**(2):366-404

[96] Ross DS. Treating hypothyroidism is not always easy: When to treat subclinical hypothyroidism, TSH goals in the elderly, and alternatives to levothyroxine monotherapy. Journal of Internal Medicine. 2022;**291**(2):128-140

[97] Behura SS, Nikhila GP, Panda SK. Screening and management of congenital hypothyroidism—Guidelines by American academy of pediatrics, 2023. Indian Pediatrics. 2023;**60**(10):855-858

[98] Rodriguez L, Dinauer C, Francis G. Treatment of hypothyroidism in infants, children and adolescents. Trends in Endocrinology and Metabolism. 2022;**33**(7):522-532

[99] Nagasaki K et al. Guidelines for newborn screening of congenital hypothyroidism (2021 revision). Clinical Pediatric Endocrinology. 2023;**32**(1):26-51

[100] Zwaveling-Soonawala N, van Trotsenburg AS, Verkerk PH. The severity of congenital hypothyroidism of central origin should not be underestimated. The Journal of Clinical Endocrinology and Metabolism. 2015;**100**(2):E297-E300

[101] Martinez M, Derksen D, Kapsner P. Making sense of hypothyroidism. An approach to testing and treatment. Postgraduate Medicine. 1993;**93**(6):135-8-141-5

[102] Jansen HI et al. Biomarkers indicating tissue thyroid hormone status: Ready to be implemented yet? The Journal of Endocrinology. 2022;**253**(2):R21-r45

[103] Hirata Y et al. Median-lower normal levels of serum thyroxine are associated with low triiodothyronine levels and body temperature in patients with central hypothyroidism. European Journal of Endocrinology. 2015;**173**(2):247-256

[104] Kratzsch J et al. Global FT4 immunoassay standardization: An expert opinion review. Clinical Chemistry and Laboratory Medicine. 2021;**59**(6):1013-1023

[105] Esfandiari NH, Papaleontiou M. Biochemical testing in thyroid disorders. Endocrinology and Metabolism Clinics of North America. 2017;**46**(3):631-648

[106] Ettleson MD, Papaleontiou M. Evaluating health outcomes in the treatment of hypothyroidism. Frontier Endocrinology (Lausanne). 2022;**13**:1026262

[107] Komur M et al. Neurodevelopment evaluation in children with congenital hypothyroidism by Bayley-III. Brain Development. 2013;**35**(5):392-397

[108] Wassner AJ. Pediatric hypothyroidism: Diagnosis and treatment. Paediatric Drugs. 2017;**19**(4):291-301

[109] Wheeler SM et al. Hippocampal size and memory functioning in children and adolescents with congenital hypothyroidism. The Journal of Clinical Endocrinology and Metabolism. 2011;**96**(9):E1427-E1434

[110] Razón-Hernández KC et al. Neuropsychological alterations in patients with congenital hypothyroidism treated with levothyroxine: Linked factors and thyroid hormone hyposensitivity. Journal of Clinical Medicine. 15 Jun 2022;**11**(12):3427

[111] Kotwal A et al. Treatment of thyroid dysfunction and serum lipids: A systematic review and meta-analysis. The Journal of Clinical Endocrinology and Metabolism. 1 Dec 2020;**105**(12):dgaa672

[112] Uthayaseelan K et al. Congenital anomalies in infant with congenital hypothyroidism: A review of pathogenesis, diagnostic options, and management protocols. Cureus. 2022;**14**(5):e24669

[113] Khan L. Thyroid disease in children and adolescents. Pediatric Annals. 2021;**50**(4):e143-e147

[114] Hammond KR et al. Gestational hypothyroidism: Development of mild hypothyroidism in early pregnancy in previously euthyroid women. Fertility and Sterility. 2015;**103**(6):1532-6.e1

[115] Lage MJ et al. Levothyroxine treatment of pregnant women with hypothyroidism: Retrospective analysis of a US claims database. Advances in Therapy. 2020;**37**(2):933-945

[116] Teng W et al. Hypothyroidism in pregnancy. The Lancet Diabetes and Endocrinology. 2013;**1**(3):228-237

[117] Soto-García AJ et al. Carotid intima-media thickness in patients with subclinical hypothyroidism: A prospective controlled study. Clinical and Investigative Medicine. 2021;**44**(4):E39-E45

[118] Feldt-Rasmussen U, Klose M, Benvenga S. Interactions between hypothalamic pituitary thyroid axis and

other pituitary dysfunctions. Endocrine. 2018;**62**(3):519-527

[119] Cabral MD et al. Effects of thyroxine replacement on endothelial function and carotid artery intima-media thickness in female patients with mild subclinical hypothyroidism. Clinics. 2011;**66**(8):1321-1328

[120] Hanley P, Lord K, Bauer AJ. Thyroid disorders in children and adolescents: A review. JAMA Pediatrics. 2016;**170**(10):1008-1019

Chapter 9

Immunotherapy-Related Hypothyroidism: Mechanisms and Management

Selin Çakmak Demir and Dilek Yazıcı

Abstract

Immunotherapy has recently emerged as an important tool in the treatment of various malignancies. However, increased use of immune checkpoint inhibitors (ICIs) has brought attention to the associated adverse events, with hypothyroidism being a noteworthy complication. This review explores the mechanisms underlying immunotherapy-induced hypothyroidism and its management. The importance of distinguishing between primary and secondary hypothyroidism in the context of immunotherapy is emphasized, as timely intervention is critical in preventing adrenal crises. Not all patients with immune-related hypothyroidism are treated with levothyroxine. Additionally, only in severe toxicities, ICIs are hold. So, determining the management strategy is important for endocrinologists and oncologists. Therefore, multidisciplinary approach is crucial for immune-related adverse reactions (irAEs). In conclusion, this review provides a comprehensive overview of immunotherapy-induced hypothyroidism, encompassing its mechanisms, diagnostic considerations, and management strategies. By enhancing our understanding of this adverse event, endocrinologists can manage potential complications associated with immunotherapy.

Keywords: malignancy, immunotherapy, immune-related adverse events, hypothyroidism, immunotherapy-induced hypothyroidism, immune checkpoint inhibitors

1. Introduction

Immunotherapy-based regimens are widely used in solid organs and hematological malignancies. By modulating immune mechanisms, immunotherapies increase progression-free survival (PFS) and overall survival (OS) in aggressive cancers. Immune check point inhibitors (ICIs) constitute an important group of immunotherapy-based regimens [1, 2].

Extensively studied immune check point inhibitors (ICIs) include monoclonal antibodies that target programmed death 1 (PD-1), its ligand-programmed death ligand (PD-L1), and cytotoxic T-lymphocyte antigen-4 (CTLA-4). Lymphocyte activation gene protein 3 (LAG-3) is a novel ICI, used mainly in combination with other immunotherapies in the treatment of metastatic malign melanoma [1–3]. ICIs are administered as monotherapy or in combination and aim to restore the inhibitory

Immune-checkpoint inhibitors	Frequent immune-related endocrine adverse events
CTLA-4 inhibitors	
İpilimumab	Hypophysitis, hypothyroidism, and hyperthyroidism
PD-1 inhibitors	
Nivolumab Pembrolizumab Atezolizumab Cemiplimab	Hypothyroidism and hyperthyroidism Hypothyroidism, hyperthyroidism, type 1 diabetes mellitus, adrenal insufficiency, and hypophysitis
PD-L1 inhibitors	
Avelumab Durvalumab Dostarlimab	Hypothyroidism
LAG-3 inhibitors	
Relatlimab	

Table 1.
Immune-checkpoint inhibitors.

effects of T-regulatory cells. **Table 1** outlines the most used ICIs and their most frequent immune-related endocrine adverse events.

2. Mechanism of action

To comprehend the pathophysiology of immunotherapy-related hypothyroidism, thorough exploration of immune system physiology is essential.

The journey of a T-cell is complicated but must be fully understood before getting into the mechanisms of immunotherapies. Following selection in thymus, naïve T cells get into blood circulation and search for different foreign or mutated antigens. Getting past through spleen and lymph nodes antigens are presented to T cells by professional antigen-presenting cells. It is noteworthy that some T cells may identify self-antigens as foreign and may result in the activation of immune process which results in autoimmunity.

Immune check point inhibitors play a crucial role in preventing aberrant response. Key pathways in this regulation involve immune checkpoint inhibitors such as CTLA-4 (also known as CD152) and PD-1 (also known as CD279), which exert negative control at distinct stages of the immune system. CTLA-4 regulates the early stages of T-cell activation, immune priming phase especially in lymph nodes. On the other hand, PD-1 inhibits the activated T cells in peripheral tissues. Therefore, combination treatments are preferred strategies to enhance the immune response on malignant cells.

CD28 is a molecule found on T cells and binds to T-cell co-stimulatory factors (CD80/B7–1 and CD86/B7–2) on antigen-presenting cells (APCs). Proliferation and activation of T cells result in interleukin-2 (IL-2) production which occurs after this stimulatory signal.

CTLA-4 is also presented on $CD4^+$ and $CD8^+$ lymphocytes and competes with CD28 to bind to CD80 or CD86. CTLA-4 inhibits this signaling pathway which results in the inhibition of T cells. This competition decreases the immune response, and anergy occurs. **Figure 1** illustrates the pathways explained above and shows the

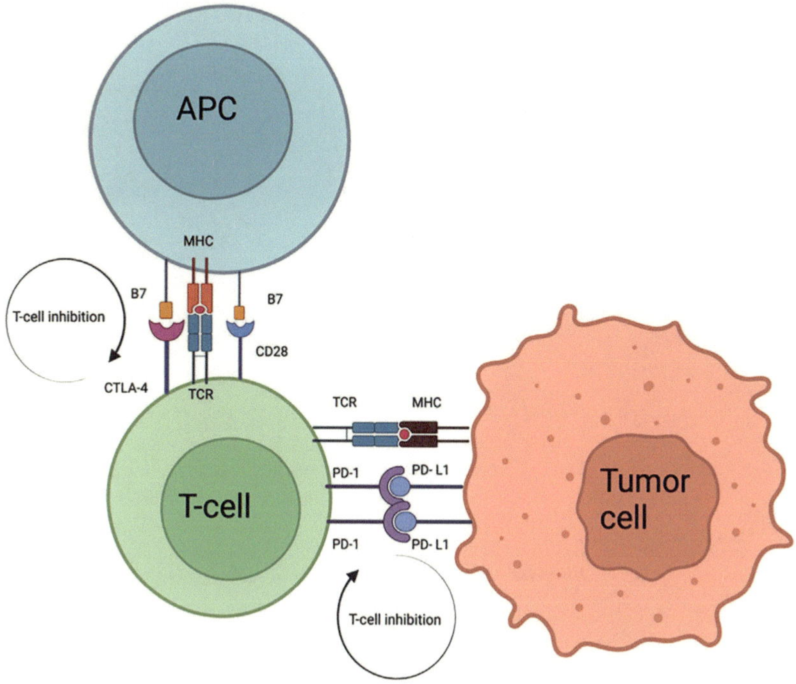

Figure 1.
Immune checkpoint inhibitors mechanism of action (created by BioRender.com). APC: Antigen presenting cells.

dual mechanism that decides whether T cells are going to be activated or inhibited. Although CTLA-4 is located intracellularly on most of the T cells, it is found on the cell surface of T-regulatory (T-reg) cells. This gives the ability to routinely suppress unwanted activation of the immune system [1].

PD-1 molecule is expressed on most of the immune cells such as T cells, B cells, and NK cells. As seen in **Figure 2**, its ligands PD-L1 or PD-L2 are presented on peripheral tissues, like CTLA-4, and B7 signaling inhibits T cells. Different from the CTLA-4 pathway, PD-1 signals only act on activated T cells. This results in self-tolerance in peripheral tissues [2].

LAG-3 is another checkpoint molecule found on T cells and contributes to T-cell exhaustion as in other ICIs discussed before [3].

In the healthy immune system, perforin and granzyme, produced by natural killer and cytotoxic $CD8^+$ T-cells along with interferon gamma secreting $CD4^+$ T cells, promote cell death [4]. Escape mechanisms of tumor cells help them to get through this elimination process. These mechanisms involve the loss of antigenicity and immunogenicity, allowing tumor antigens to evade immune detection. Additionally, overexpression of PDL-1 also induces the immunogenicity of the tumor cells [2, 4, 5].

Targeting these molecules enhances immune response and helps apoptosis and necrosis of tumoral tissues. However, blockage of these signaling pathways by monoclonal antibodies triggers the immune system leading to the elimination of tumor cells causing immune system disbalance. Harnessing immune system with ICIs leads to activation of pro-inflammatory conditions and self-tolerance triggering inflammatory-mediated adverse reactions [6, 7]. Studies show that patients with irAEs have improved survival rates, and this may be used as a predictor of response to the treatment [8].

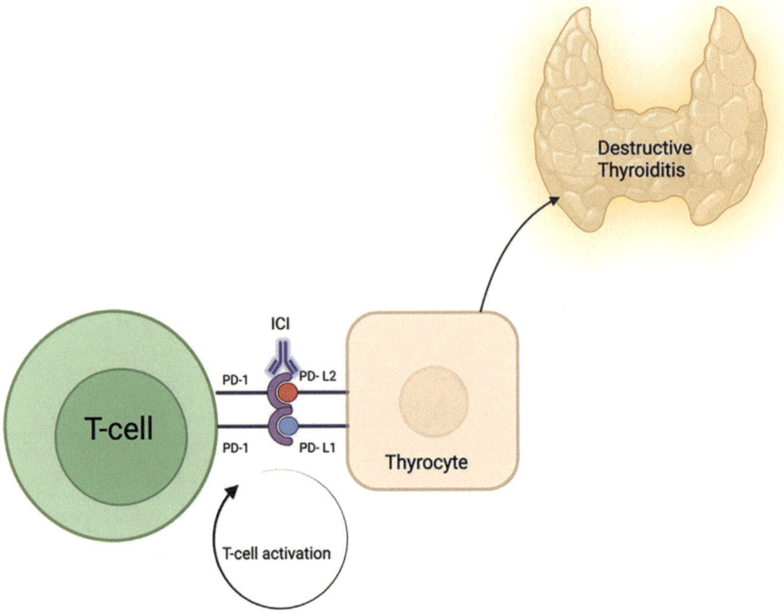

Figure 2.
Immunotherapy related destructive thyroiditis mechanism of action (created by BioRender.com).

The main mechanism of irAEs is peripheral self-tolerance and accumulation of cytotoxic $CD8^+$ T cells in tissues. In a single-center study, thyroid fine needle aspiration was performed in patients with ICI-induced thyroiditis and intra-thyroidal predominance of $CD8^+$ and $CD4^-$ $CD8^-$ T lymphocytes were linked with thyroid dysfunction [8, 9]. In addition to the activation of $CD4^+$ and $CD8^+$ T cells, atypical B-cell proliferation is enhanced with ICIs. B-cell changes occur as soon as the first cycle and are shown to predict and correlate with irAEs [10]. Recently, PD-L1 and PD-L2 molecules have been identified in normal thyroid glands. ICIs, monoclonal antibodies, can potentially bind directly to the thyroid cells, disrupting and infiltrating the thyroid gland with autoreactive T and B lymphocytes, leading to thyroiditis [11, 12].

Increase in immune activity results in a wide range of clinical manifestation. Adverse events (AEs) are potentially immune-mediated disorders due to activation of the immune system response. Most common irAEs are skin abnormalities (e.g., rash and pruritus), gastrointestinal disturbances (e.g., colitis), and endocrinopathies (e.g., thyroid function disturbances and hypophysitis), but all organs can be involved [6]. These AEs may occur de novo or may exacerbate the underlying autoimmune or inflammatory conditions [13].

Although all checkpoint inhibitors have adverse events, when compared, PD-1 inhibitors have less severe ones. This may be due to the restricted peripheral effects of PD-1. As discussed before, CTLA-4 inhibits T-cell activation in early phases, whereas PD-1 inhibits only activated T cells. Ipilimumab, a CTLA-4 inhibitor, accounts for 20% of all severe AEs compared to 10–13% with pembrolizumab, a PD-1 inhibitor [14]. Increased T-cell response with dual immune check point inhibitors may cause an increased adverse reaction. Postow et al. showed that the severe adverse events were seen in 23.9% of the patients receiving ipilimumab treatment alone and 54.3% with nivolumab and ipilimumab combination group [15]. In another study by Arnaud-Coffin et al., 16,485 patients were analyzed, and severe AEs were seen in 14.0% of patients treated with PD-L1 inhibitors, 34.0% of patients with CTLA-4 inhibitors, 55.0% of patients with immunotherapy combinations, and 46.0% of patients with immunotherapy and chemotherapy combinations [16].

Among all endocrinopathies, the most commonly seen irAEs are hypothyroidism and thyroiditis [17]. Although the irAEs are not predictable and may persist after the cessation of the drugs, Patrizio et al. investigated the ICIs adverse effects and found that thyroid disorders occurred mostly in female patients. In this study, the median occurrence was 9 weeks after the initial treatment [16, 18]. In general, irAEs may occur at any time during and after cessation of the treatment [19]. Still, the predictors of risk factors are an ongoing investigation [20].

3. Primary hypothyroidism

Many endocrinopathies may be seen due to organ destruction by the activation of immune system. The true incidence of immunotherapy-induced endocrinopathies is not known, but it occurs approximately in up to 20.0% of patients; 3.0–8.0% of patients receiving ICI monotherapy and in 15.0% of patients with combination [16, 21]. The most common endocrinopathy is destructive thyroiditis, mostly resulting in hypothyroidism, with an incidence of 5.5–7.8% [22]. Thyrotoxicosis can initially be seen in 4.0–5.0% of patients due to destructive thyroiditis, and in 90.0% of these patients, the destruction and necrosis of thyroid follicles result in hypothyroidism [23]. Immunotherapy-related thyroiditis is painless, and the thyrotoxicosis phase, if occurs, is much shorter (approximately 3 months) compared to other thyroiditis [8]. Thyroid toxicity especially hypothyroidism is much more common in patients on PD-1 inhibitors than CTLA-4 and PD-L1 monotherapies [23–26]. Osorio et al. included 35 clinical trials in a meta-analysis, with a total of 7318 patients, and the incidence of thyroid dysfunction was significantly higher in melanoma patients treated with anti-PD-1 (7.5%) than in those treated with anti-CTLA-4 antibody (3.6%), while no thyroid dysfunction was observed with anti-PD-L1 agents [22].

Regarding the risk factors for hypothyroidism in patients on immunotherapy, data about the association of age and gender are inconsistent. In a small cohort, the male-to-female ratio of hypothyroidism is 6/9, incidences being 4.0 to 10.0% respectively [21]. Lee et al. demonstrated similar incidence of hypothyroidism in 45 patients treated with ICI. Median age was 58 in patients treated with both PD-1 and CTLA-4 inhibitors and 55 in those receiving monotherapy with no statistically significant difference between them [27]. Storm et al. observed irAEs in older patients, but no difference was noted between different age groups [28]. In a multi-ethnic cohort, Caucasian and Hispanic races were found to have increased incidence of hypothyroidism [29]. Recent studies have assessed the heightened risk of obesity with immune-related adverse events (irAEs). In two studies conducted by Pollack et al. an increase in body mass index was found to be associated with thyroid dysfunction [30, 31]. However, the increased risk was specifically linked to thyrotoxicosis rather than hypothyroidism.

Many studies have investigated the time of occurrence of hypothyroidism, and it is observed as early as 3.4 weeks or be delayed until 48.71 weeks [28]. The onset time of biphasic thyroiditis, starting with thyrotoxicosis and then conversion to hypothyroidism, occurs earlier than hypothyroidism alone, with a median of 3.4 weeks. Sabbagh et al. demonstrated an earlier incidence in patients on combination treatments [23].

Primary hypothyroidism usually appears after 10 or 20 weeks of ICI treatment [11, 12]. In the study where 822 patients treated by ICIs were investigated, de novo hypothyroidism occurred as early as 2 weeks [24–26, 32]. The need for change in the levothyroxine replacements dose in patients with pre-existing hypothyroidism occurred later in the course, approximately in the 6th week. Patients with pre-existing hypothyroidism may develop transient hyperthyroidism during ICI treatment [27]. Although most of these patients require an increase in levothyroxine dosage, prophylactic increase is not suggested.

Most patients with hypothyroidism are asymptomatic but may present with nonspecific symptoms like fatigue and weight gain which can be overlapped by the progressing symptoms of the underlying disease [33]. Regularly checking thyroid function tests allow the clinician to detect and treat irAEs in early phases. While there are different recommendations, all involve monitoring thyroid function tests before starting the treatment, before each cycle and continue monitoring after cessation. Existing guidelines recommend checking thyroid function tests every 4–6 weeks during ICI treatment and continuing testing every 6–12 months following the cessation of ICIs [34]. As after the cessation of the treatment, the immune reactivation starts to resolve, but new occurrences of thyroid dysfunction can be observed even after 36 months. Additionally, in patients with thyroid antibodies, the dysfunction may persist [17, 21]. Anti-thyroid peroxidase (anti-TPO) antibody and to a lesser degree anti-thyroglobulin (anti-Tg) positivity were linked with persistent thyroid dysfunction at rates of 11.6 and 8.0%, respectively [28].

Primary hypothyroidism is defined as low free thyroxine (fT4), regardless of thyrotropin (TSH), which may be seen in resolution phases of thyroiditis, or a high TSH, with a low or normal fT4 [23]. In patients with normal fT4 and elevated TSH, cortisol deficiency must be excluded to exclude concurrent adrenal insufficiency and avoid adrenal crisis [22]. Checking autoantibodies, such as anti-TPO and anti-Tg, prior to the treatment is still controversial. Some recommend checking antibodies only in patients with a family or self-history of autoimmunity, while the others suggest checking in all patients prior to immunotherapies [6]. Elevated baseline antibodies may pose a potential risk, but further studies are required to confirm this. In patients with immune-related hypothyroidism, antibody positivity was observed in 80.0%, whereas in patients without thyroid dysfunction, antibody positivity was only 8.0% [35]. Maekura et al. demonstrated that hypothyroidism developed in 44.0% of the patients with antibody positivity at baseline but in only 2.0% of the patients with negative antibody levels [36]. Studies suggest that pre-existing antibodies are risk factors for thyroid dysfunction [24–26, 32]. Not all studies correlate antibodies with ICI-related hypothyroidism and not all patients with antibodies develop hypothyroidism. Anti-TPO positivity was higher than anti-Tg positivity in general.

Thyroid ultrasound can reveal the underlying thyroid disease and help to distinguish diffuse or localized thyroiditis. The use of thyroid scintigraphy and PET scan is useful in hyperthyroidism but have minimal contribution in hypothyroidism [17].

It is also found that the median survival of patients with endocrinologic irAEs is longer [28]. This has been attributed to the increased immune system stimulation, which strengthens the fight against cancer cells by activating the immune response.

Autoimmune thyroid disorders tend to be seen along with other autoimmune diseases [37]. Lee et al. examined this hypothesis in patients with ICI-related hypothyroidism. Among 27 patients receiving combination treatment, 10 patients with thyroid dysfunction had either hypophysitis or secondary adrenal insufficiency. Additionally, 22.0% of patients on anti-PD-1 monotherapy presented with metachronous endocrine toxicities (hypophysitis, secondary adrenal insufficiency, and diabetes mellitus) [27].

4. Secondary hypothyroidism

Secondary hypothyroidism can manifest as a component of hypophysitis. In hypophysitis, reduced production of one or more hormones in the pituitary gland leads to hypopituitarism. Adrenocorticotropic hormone (ACTH), TSH, follicle-stimulating hormone (FSH), luteinizing hormone (LH), growth hormone (GH), and prolactin are the affected hormones. It is important to distinguish primary hypothyroidism from secondary hypothyroidism because when levothyroxine is initiated before the evaluation of secondary adrenal insufficiency, adrenal crisis may develop. Primary hypothyroidism generally is asymptomatic, but in secondary hypothyroidism due to panhypopituitarism, patients tend to be more symptomatic; fatigue, muscle weakness, headache, anorexia, nausea, weight loss, visual changes, intolerance of temperatures, arthralgias, and electrolyte disturbances may be observed [38].

As seen in primary hypothyroidism, hypophysitis is more common with combination treatments. A study involving 6472 patients reported the incidence of hypophysitis as 6.4% with combination therapies, 3.2% with CTL4 inhibitors, 0.4% with PD-1 inhibitors, and 0.1% PD-L1 inhibitors [39]. While primary hypothyroidism is common in PD-1 inhibitor monotherapies, hypophysitis is more frequently observed in CTLA-4 inhibitor monotherapy [38]. Risk factors are still debatable for secondary hypothyroidism. Cumulative dose, gender, and age data are controversial, and new studies are needed to clarify this [40]. ICI-related hypophysitis tends to be more prevalent in old male patients, whereas hypophysitis is more commonly observed in young female patients [38].

Time of onset is 2–3 months after initiation of ICIs, but the duration may be as long as 19 months. It is observed earlier with CTLA-4 inhibitors and in combination with PD-1 inhibitors, than with PD-1 inhibitors alone, with durations of 12.5 weeks, 9.3 weeks, and 25.8 weeks, respectively [40].

In secondary hypothyroidism, TSH levels are low or normal with low fT4. Morning assessment of ACTH and cortisol levels are necessary to rule out coexisting ACTH insufficiency. Increased heterogenicity and enlarged hypophyseal gland are the radiological findings that support hypophysitis in magnetic resonance imaging.

5. Management

The treatment of irAEs must be multidisciplinary, and patients should be evaluated thoroughly by endocrinologists. The severity of toxicity is crucial for the treatment and determining whether to continue ICIs. The degree of elevation in TSH and patients' symptoms must be carefully evaluated before deciding on the treatment [41]. **Table 2** summarizes the definitions of grading and management of hypothyroidism induced by ICIs. The treatment of hypothyroidism induced by immunotherapies typically involves levothyroxine. Common Terminology Criteria for Adverse Events (CTCAE) points out that Grade 4 toxicity entails life-threatening consequences which requires urgent investigation, and Grade 5 toxicity denotes death resulting from AEs [42].

Grade of Toxicity	Evaluation	Management
Grade 1	Asymptomatic patient TSH > 4,5 mIU/L but <10 mIU/L	• ICIs may be continued • Thyroxine replacement is controversial • Monitoring TSH (+ fT4) every 4–6 weeks
Grade 2	Moderate symptoms TSH > 10 mIU/L	• Endocrine evaluation o Adrenal insufficiency should be excluded • ICIs may be stopped until recovery or continued • Initiation of thyroxine treatment o Monitoring TSH (+ fT4) every 4–6 weeks o Aim TSH in the reference range
Grade 3 - Grade 4	Severe symptoms, cannot perform daily activities	• Endocrine evaluation is necessary • ICIs should be discontinued until recovery • Initiation of thyroxine treatment o Monitoring TSH (+ fT4) every 4–6 weeks o Aim TSH in the reference range • If central hypothyroidism or adrenal insufficiency suspected hydrocortisone should be given • Myxedema coma (bradycardia, hypothermia, and altered mental status) o Life-threatening condition o Follow-up in ICU setting o IV thyroxine treatment should be evaluated

Table 2.
Management of ICIs-induced hypothyroidism.

Grade 1 and 2 toxicities are mild and self-limiting. Patients with subclinical hypothyroidism, where thyroid hormones are normal, but TSH is elevated (<10 mU/L) and evaluated as having Grade 1 toxicity, and thyroid hormone supplementation is not crucial [43]. Toxicities greater than grade 2 should be evaluated by endocrinologists, and levothyroxine treatment should be initiated. Depending on the age and comorbidities of the patient, suggested replacement dose is 1–1.5mcg/kg/day. Preferred starting dose is 75 mcg/day in otherwise healthy patients and in old (>65 years) and frail patients. The starting dosage should be 25–50 mcg/day and titrated slowly [33]. Iyer et al. calculated the median levothyroxine dose in patients treated with ICIs to be 1.2 mcg/kg, which is lower than the usual replacement dose for non-malignant total thyroidectomy cases, which is 1.6 mcg/kg daily [23, 44]. ICIs can be continued in mild settings, whereas in Grade 3 and 4 toxicities, where severe and symptomatic hypothyroidism and myxedema coma ensue, they may be indications for discontinuation [33].

In patients with altered mental status, bradycardia, generalized edema, and hypotension, the life-threatening condition "myxedema coma," should be taken into consideration [22]. Patients should be admitted to intensive care units and monitored closely for requirement of intravenous levothyroxine treatment [41].

Patients must be followed up throughout and after cessation of the treatment. TSH must be monitored every 4–6 weeks and low TSH levels, while taking levothyroxine supplement may suggest recovery or overtreatment. American Society of Clinical Oncology (ASCO) 2018 guidelines suggest continuing monitorization of TSH levels annually after cessation of ICIs. ASCO recommends titrating the levothyroxine dose every 6–8 weeks by monitoring TSH levels until TSH reaches the normal range. For patients with overt hypothyroidism, free T4 may be monitored every 2 weeks to assess short-term responses. The European Society for Medical Oncology (ESMO) 2017 guidelines differentiate hormonal screening for patients using CTLA-4 inhibitors and PD-1/PD-L1 inhibitors. It is recommended that patients treated with CTLA-4 inhibitors should undergo monitoring after each cycle and every 4 weeks after the fourth cycle. For patients receiving PD-1/PD-L1 inhibitors, screening should occur after every cycle for the first 3 months and subsequently every second cycle. As mentioned earlier, some guidelines do not recommend screening for antibodies before initiating treatment. The French Society of Endocrinology (SFE) 2018 advocates against screening for antibodies before initiating treatment. Their recommendation is to monitor thyroid function every cycle for the first 6 months and then every 2 months for a year. Following the first year, routine monitoring of TSH levels is not recommended. However, in the presence of symptomatic hypothyroidism, they suggest checking thyroid function tests [41].

The importance of anti-thyroid peroxidase antibodies (anti-TPO) and anti-thyroglobulin antibodies (anti-Tg) in the pathogenesis is not fully understood. However, levothyroxine dose requirement during treatment seemed to be increased in patients with pre-treatment antibody positivity [23, 34, 44].

Treatment of ICIs-induced hypophysitis (secondary hypothyroidism) resembles that for any other cause of hypopituitarism. Hydrocortisone replacement is the initial step. TSH levels are not reliable for central hypothyroidism and cannot be used as a guide. Thus, thyroid hormone replacement is based on fT4 levels. The treatment objective is maintaining fT4 being in the mid to upper half of the reference range and with a suggested dose of 1.6 mcg/kg/day [30]. In the study by Kristan et al. the required dose was 0.9 mcg/kg/day [34]. The study emphasized that the patients with secondary hypothyroidism tend to be older, and lower doses of replacement therapy were administered due to comorbidities. In older patients with multiple comorbidities such as coronary heart disease, the starting dose should be 25–50 mcg/day, and the dose should be titrated slowly [10].

In conclusion, primary hypothyroidism can be observed during the treatment with immunocheckpoint inhibitors. This may be due to an immune destruction of the thyroid tissue and is usually seen as a consequence of thyroiditis. Secondary hypothyroidism is another thyroid problem seen due to hypophysitis induced by these agents. For both conditions, there is no consensus on which individuals are at risk of developing thyroid toxicity. Nevertheless, routine monitorization of thyroid function tests during and even after cessation of therapies are recommended. Although discrepancies exist between guidelines, checking thyroid antibody levels before immunotherapy commencement may be of help in predicting the development of immunotherapy-induced hypothyroidism. Management by treatment with levothyroxine according to severity of hypothyroidism and referral to endocrinology are advocated.

Acknowledgements

All figures were created by BioRender.com.

Author details

Selin Çakmak Demir and Dilek Yazıcı*
Section of Endocrinology and Metabolism, Koç University School of Medicine, Istanbul, Turkey

*Address all correspondence to: dyazici@ku.edu.tr

References

[1] Buchbinder EI, Desai A. CTLA-4 and PD-1 pathways: Similarities, differences, and implications of their inhibition. American Journal of Clinical Oncology. 2016;**39**(1):98-106. DOI: 10.1097/COC.0000000000000239

[2] Taube JM, Klein A, Brahmer JR, Xu H, Pan X, Kim JH, et al. Association of PD-1, PD-1 ligands, and other features of the tumor immune microenvironment with response to anti-PD-1 therapy. Clinical Cancer Research. 2014;**20**(19):5064-5074. DOI: 10.1158/1078-0432.CCR-13-3271. Epub 2014 Apr 8

[3] Tawbi HA, Schadendorf D, Lipson EJ, Ascierto PA, Matamala L, Castillo Gutiérrez E, et al. Long GV; RELATIVITY-047 investigators. Relatlimab and nivolumab versus nivolumab in untreated advanced melanoma. The New England Journal of Medicine. 2022;**386**(1):24-34. DOI: 10.1056/NEJMoa2109970

[4] Ferrone C, Dranoff G. Dual roles for immunity in gastrointestinal cancers. Journal of Clinical Oncology. 2010;**28**(26):4045-4051. DOI: 10.1200/JCO.2010.27.9992. Epub 2010 Jul 19

[5] Beatty GL, Gladney WL. Immune escape mechanisms as a guide for cancer immunotherapy. Clinical Cancer Research. 2015;**21**(4):687-692. DOI: 10.1158/1078-0432.CCR-14-1860. Epub 2014 Dec 12

[6] Tison A, Garaud S, Chiche L, et al. Immune-checkpoint inhibitor use in patients with cancer and pre-existing autoimmune diseases. Nature Reviews Rheumatology. 2022;**18**:641-656. DOI: 10.1038/s41584-022-00841-0), 10.1038/s41584-022-00841-0)

[7] Postow MA, Sidlow R, Hellmann MD. Immune-related adverse events associated with immune checkpoint blockade. The New England Journal of Medicine. 2018;**378**(2):158-168. DOI: 10.1056/NEJMra1703481

[8] Kotwal A, Gustafson MP, Bornschlegl S, Kottschade L, Delivanis DA, Dietz AB, et al. Immune checkpoint inhibitor-induced thyroiditis is associated with increased intrathyroidal T lymphocyte subpopulations. Thyroid. 2020;**30**(10):1440-1450. DOI: 10.1089/thy.2020.0075. Epub 2020 May 21

[9] Basak EA et al. Overt thyroid dysfunction and antithyroid antibodies predict response to anti-PD-1 immunotherapy in cancer patients. Thyroid. 2020;**30**(7):966-973. Epub 2020 Mar 10

[10] Das R, Bar N, Ferreira M, Newman AM, Zhang L, Bailur JK, et al. Early B cell changes predict autoimmunity following combination immune checkpoint blockade. The Journal of Clinical Investigation. 2018;**128**(2):715-720. DOI: 10.1172/JCI96798. Epub 2018 Jan 8

[11] Abdel-Wahab N, Shah M, Lopez-Olivo MA, Suarez-Almazor ME. Use of immune checkpoint inhibitors in the treatment of patients with cancer and preexisting autoimmune disease: A systematic review. Annals of Internal Medicine. 2018;**168**(2):121-130. DOI: 10.7326/M17-2073. Epub 2018 Jan 2

[12] Yamauchi I, Sakane Y, Fukuda Y, Fujii T, Taura D, Hirata M, et al. Clinical features of nivolumab-induced thyroiditis: A case series study. Thyroid. 2017;**27**(7):894-901. DOI: 10.1089/thy.2016.0562

[13] Chalan P, Di Dalmazi G, Pani F, De Remigis A, Corsello A, Caturegli P. Thyroid dysfunctions secondary to cancer immunotherapy.JournalofEndocrinological Investigation. 2018;**41**(6):625-638. DOI: 10.1007/s40618-017-0778-8. Epub 2017 Dec 13

[14] Farolfi A, Ridolfi L, Guidoboni M, et al. Ipilimumab in advanced melanoma: Reports of long-lasting responses. Melanoma Research. 2012;**22**:263-270

[15] Postow MA, Chesney J, Pavlick AC, Robert C, Grossmann K, McDermott D, et al. Nivolumab and ipilimumab versus ipilimumab in untreated melanoma. The New England Journal of Medicine. 2015;**372**(21):2006-2017. DOI: 10.1056/NEJMoa1414428. Epub 2015 Apr 20. Erratum in: N Engl J Med. 2018;379(22):2185

[16] Arnaud-Coffin P, Maillet D, Gan HK, Stelmes JJ, You B, Dalle S, et al. A systematic review of adverse events in randomized trials assessing immune checkpoint inhibitors. International Journal of Cancer. 2019;**145**(3):639-648. DOI: 10.1002/ijc.32132. Epub 2019 Feb 4

[17] Baraka B, Abosheaishaa H, Nassar M. Immunotherapy-induced thyroid dysfunction: An updated review. The Egyptian Journal of Internal Medicine. 2023;**35**:48. DOI: 10.1186/s43162-023-00210-7

[18] Patrizio A, Fallahi P, Antonelli A, Ferrari SM. Immune checkpoint inhibitor-induced thyroid disorders: A single center experience. Current Pharmaceutical Design. 2023;**29**(4):295-299. DOI: 10.2174/13816128286 66220518151509

[19] Couey MA, Bell RB, Patel AA, Romba MC, Crittenden MR, Curti BD, et al. Delayed immune-related events (DIRE) after discontinuation of immunotherapy: Diagnostic hazard of autoimmunity at a distance. Journal for Immunotherapy of Cancer. 2019;**7**(1):165. DOI: 10.1186/s40425-019-0645-6

[20] Brahmer JR, Abu-Sbeih H, Ascierto PA, Brufsky J, Cappelli LC, Cortazar FB, et al. Society for immunotherapy of cancer (SITC) clinical practice guideline on immune checkpoint inhibitor-related adverse events. Journal for Immunotherapy of Cancer. 2021;**9**(6):e002435. DOI: 10.1136/jitc-2021-002435

[21] Ryder M, Callahan M, Postow MA, Wolchok J, Fagin JA. Endocrine-related adverse events following ipilimumab in patients with advanced melanoma: A comprehensive retrospective review from a single institution. Endocrine-Related Cancer. 2014;**21**(2):371-381. DOI: 10.1530/ERC-13-0499

[22] Barroso-Sousa R, Barry WT, Garrido-Castro AC, Hodi FS, Min L, Krop IE, et al. Incidence of endocrine dysfunction following the use of different immune checkpoint inhibitor regimens: A systematic review and meta-analysis. JAMA Oncology. 2018;**4**(2):173-182. DOI: 10.1001/jamaoncol.2017.3064

[23] Iyer PC, Cabanillas ME, Waguespack SG, Hu MI, Thosani S, Lavis VR, et al. Immune-related thyroiditis with immune checkpoint inhibitors. Thyroid. 2018;**28**(10):1243-1251. DOI: 10.1089/thy.2018.0116

[24] El Sabbagh R, Azar NS, Eid AA, Azar ST. Thyroid dysfunctions due to immune checkpoint inhibitors: A review. International Journal of General Medicine. 2020;**13**:1003-1009. DOI: 10.2147/IJGM.S261433

[25] Kristan MM, Toro-Tobon D, Francis N, Desale S, Bikas A, Jonklaas J, et al. Immunotherapy-associated hypothyroidism: Comparison of the pre-existing with de-novo hypothyroidism. Frontiers in Endocrinology (Lausanne). 2022;**13**:798253. DOI: 10.3389/fendo.2022.798253

[26] Chang L-S, Barroso-Sousa R, Tolaney SM, Hodi FS, Kaiser UB, Min L. Endocrine toxicity of cancer immunotherapy targeting immune checkpoints. Endocrine Reviews. 2019;**40**(1):17-65. DOI: 10.1210/er.2018-00006

[27] Osorio JC, Ni A, Chaft JE, et al. Antibody-mediated thyroid dysfunction during T-cell checkpoint blockade in patients with non-small-cell lung cancer. Annals of Oncology. 2017;**28**(3):583-589. DOI: 10.1093/annonc/ mdw640

[28] Lee H, Hodi FS, Giobbie-Hurder A, Ott PA, Buchbinder EI, Haq R, et al. Characterization of thyroid disorders in patients receiving immune checkpoint inhibition therapy. Cancer Immunology Research. 2017;**5**(12):1133-1140. DOI: 10.1158/2326-6066.CIR-17-0208. Epub 2017 Oct 27

[29] Storm BN, Abedian Kalkhoran H, Wilms EB, Brocken P, Codrington H, Houtsma D, et al. Real-life safety of PD-1 and PD-L1 inhibitors in older patients with cancer: An observational study. The Journal of Geriatric Oncology. 2022;**13**:997-1002. DOI: 10.1016/j.jgo.2022.05.013

[30] D'Aiello A, Lin J, Gucalp R, Tabatabaie V, Cheng H, Bloomgarden NA, et al. Thyroid dysfunction in lung cancer patients treated with immune checkpoint inhibitors (ICIs): Outcomes in a multiethnic urban cohort. Cancers. 2021;**13**:1464. DOI: 10.3390/cancers13061464

[31] Pollack R, Ashash A, Cahn A, Rottenberg Y, Stern H, Dresner-Pollak R. Immune checkpoint inhibitor-induced thyroid dysfunction is associated with higher body mass index. The Journal of Clinical Endocrinology and Metabolism. 2020;**105**:1-8. DOI: 10.1210/clinem/dgaa458

[32] Ruggeri RM, Campennì A, Giuffrida G, Trimboli P, Giovanella L, Trimarchi F, et al. Endocrine and metabolic adverse effects of immune checkpoint inhibitors: An overview (what endocrinologists should know). Journal of Endocrinological Investigation. 2019;**42**(7):745-756. DOI: 10.1007/s40618-018-0984-z

[33] Pollack RM, Kagan M, Lotem M, Dresner-Pollak R. Baseline TSH level is associated with risk of anti–PD-1–induced thyroid dysfunction. Endocrine Practice. 2019;**25**:824-829. DOI: 10.4158/EP-2018-0472

[34] Ross DS, Burch HB, Cooper DS, Greenlee MC, Laurberg P, Maia AL, et al. 2016 American Thyroid Association guidelines for diagnosis and Management of Hyperthyroidism and Other Causes of thyrotoxicosis. Thyroid. 2016;**26**(10):1343-1421. DOI: 10.1089/thy.2016.0229. Erratum in: Thyroid. 2017;27(11):1462

[35] Chieng JHL, Htet ZW, Zhao JJ, Tai ES, Tay SH, Huang Y, et al. Clinical presentation of immune-related endocrine adverse events during immune checkpoint inhibitor treatment. Cancers (Basel). 2022;**14**:2687. DOI: 10.3390/cancers14112687

[36] Hattersley R, Nana M, Lansdown AJ. Endocrine complications of immunotherapies: A review. Clinical Medicine (London, England). 2021;**21**:e212-e222. DOI: 10.7861/clinmed.2020-0827

[37] Maekura T, Naito M, Tahara M, Ikegami N, Kimura Y, Sonobe S, et al. Predictive factors of nivolumab- induced hypothyroidism in patients with non-small cell lung cancer. In Vivo. 2017;**31**(5):1035-1039

[38] Chera A, Stancu AL, Bucur O. Thyroid-related adverse events induced by immune checkpoint inhibitors. Frontiers in Endocrinology. 2022;**13**:1010279. DOI: 10.3389/fendo.2022.1010279

[39] Jonklaas J, Bianco AC, Bauer AJ, Burman KD, Cappola AR, Celi FS, et al. American Thyroid Association task force on thyroid hormone replacement. Guidelines for the treatment of hypothyroidism: Prepared by the american thyroid association task force on thyroid hormone replacement. Thyroid. 2014;**24**(12):1670-1751. DOI: 10.1089/thy.2014.0028

[40] Stelmachowska-Banaś M, Czajka-Oraniec I. Management of endocrine immune-related adverse events of immune checkpoint inhibitors: An updated review. Endocrine Connections. 2020;**9**(10):R207-R228. DOI: 10.1530/EC-20-0342

[41] Illouz F. Expert opinion on thyroid complications in immunotherapy. Annales d'endocrinologie. 2018;**79**(5):555-561. DOI: 10.1016/j.ando.2018.07.007

[42] National Cancer Institute. Common terminology criteria for adverse events (CTCAE) v5.0. 2017. Available from: https://ctep.cancer.gov/protocoldevelopment/electronic_applications/docs/CTCAE_v5_Quick_Reference_5x7.pdf [Accessed: August 19, 2022]

[43] Garber JR, Cobin RH, Gharib H, Hennessey JV, Klein I, Mechanick JI, et al. Clinical practice guidelines for hypothyroidism in adults: Cosponsored by the American Association of Clinical Endocrinologists and the American Thyroid Association. Endocrine Practice. 2012;**18**(6):988-1028. DOI: 10.4158/EP12280.GL. Erratum in: Endocr Pract. 2013;19(1):175

[44] Wall CR. Myxedema coma: diagnosis and treatment. American Family Physician. 2000;**62**(11):2485-2490

Chapter 10

Hashimoto Thyroiditis and Type 2 Diabetes Mellitus: Risk Factors Involved in the Association of These Pathologies

Oana-Andreea Parliteanu, Octavian Alexe, Corina Risca (Popazu), Dan Mircea Cheta and Cristiana Voineag

Abstract

This is a retrospective study that has had the objective to establish if there are any risk factors for developing Hashimoto thyroiditis (HT) in a type 2 diabetes (T2DM) population and also to determine if the prevalence of HT is higher in the population of T2DM, comparing with the European population. In the beginning, 5064 patients were evaluated and after that three groups were analysed, one of patients having only type 2 diabetes, one having only Hashimoto thyroiditis and one in which the patients had both of this diseases; each group had 50 patients in it. All patients were analysed using the same clinical and biological parameters. Results showed an increased prevalence of Hashimoto thyroiditis among the type 2 diabetes population, three times higher than in the European population ($789.89/10^5$ per year versus $259.12/10^5$ per year). The second part of the study established that female gender, insulin resistance, overweight, high value of glycaemia, hepatic steatosis, cardiac ischemic disease, hypothyroidism, smoking and alcohol intake are risk factors for the onset of HT in T2DM population.

Keywords: Hashimoto thyroiditis (HT), type 2 diabetes mellitus (T2DM), insulin resistance, obesity, risk factors

1. Introduction

Our goal with this research was to demonstrate if the association between type 2 diabetes mellitus (T2DM) and Hashimoto's autoimmune thyroiditis (HT) is a real or just it was just a random coincidence. In our practice, we noticed an increased prevalence of chronic lymphocytic thyroiditis in patients with T2DM. After searching the literature, we noticed that this association had not been studied and only type 1 diabetes mellitus (T1DM) and HT were known to associate, both of which are autoimmune diseases and the association between them was logical.

We designed an observational, retrospective study on patients from "Sanamed Hospital" clinic in Bucharest; this clinic mainly treats diabetes patients, both type 1 and type 2 diabetes.

Using the data from the patient database, we analysed firstly the incidence of the association of the two diseases, comparing it with the European dates, and we proved that our incidences were significantly and statistically higher, showing that our initial hypothesis was right, and there is an association between T2DM and HT.

The second phase of our research was focused on clinical and paraclinical elements that can explain the abovementioned association, risk factors involved and finding the population at risk for developing both this diseases.

2. Research methodology

We used the data collected from the database of the clinic "Sanamed Hospital" based in Bucharest during 01 January 2016–2031 December 2018 to identify the possible correlations in patients with T2DM and thyroid impairment.

First, we evaluated 5064 patients with T2DM that were examined during that period of time; this patients were used in an initial study that was called Study 1 Determining the incidence of chronic autoimmune lymphocytic thyroiditis in the population of patients diagnosed with T2DM.

Second, we designed another study—Study 2: Clinicometabolic and therapeutic features in patients with T2DM and HT, in which we evaluated 150 patients divided into three groups: 50 patients had only T2DM, 50 patients had only HT and 50 patients had both T2DM and HT (referred to as Lot 1, Lot 2 and Lot 3).

The database and processing of own data was performed in Microsoft Office Excel 2010 and SPSS.

2.1 Purpose of the research

2.1.1 Main objectives

- to determine the incidence of HT in a population with T2DM,
- to determine the existence of independent predictors of the association, if any, between the two pathologies.

As secondary objectives we proposed:

- to determine if insulin resistance (IR) is in any way involved in this association by determining by surrogate indices of IR;
- to determine if the presence or absence of obesity is correlated with the association of T2DM and HT;
- to determine if the presence or absence of dyslipidaemia is correlated with the association of T2DM and HT;
- to determine if the presence or absence of metabolic syndrome is correlated with the association of T2DM and HT;

- to determine if the existence of clinicometabolic features of micro- and macrovascular complications of T2DM in patients are a risk factor for developing HT.

2.1.2 Criteria for inclusion in study 1

- age over 16 years,
- previous diagnosis of T2DM established according to the criteria listed below:
- previous diagnosis of HT established according to the criteria listed below for patients in Group 2,
- previous diagnosis of HT established during the follow-up period of the study established according to the criteria listed below for patients in Group 3,
- patients who have agreed to the processing of their personal data by signing the informed consent form of the clinic in which they were investigated.

2.1.3 Exclusion criteria in study 1

- diagnosis of T1DM,
- presence of anti-GAD antibodies in patients' serum.

2.1.4 Inclusion criteria in study 2

- age over 16 years,
- previous diagnosis of T2DM established according to the criteria listed below,
- previous diagnosis of HT established according to the criteria listed below for patients in Group 2,
- diagnosis established during the follow-up period of the HT study established according to the criteria listed below for patients in Group 3,
- patients who agreed to the processing of their personal data by signing the informed consent form of the clinic where they were investigated.

2.1.5 Exclusion criteria in study 2

- patients with other associated autoimmune pathologies (Graves-Basedow disease, rheumatoid polyarthritis, Lupus, inflammatory bowel disorders, multiple sclerosis, psoriasis, vitiligo, Guillain-Barre syndrome, vasculitis, Sjogren's syndrome, celiac disease, autoimmune hepatitis, spondyloarthropathies, antiphospholipid syndrome, etc.)
- presence of anti-TPO antibodies in the serum of patients in Group 1,
- pregnant or breastfeeding patients,

- patients with severe psychiatric pathologies that prevent from discerning,
- patients with physical disabilities or severe cognitive impairment that may affect their mobility and therefore their ability to move for further investigations necessary to complete the database in this study,
- patients who have refused to sign the clinic's informed consent to the processing of personal data,
- patients who refused to continue further investigations necessary to collect data for this study.

Patients included in the study were additionally analysed for the following clinical and paraclinical parameters: total cholesterol, triglycerides, serum creatinine, estimated glomerular filtration rate (eGFR), uric acid, oxalacetic transaminase (TGO), pyruvic transaminase (TGP), height, weight, abdominal circumference, body mass index (BMI) and blood pressure. These parameters were used to identify possible correlations and possible risk factors.

Patients were also clinically assessed; the presence or absence of the following conditions was sought: obesity, dyslipidaemia, atrial hypertension, chronic micro- and/or macrovascular complications of DM, ischemic heart disease, congestive heart failure, metabolic syndrome, hepatic steatosis, hyperuricemia/gout, cataracts, glaucoma, depression and pre-existing thyroid pathology, each was defined according to international diagnostic criteria.

We calculated surrogate markers for the determination of IR. We used the value of Triglycerides and Glucose Index (TyG Index), Visceral Adiposity Index (VAI), Lipid Accumulation Product (LAP) and Triglycerides Ratio on HDL Cholesterol (TG/HDL). We also calculated variants of TyG, more exactly TyG in relation to BMI (TyG-BMI) and in relation to abdominal circumference (TyG-WC) [1, 2].

2.1.6 Research hypotheses

In this regard, we formulated the following hypotheses:

- Patients diagnosed with T2DM have a higher risk of developing HT compared to the general population;
- Patients with a certain degree of high risk for T2DM and HT will have a high degree of association with medical laboratory values in relation to the associated thyroid disfunction and metabolic syndrome.

2.2 Study 1: determination of the incidence of chronic autoimmune lymphocytic thyroiditis in a population of patients diagnosed with type 2 diabetes mellitus

2.2.1 Introduction

Based on a finding from our daily practice with patients, we aimed to assess the incidence of HT in patients with T2DM. Among patients diagnosed with T2DM, we observed a large number of new cases of HT. Previously in the literature, only the association between T1DM and HT was described in terms of the underlying

DOI: http://dx.doi.org/10.5772/intechopen.1004796

autoimmune pathophysiological mechanism of the two pathologies; thus, our findings were either mere coincidences or there is a link between T2DM and HT.

2.2.2 Objectives of study 1

In the first phase of our research, we aimed to assess the incidence of HT in patients with T2DM, to determine what we had previously found, namely an increased proportion of thyroiditis in patients with T2DM, was confirmed or was just a chance finding without clinical significance.

2.2.3 Purpose

The main purpose of this first study was to determine the incidence of HT in the population with T2DM from "Sanamed Hospital" clinic in Bucharest, through a retrospective observational study for over 3 years, between 1 January 2016 and 31 December 2018.

2.2.4 Materials and methods

A total number of 5064 patients with T2DM were evaluated using patient details from "Sanamed Hospital" clinic, which were collected over 3 years, between 1 January 2016 and 31 December 2018. Subsequently, the incidence per 100,000 inhabitants was calculated and the data were compared with those found in the European population; at the national level such data are not available, so the comparison with the Romanian population was not possible.

2.2.5 Results of study 1

Of the 5064 subjects analysed in the initial phase of our study, 2383 were men, representing 47.05%, and 2681 (52.94%) were female. We can say that the initial sample was divided into almost two equal parts which did not create a research bias (**Figure 1**).

Regarding the mean age in the initial group, we had 67.545 ± 11.701 years, with an older age for the patients evaluated in the Diabetes Mellitus section (68.508 ± 10.653 years) compared to those evaluated in the Endocrinology ward

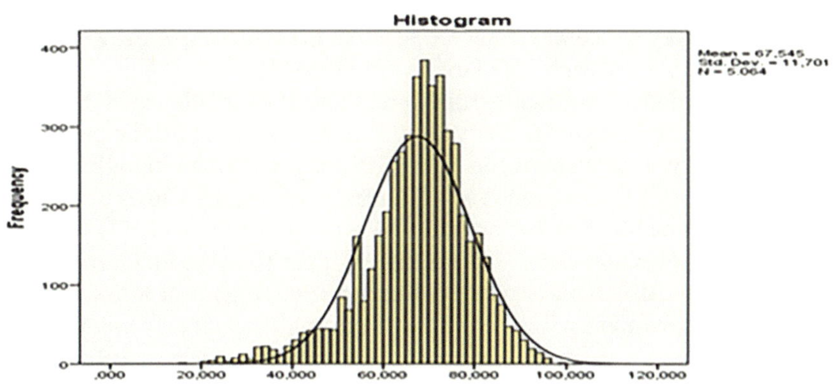

Figure 1.
Average age in the initial lot.

	Total subjects (n = 5064)	Men (n = 2383)	Women (n = 2681)	Total incidence per year 10^5	Incidence in men per year 10^5	Incidence in women per year 10^5
With HT acquired after the diagnosis of T2DM in the present study	80	11	69	789.89	230.80	1286.83
Incidence of HT in the general population of Europe*				259.12	85.36	419.72

Table 1.
Incidence of patients diagnosed with HT after acquisition of T2DM in the study group and incidence at European level [3].

(57.058 ± 16.432 years). This was natural, given that the average age at the onset of patients with T2DM is older.

During the three-year period of the study, the incidence of HT in the group of 5064 patients diagnosed with T2DM was $789.89/10^5$ per year, with an incidence of $230.80/10^5$ per year among diabetic men and an incidence of $1286.83/10^5$ per year among women. Comparing European wide reports of HT incidence in the general European population [3] ($259.12/10^5$ per year, $85.36/10^5$ per year in men and $419.72/10^5$ per year in women), there is a highly significant difference between the incidence in the general population and the incidence among patients diagnosed with T2DM (**Table 1**). This confirms the original hypothesis of the study. Remarkably, a patient with T2DM has a threefold higher risk of developing chronic lymphocytic thyroiditis (HT), and also, female patients with T2DM have an almost sixfold higher prevalence of Hashimoto's thyroiditis than men diagnosed with T2DM.

2.2.6 Analytical discussions: Study 1

Comparing our incidence studies of HT in a population with T2DM with incidence studies of HT in the general population published in the literature, we found similarities. A study conducted by Wiersinga et al. showed a prevalence of HT of 10–12% in the general population, making it the most common autoimmune disease encountered. The higher prevalence was observed in women, increasing with age and being higher in the white versus black population worldwide [4].

In terms of incidence worldwide, this study showed an incidence of 350 per 10^5 per year in women and 60 per 10^5 per year in men in non-iodine-deficient areas and 44 per 10^5 per year in women and 12 per 10^5 per year in men in iodine-deficient areas. [4] In our study, the incidence was 789.89 per 10^5, which allows us to conclude that T2DM may be a risk factor involved in the occurrence of HT, since the incidence in the population with T2DM is much higher than the incidence in the general population. Also in our study, the incidence was higher in women than in men, which is in agreement with the results of the study previously mentioned. The population in our study, the initial sample of 5064 patients, were mainly patients from Bucharest and from vicinity of the country's capital, so from areas without iodine deficiency, also the patients were white (Caucasian). Comparing with the results of the aforesaid study, in which the highest incidence was in white patients

DOI: http://dx.doi.org/10.5772/intechopen.1004796

from areas without iodine deficiency, we can say that the results of our study are in agreement with those described in the study by Wiersinga et al. In our study, the highest incidence was in females, almost six times higher than in males; in females, it was 1286.83 per 10^5 per year, while in males, it was 230.80 per 10^5 per year, and these data agree with the previously mentioned results, where a higher incidence was shown in females versus males.

Another study led by Lee et al. showed an HT incidence in the US population of 350 per 10^5 per year in women and 80 per 10^5 per year in men, with an incidence of nearly 600 per 10^5 from the Appalachian Mountain region. In this study, a global incidence of HT was estimated at 30–150 per 10^5, 10–15 times higher in women than in men, occurring most frequently in the 30–50 age group in women, with a peak incidence in men 10–15 years later [5]. The results of our study agree with those of this study, with a higher incidence among women than men of six times higher. The age group in which occurred most frequently in our study HT in the population with T2DM studied was in women between 60 and 70 years, and for men it was the same age category. These results are not in agreement with those of the study conducted by Lee et al., with the peak incidence in that study being at age of 30–50 years for women and 45–60 years for men. We can say that our population being composed of patients with T2DM had an older age than the general population studied in that study of HT incidence; thus, these results are in agreement with the average age of the people studied by us. We notice, however, that the proportion in relation to the predominant gender, female, is preserved.

In another study conducted by Dong et al. in the US army, on 20.270688 soldiers, predominantly male 85.8%, an incidence of HT of 758 cases in females and 548 cases in males was described. This study showed that the highest incidence was in the white Caucasian population, and the lowest incidence was in black females (IRR, 0.33; 95% Cl, 0.21–0.51) and black males (IRR, 0.22; 95% Cl, 0.11–0.47), in Asian Pacific Islander females (IRR, 0.31; 95% Cl, 0.17–0.56) and in Asian Pacific Islander males (IRR, 0.23; 95% Cl, 0.07–0.72) [6]. The results of this study are mainly determined by the preponderantly male gender of the study participants (85.8% were male), but even so we can observe that the number of HT cases in females is higher, 758, than in males, 548. Considering that the female population of the study was 14.2%, we can say that the incidence in the female population is much higher than in the male population. These results were also obtained by us in our study, a much higher incidence in women. Our study evaluated only white, Caucasian population, which, by comparison to the increased incidence in the study conducted by Dong et al. in the white population, could explain a high incidence rate in our study population as well.

2.2.7 Conclusions of study 1

As a conclusion of Study 1 "Determining the incidence of chronic autoimmune lymphocytic thyroiditis in a population of patients diagnosed with Type 2 Diabetes Mellitus," we can state that we have demonstrated our main objective: we have shown that T2DM is a risk factor for the development of autoimmune thyroiditis through a higher incidence of HT among patients with T2DM versus the general European population (789.89/10^5 per year, with an incidence of 230.80/10^5 per year among diabetic men respectively an incidence of 1286.83/10^5 per year among women versus 259.12/10^5 per year, 85.36/10^5 per year among men and 419.72/10^5 per year among women in the general European population).

2.3 Study 2: clinicometabolic and therapeutic features in patients with type 2 diabetes mellitus and Hashimoto's autoimmune thyroiditis

2.3.1 Introduction

After demonstrating the main objective of this research thesis, proving the statistically significant association between T2DM and HT, by means of Study 1, through determining the incidence of chronic autoimmune lymphocytic thyroiditis in a population of patients diagnosed with type 2 diabetes mellitus, we set out to evaluate the possible causes for this association: we aimed to detect the clinicometabolic and therapeutic features in patients with type 2 diabetes mellitus and Hashimoto's autoimmune thyroiditis.

2.3.2 Objectives of study 2

The objectives of Study 2 are as follows:

- to determine the weights of associated pathologies impacting the two studied pathologies in the three groups,
- to determine the implications of IR assessed by surrogate indices of IR, that is, whether it correlates with the presence or absence of the studied association,
- to determine the correlation of obesity with the presence or absence of HT in the group of patients with T2DM,
- to determine the correlation of dyslipidaemia with the presence or absence of HT in the T2DM group of patients,
- to determine whether metabolic syndrome correlates with the presence of absence of HT in the T2DM group of patients,
- to determine the existence of clinicometabolic features of micro- and macrovascular complications of T2DM in patients with HT.

2.3.3 Purpose

We aimed to:

- evaluate the relationship between the clinicometabolic factors in the groups of patients with T2DM, HT, T2DM and HT,
- determine independent predictors of the association of the two pathologies studied,
- evaluate the risk factors or the protection factors involved in the occurrence of HT in patients with T2DM.

After evaluating the 5064 patients diagnosed with T2DM and determining the incidence of HT in the study population, we developed a new study, Study

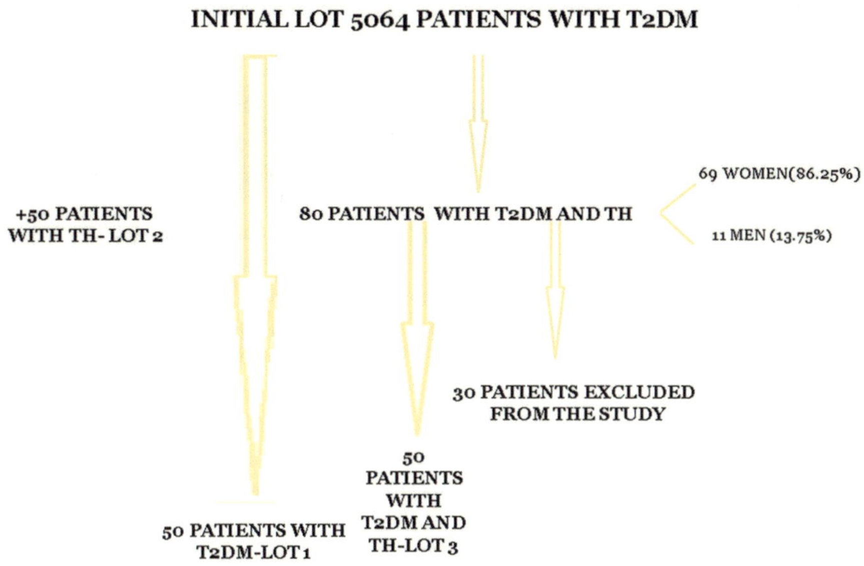

Figure 2.
Design of Study 2.

2—Clinicometabolic and therapeutic features in patients with type 2 diabetes mellitus and Hashimoto's autoimmune thyroiditis study, to try to better understand the association between the two pathologies. We selected from the group of patients with T2DM and HT a number of 50 patients who were eligible to participate in our study. Of the initial 80 patients diagnosed with HT, 11 also suffered from other autoimmune diseases (Graves Basedow disease—5, rheumatoid polyarthritis—4, vitiligo—1 and ankylosing spondylitis—1), 7 had advanced chronic diseases or physical disabilities that prevented them from continuing the investigations needed to complete the study database, 3 had severe mental illnesses that prevented them from making judgements and 9 refused to continue the investigations needed to complete the study database. Thus, out of the total of 80 patients diagnosed with HT, only 50 were eligible after applying the exclusion criteria for the study, thus forming Group 3. Group 1 was made up of patients with only T2DM, also from the initial group followed in Study 1, out of 5064 patients with T2DM of the clinic, this being the control group. Group 2 included 50 patients with HT from the Endocrinology department's records, also a control group. The selection of patients was consecutive; initially, patients were selected from Group 3, subsequently, from the same time period; consecutively, as they presented to the clinic, patients were selected for groups 1 and 2.

2.3.4 Materials and methods

See **Figure 2**.

2.3.5 Results of study 2

The mean age of the patients in the three groups was 58.1 years.

The study sample consisted predominantly of 122 (81.3%) female and (18.7%) male patients [7].

We found statistically significant differences between groups 1 and 2 and between groups 2 and 3 for the parameters: abdominal circumference, weight, BMI, obesity, dyslipidaemia and SM; and between groups 1 and 3 for TAD, cholesterol, macro- and microvascular complications, depression, visceral adiposity index (VAI), trigliceride glucose index (TyG), trigliceride glucose-body mass index (TyGBMI), trigliceride glucose-waist circumference index (TyGWC) and lipid accumulation product (LAP).

Univariate analysis revealed the following risks factors for HT in patients with T2DM: weight over 83.5 kg, BMI over 29.6 kg/m^2, HbA1c over 5.85%, blood glucose over 122 mg/dl, thyroid-stimulating hormone (TSH) over 1.1 pmol/L, TyG over 4.7, TyG BMI over 140.8, and TyGWC, female gender, alcohol consumption, smoking, BCI, hypothyroidism, goitre, microvascular complications of T2DM, depression and insulin treatment.

After multivariate analysis, it was found that the protective factor TAD was retained and BMI, blood glucose and surrogate index of insulin resistance TyG, female gender, alcohol, smoking, hepatic steatosis, BCI, hypothyroidism and insulin treatment remained as risk factors.

Table 2 Values obtained in all three groups for surrogate markers: Group 1, Group 2 and Group 3.

See (**Table 3**).

In the three groups studied, a TyG value of more than 4.7 was observed, but the highest value was detected in the combined group 5.02 (standard deviation 0.32335).

2.3.6 Analytical discussions: Study 2

2.3.6.1 Insulin resistance in patients with Hashimoto's thyroiditis and euthyroidism

The relationship between IR and clinical and subclinical hypothyroidism is well-documented. Hashimoto's thyroiditis (HT) is the most common cause of hypothyroidism.

Hashimoto's thyroiditis is a chronic autoimmune inflammatory disease and the most common cause of hypothyroidism in adults. It is characterised by histological infiltration of T- and B-cells in the thyroid gland. Autoimmune diseases detect the body's own tissue as foreign and work to destroy it. Therefore, the immune system starts producing anti-thyroid antibodies (anti-TPO) and anti-thyroglobulin antibodies (anti-Tg) to destroy the thyroid gland. It is not known why the body starts behaving this way. Perioxidase thyroid antibodies are positive in 95% of Hashimoto's thyroiditis and 85% of Graves' disease [8].

2.3.6.2 Personal discussion

In order to try to demonstrate a definitive link between IR and the association of the two pathologies studied in the present study, we used surrogate indices of IR,

TyG	TyGBMI	TyGWC	LAP	VAI	TG/HDL
4.8886	149.6063	449.84	57.11	1.8315	3.0914

Table 2.
Results of surogate markers for insulin resistance.

Group		TyG	TyGBMI	TyGWC	LAP	VAI	TG/HDL
Group 1T2DM	Average	4.9461	157.3483	496.8141	67.3173	2.2955	3.2615
	N	50	50	50	50	50	50
	Standard Dev.	.23133	25.43355	96.40244	37.51971	1.71620	1.55994
	Median	4.9766	153.8312	480.6573	65.6570	2.1656	2.9156
Group 3T2DM + HT	Average	5.0245	161.8517	479.7390	69.9242	1.6783	3.4651
	N	50	50	50	50	50	50
	Standard Dev.	.32335	34.00789	114.08299	52.19408	1.27814	1.99627
	Median	4.9746	158.2189	463.1977	61.6378	1.5874	3.0291
Group 2HT	Average	4.6951	129.6190	372.9825	34.1159	1.5208	2.5476
	N	50	50	50	50	50	50
	Standard Dev.	.25271	28.41573	76.98818	28.70756	1.55027	1.56256
	Median	4.6625	124.8493	378.8840	24.5896	1.1877	2.0793
TotalGroups 1,2 and 3	Average	4.8886	149.6063	449.8452	57.1191	1.8315	3.0914
	N	150	150	150	150	150	150
	Standard Dev.	.30473	32.60511	110.94231	43.55847	1.55201	1.75201
	Median	4.8828	149.3270	428.8168	47.8244	1.5352	2.6170

Table 3.
Surrogate indices of IR for each group, group 1, group 2 and group 3.

indices that have demonstrated their accuracy and precision in establishing the presence of IR in many other studies [9–13].

According to the study by Kim et al., the surrogate IR marker TyG was a better predictor for T2DM than Homa-IR, and VAI and LAP also had prediction for T2DM, but a more modest one than TyG. The conclusion of this study was that this TyG marker may be a useful additional tool to determine which patients are at risk of IR and T2DM [1].

The results of this study for the surrogate markers were TyG 4.7 +/− 0.2, VAI 2.5 +/−1.9 and LAP 38.5 +/−31.9. In our study, we obtained similar values TyG 4.88, VAI 1.83 and LAP 57.11, values for the whole group of 150 patients cumulated from groups 1, 2 and 3.

The cut-off values from the study by Kim et al. were 4.69 for TyG, 2.54 for VAI and 36.6 for LAP. In our study, we obtained cut-off values of 4.7 for TyG, 1.4 for VAI and 27.19 for LAP.

In the study by Guerrero-Romano et al., a cut-off value for the IR determination of TyG of 4.68 was established [14]. Considering that the results of the two mentioned studies were similar to the results of our study, we can conclude that a TyG of 4.7, obtained by us, is diagnostic for IR.

Correlating the results obtained in the two studies conducted by Kimm et al. and Guerrero-Romano et al. with the results obtained in our study, we can state that the values obtained by us were diagnostic for IR.

In the study conducted by Kim et al., a strong relationship was established between the surrogate marker of IR, TyG and the occurrence of T2DM, which was found to be a better predictor of T2DM than HOMA-IR [1].

In a meta-analysis conducted by Song et al., obesity was shown to be a risk factor for HT occurrence, with odds ratio (OR) of 1.91 (Cl 95% 1.10–3.32) and $p = 0.022$ [15]. In our study, after risk analysis, obesity was not retained as a risk factor, but an increased BMI at the upper limit of overweight, 29.6 kg/m^2, close to the limit of obesity, with $p = 0.008$ and an odds ratio of 1.230 (CL 95% 1.056–1.432), was found to be a risk factor in the occurrence of HT in patients with T2DM. Thus, our data are in agreement with those stated by Song et al.

We also found similar results to our study in the publication by Du et al., where it was shown that in diabetic patients, a high blood glucose was a risk factor involved in the occurrence of thyroid pathologies, with OR of 2.653 (Cl 95% 1.18–5.9) and $p = 0.019$ [16]. Our results were also in agreement with what Du et al. presented, and a blood glucose value over 122 mg/dL was also in our case an independent predictor of HT occurrence in diabetic patients, with OR of 1.023 (Cl 95% 1.007–1.040) and $p = 0.004$.

The study led by Choi et al. was the first to indicate TyG as a surrogate marker of IR in its evaluation in relation to thyroid dysfunction. It showed higher predictive values for the thyroid pathology including HOMA-IR, with OR of 1.81 and $p = 0.031$ [17]. Our study showed that at a TyG over 4.7, the risk of developing HT among patients with T2DM is 65-fold higher, with OR of 65.344 (Cl 5.067–842.607) and $p = 0.001$. We can state as a conclusion that our study is the second to demonstrate the predictive value of TyG for thyroid pathologies and the first that demostrates this in regards to Hashimoto's autoimmune thyoriditis.

In the study led by Lee et al. [5], a 10–15-fold higher incidence of HT among females was shown, and similar results were also found in our study, which allows us to comment the result obtained that the female gender is at a risk factor of occurrence of HT in the patients with T2DM. For female gender, we obtained OR of 23.176 (Cl 4.530–118.572) and $p = 0.0001$ after multivariate analysis performed comparing the groups of patients with T2DM and with HT and T2DM. This result is not surprising in the context of the high incidence of HT among the female population.

Another risk factor for developing HT in patients with T2DM, comparing groups 1 and 3, is that our study found was alcohol consumption, with OR of 7.048 (Cl 95% 2.187–22.720) and $p < 0.001$. From our results, we can state that alcohol increases risk of developing HT, among the diabetic patients by 7 times, which is statistically significant. Comparing with the literature, we did not find another study attesting the risk; therefore, we can state that our study is the first to certify the causal relationship between the two. Moreover, a study conducted by Efferaimidis et al. showed that there is no association between alcohol consumption and *de novo* development of TPO antibodies. The results of this study are not in agreement with the results of our study [18].

Univariate analysis between groups 1 and 3 showed that BCI is also a risk factor for developing HT in patients with T2DM, with OR of 5.318 (Cl 95% 2.214–12.774) and $p < 0.001$. We found no other studies in the literature that addressed this relationship, but we did find one study that addressed the inverse relationship, and it described a twofold increased risk in HT patients to develop BCI, with OR of 2.06 (Cl 95% 1.46–2.92) [19]. Interpreting the results inversely, we can say that BCI may also be a risk factor involved in the development of HT, even with a higher prediction value, the risk being in this case five times higher in the population with T2DM. The higher result is somewhat normal, given that the population we studied was composed of diabetics, who have a higher proportion of associated BCI. Again our study is the first to demonstrate a positive independent predictor relationship for BCI in terms of the occurrence of HT in patients with T2DM.

DOI: http://dx.doi.org/10.5772/intechopen.1004796

The study conducted by Ogbonna et al. [20] showed a higher risk of patients with thyroid pathologies to develop diabetic nephropathy, with OR of 4.8 and $p = 0.001$. Considering diabetic nephropathy a part of microvascular complications of diabetes we can say that the results of our study are so similar to those of the above-mentioned study. In our case, after analysis of the comparison between groups 1 and 3, it was shown that there is a four times higher risk of developing HT among patients with microvascular complications among the population with T2DM; in other words, the presence of microvascular complications is a risk factor for the development of the association between the two pathologies, with OR of 4.571 (Cl 95% 1.963–10.646) and $p < 0.001$.

Another parameter that had statistical significance as a risk factor for the association between HT and T2DM was depression, this time in the comparison between the groups 2 and 3, with OR of 9.333 (Cl 1.121–77.204) and $p < 0.001$. In the study conducted by Bode et al., a positive predictive value for hypothyroidism was demonstrated for depression, with OR 1.30 (Cl 95% 1.08–1.57), while for autoimmune thyroid pathologies the results were inconclusive, with OR 1.24 (Cl 95% 0.89–1.74) [21]. Unfortunately, this situation is also confirmed by us, and the depression parameter maintains statistical significance for the other groups and not even after multivariate analysis of the data.

2.3.7 Conclusions of study 2

The univariate analysis revealed the following risk factors for developing HT in patients with T2DM: weight over 83.5 kg, BMI over 29.6 kg/m^2, HbA1c over 5.85%, blood glucose over 122 mg/dl, TSH over 1.1 pmol/L, TyG over 4.7, TyG BMI over 140.8, and TyGWC, female gender, alcohol consumption, smoking, BCI, hypothyroidism, Goitre, microvascular complications of T2DM, depression and insulin treatment.

After multivariate analysis, it was found that the protective factor TAD was retained and BMI, glycaemia and surrogate index of insulin resistance TyG, female gender, alcohol, smoking, hepatic steatosis, BCI, hypothyroidism and insulin treatment remained as risk factors.

3. General conclusions

1. T2DM is a risk factor for the development of autoimmune thyroiditis through a higher incidence of HT among patients with T2DM versus general European population.

2. Female gender was found to be a risk factor involved in the occurrence of HT in patients with T2DM, probably determined by the high incidence of thyroid pathology in female population.

3. Insulin resistance seems to be the vector linking HT and T2DM. A value of TyG, a calculated insulin resistance surrogate index, above 4.7 was found to be a risk factor involved in the occurrence of HT in patients with T2DM, and TyG increased the risk of occurrence of HT in the T2DM population by 65-fold.

4. Insulin resistance seems to be the vector linking HT and T2DM.

5. Overweight is a risk factor involved in the association of HT in patients with T2DM most likely through a week metabolic control, since it is known that overweight and obesity is a cause of glycaemic imbalance.

6. Abdominal obesity, above 88,5 cm, increases the risk of HT association with T2DM 6-fold, and this is caused also by a metabolic imbalance.

7. Blood glucose above 122 mg/dl was found to be an independent predictor of association of HT with T2DM, proving once more that a week metabolic control is the probable cause of the association between the two studied pathologies.

8. Insulin treatment increased the risk of developing HT in patients with T2DM over seven times, showing once again the involvement of the metabolic control in this association.

9. The correlation between elevated HbA1c, metabolic syndrome and elevated ATPO values was shown with increased statistical significance ($p < .001$) to be the pathophysiological link between T2DM and HT.

10. High systolic blood pressure increases the risk of HT in patients with T2DM almost threefold, and this is explained through the pathophysiological mechanism of cerebral insulin resistance involved in the pathology of arterial hypertension, mechanism which was proven by high values of insulin resistance markers; this allows us to conclude that insulin resistance is the real risk factor.

11. Diastolic blood pressure below 77.5 mmHg seems to have a protective effect on the occurrence of HT in patients with T2DM, because the normal or low values of diastolic blood pressure do not associate with insulin resistance, and this does not only elevate the risk, but gives a protective effect against the association of the two pathologies.

12. Hepatic steatosis is a risk factor for HT association in patients with T2DM, due to the high level of insulin resistance that low metabolic control patients have, as we have shown already.

13. The presence of ischemic heart disease increased the risk of HT association with T2DM twice, the pathophysiological mechanism to blame for this looks to be insulin resistance, especially the cardiac one, correlated with a low metabolic control.

14. Hypothyroidism was found to be risk factor for the association of HT with T2DM, and an association of high values of TSH in patients with type 2 diabetes can lead to a metabolic disorder, which seems to be the real risk factor for the association of Hashimoto thyroiditis with type 2 diabetes.

15. Smoking increased T2DM patient's risk of developing HT sevenfold, it is known that smoking is a risk factor for autoimmune thyroid disorders, and in our study, it was also confirmed to be a risk factor for developing HT.

16. Alcohol consumption increased T2DM patient's rick of developing HT by almost 3.5-fold; the probable cause is the destruction of the gland due to the increased

toxicity associated with alcohol intake, this being probably followed by an autoimmune destruction.

17. This is the *first* study to demonstrate the predictive value of TyG for Hashimoto's autoimmune thyroiditis.

18. Our study is the *first* to certify the causal relationship between alcohol consumption and the occurrence of HT in patients with T2DM.

19. Again our study is the *first* to demonstrate a positive independent predictive factor relationship for BCI with respect to the occurrence of HT in patients with T2DM.

20. The results of our study attest the need to introduce screening for the autoimmune thyroid pathologies among patients with T2DM.

Author details

Oana-Andreea Parliteanu[1*], Octavian Alexe[2], Corina Risca (Popazu)[2], Dan Mircea Cheta[3] and Cristiana Voineag[4]

1 National Institute of Pneumoftiziology "Marius Nasta" Bucharest, Romania

2 "Dunarea de Jos" University Galati, Romania

3 "Carol Davila" University of Medicine and Pharmacy, Bucharest, Romania

4 Emergency County Clinical Hospital Braila, Romania

*Address all correspondence to: oana_andreea@yahoo.com

References

[1] Kim B, Choi HY, Kim W, Ahn C, Lee J, Kim JG, et al. The cut-off values of surrogate measures for insulin resistance in the Korean population according to the Korean genome and epidemiology study (KOGES). PLoS One. 2018;**13**(11): e0206994. DOI: 10.1371/journal.pone.0206994

[2] Lim J, Kim J, Koo SH, Kwon GC. Comparison of triglyceride glucose index, and related parameters to predict insulin resistance in Korean adults: An analysis of the 2007-2010 Korean National Health and nutrition examination survey. PLoS One. 2019;**14**(3):e0212963

[3] Madariaga AG, Palacios SS, Guillen-Grima F, Galofre JC. The incidence and prevalence of thyroid dysfunction in Europe: A meta-analysis. The Journal of Clinical Endocrinology and Metabolism. 2014;**99**(3):923-931

[4] Wiersinga WM. Hashimoto's Thyroiditis. In: Vitti P, Hegedüs L, editors. Thyroid Diseases. Endocrinology. Cham: Springer; 2018. DOI: 10.1007/978-3-319-45013-1_7 [Accessed: May 31, 2018]

[5] Lee SL, Griffing GT. What is the incidence of Hashimoto's thyroiditis in the US?. 2020. Available from: https://www.medscape.com/answers/120937-122448/what-is-the-incidence-of-hashimoto-thyroiditis-in-the-us

[6] McLeod DSA, Caturegli P, Cooper DS, Matos PG, Hutfless S. Variation in rates of autoimmune thyroid disease by race/ethnicity in US military personnel. Journal of the American Medical Association. 2014;**311**(15):1563-1565. DOI: 10.1001/jama.2013.285606

[7] Parliţeanu O, Cheţa D. Type 2 diabetes and Hashimoto's thyroiditis-possible associations and clinical correlations - preliminary results. Romanian Journal of Diabetes Nutrition and Metabolic Diseases. 2018;**25**(3):297-301

[8] Ozkardes A, Ozata M, Beyhan Z, Vural O, Yardim M, Gundogan MA. Acute hypothyroidism leads to reversible alterations in central nervous system as revealed by somatosensory evoked potentials. Electroencephalography and Clinical Neurophysiology. 1996;**100**(6):500-504

[9] Ji B, Qu H, Wang H, Wei H, Deng H. Association between the visceral adiposity index and homeostatic model assessment of insulin resistance in participants with normal waist circumference. Angiology. 2017;**68**:716-721

[10] Oh JY, Sung YA, Lee HJ. The visceral adiposity index as a predictor of insulin resistance in young women with polycystic ovary syndrome. Obesity (Silver Spring). 2013;**21**:1690-1694

[11] Khan HS. The lipid accumulation product is better than BMI for identifying diabetes. Diabetes Care. 2006;**29**:151-153

[12] Simental-Mendía LE, Rodríguez-Morán M, Guerrero-Romero F. The product of fasting glucose and triglycerides as surrogate for identifying insulin resistance in apparently healthy subjects. Metabolic Syndrome and Related Disorders. 2008;**6**:299-304

[13] Vasques AC et al. TyG index performs better than HOMA in a Brazilian population: A hyperglycemic clamp validated study. Diabetes Research and Clinical Practice. 2011;**93**:e98-e100

[14] Jali MV, Kambar S, Jali SM, Pawar N, Nalawade P. Prevalence of thyroid dysfunction among type 2 diabetes mellitus patients. Diabetes and Metabolic Syndrome. 2017;**11**(Suppl. 1):S105-S108

[15] Song RH, Wang B, Yao QM, Li Q, Jia X, Zhang JA. The impact of obesity on thyroid autoimmunity and dysfunction: A systematic review and meta-analysis. Frontiers in Immunology. 2019;**10**:2349

[16] Du Wenhua WF, Meng Z, Haiqing Z, Xu Z, Jia-Jun Z, Ling G. Prevalence of thyroid disorders and associated risk factors with various glycemic status in North China. Biotechnology & Biotechnological Equipment. 2019;**33**:1244-1250. DOI: 10.1080/13102818.2019.1656106

[17] Choi W, Park JY, Hong AR, Yoon JH, Kim HK, Kang H-C. Association between triglyceride-glucose index and thyroid function in euthyroid adults: The Korea National Health and nutritional examination survey. PLoS One. 2021;**16**(7):e0254630

[18] Effraimidis G, Tijssen JG, Wiersinga WM. Alcohol consumption as a risk factor for autoimmune thyroid disease: A prospective study. European Thyroid Journal. 2012;**1**(2):99-104

[19] Chen W-H, Chen Y-K, Lin C-L, Yeh J-H, Kao C-H, Thyroiditis H's. Risk of coronary heart disease, and L-thyroxine treatment: A Nationwide cohort study. The Journal of Clinical Endocrinology & Metabolism. 2015;**100**(1):109-114

[20] Ogbonna SU, Ezeani IU. Risk factors of thyroid dysfunction in patients with type 2 diabetes mellitus. Frontiers in Endocrinology (Lausanne). 2019;**10**:440

[21] Bode H, Ivens B, Bschor T, Schwarzer G, Henssler J, Baethge C. Association of hypothyroidism and clinical depression: A systematic review and meta-analysis. JAMA Psychiatry. 2021;**78**(12):1375-1383

Section 4

Thyroid Nodules

Chapter 11

Thyroid Nodules and Biopsy

Muzaffer Serdar Deniz

Abstract

The present chapter provides an in-depth review of the prevalence, diagnostic challenges, and management strategies for thyroid nodules, emphasizing the integration of various diagnostic modalities to enhance precision and guide therapeutic decisions. Thyroid nodules are frequently encountered in clinical settings, with a significant proportion detected incidentally. While most are benign, the potential for malignancy necessitates careful evaluation, primarily through ultrasound-guided fine-needle aspiration (FNA). However, FNA has limitations, including unsatisfactory and indeterminate results, which may lead to unnecessary interventions. The chapter discusses the evolution of diagnostic techniques, including the role of ultrasonography, molecular diagnostics, and core needle biopsy, alongside traditional FNA. It highlights recent clinical experiences and studies that address diagnostic ambiguities, aiming to optimize patient outcomes by reducing unnecessary surgeries and improving diagnostic accuracy. The impact of external factors, such as the COVID-19 pandemic on thyroid nodule diagnostics, is explored. Through a comprehensive analysis, the chapter seeks to provide clinicians with updated strategies and insights into managing thyroid nodules effectively in diverse clinical contexts.

Keywords: thyroid nodules, fine-needle aspiration biopsy, thyroid cancer, Bethesda system, TIRADS, thyroid function tests, thyroid ultrasonography

1. Introduction

Thyroid nodules are commonly detected in clinical practice, with their prevalence reported to be over 60% in radiological examinations [1–3]. Although most thyroid nodules are benign, thyroid cancer remains the most prevalent endocrine malignancy, with a relatively low rate of malignancy [3–5]. Recent data indicate a rise in the incidence of thyroid cancer, making it the thirteenth most commonly diagnosed cancer globally and the sixth most common among women [6]. The primary diagnostic method for assessing thyroid nodules preoperatively is ultrasound-guided fine-needle aspiration (FNA) biopsy [7]. However, the limitations of FNA, including unsatisfactory results in up to 20% of cases, indeterminate findings in up to 30%, and significant rates of false positives and false negatives, complicate the diagnostic process [8–10]. High concordance rates among pathologists are typically seen in clearly benign or malignant cases, but variability arises in interpreting indeterminate cytology [11–13]. Moreover, there is no consensus among pathologists regarding the

 IntechOpen

precise definition of indeterminate cytology, which may include atypia of undetermined significance and follicular lesion of uncertain significance, as well as follicular neoplasm or suspicious for a follicular neoplasm, or suspicious for malignancy [14]. Due to the diagnostic uncertainties, FNA may lead to unnecessary thyroidectomies in patients where the procedure could have been avoided [15].

In light of these challenges, there has been a growing emphasis on integrating ultrasonography, molecular diagnostics, and core needle biopsy with FNA to enhance diagnostic precision and guide appropriate therapeutic decisions. This chapter assesses FNA's efficacy and explores the role of supplementary diagnostic biopsy techniques in the preoperative management of thyroid nodules. Through this comprehensive analysis, we shared our clinical experience and reviewed the current strategies employed to mitigate diagnostic ambiguities and optimize patient outcomes in the context of thyroid nodule management.

2. Thyroid nodules

2.1 Diagnosis

Globally, iodine deficiency is the primary cause of goiter and thyroid nodule formation [16]. The prevalence of this deficiency varies significantly based on dietary iodine intake, gender, and age [17]. In regions where iodine consumption is sufficient, the prevalence of thyroid nodules is relatively low [18]. Notably, women are four times more likely to develop thyroid nodules than men, with prevalence increasing in both genders after the age of 40 [19, 20]. Thyroid nodules are typically detected during routine physical examinations by healthcare providers or when patients seek medical advice due to noticeable swelling in the neck or through elective thyroid ultrasonography (USG) [21, 22]. Incidental findings of thyroid nodules can also occur during imaging studies that do not specifically target the thyroid [23, 24]. Palpation tends to identify nodules larger than 1 cm in diameter; palpation detects thyroid nodules in about 6% of women and 1.5% of men in iodine-sufficient regions. Conversely, imaging techniques have discovered thyroid nodules in up to 70% of otherwise healthy individuals [25–27].

Thyroid nodules are often multiple, although solitary nodules can occur [28]. In studies, approximately 50% of individuals with a palpably solitary nodule were found to have multiple nodules upon USG examination [29]. Most patients with thyroid nodules are euthyroid, showing normal thyroid function without other symptomatic manifestations, though signs of hyperthyroidism or hypothyroidism can occasionally be observed [30]. Recent nonsurgical data indicate that 4–6.5% of all thyroid nodules are malignant. Upon detecting a thyroid nodule, the initial diagnostic test should involve assessing thyroid status *via* a TSH measurement [31, 32]. Subsequently, all patients with a suspected nodule or nodules should undergo a thyroid USG to conduct a sonographic risk assessment [33, 34]. The primary objective must be to evaluate the risk of malignancy within these nodules [35].

2.2 Clinical evaluation

When assessing a thyroid nodule, clinicians should address three critical questions: What is the functional status of the nodule (is it hyperfunctioning)? What is the risk of malignancy? Are there any compressive symptoms or signs associated with the nodule? To effectively respond to these queries, a series of diagnostic procedures should be implemented. These include a detailed patient history and physical examination, thyroid-stimulating hormone (TSH) level measurement, ultrasound imaging, and FNA for nodules presenting a higher risk of malignancy [36]. Additionally, thyroid scintigraphy is advised only for nodules that suppress TSH and are more significant than 1.5 cm in diameter [32].

As previously outlined, the etiological causes of thyroid nodules are summarized in **Table 1**. This table serves as a reference for understanding thyroid nodules' potential origins and nature, guiding the diagnostic and management strategies.

2.2.1 History and physical examination

The initial step after detecting a thyroid nodule is a comprehensive patient history collection [37]. Nodules are often incidentally discovered and are predominantly asymptomatic [38]. Rarely, a nodule may bleed internally or undergo sudden enlargement, stretching the thyroid capsule and skin, leading to pain and sensitivity [19, 39]. Rapid and painful growth should raise concerns for aggressive conditions such as anaplastic thyroid cancer, Riedel's thyroiditis, or primary thyroid lymphoma [40, 41]. The patient history should include age, gender, body mass index (BMI), presence of metabolic syndrome, personal or family history of thyroid disease or cancer, associated syndromes such as Familial medullary thyroid cancer, endocrine neoplasia, Cowden syndrome, Carney complex, Werner syndrome, Familial adenomatous polyposis, DICER1 syndrome, previous imaging and biopsies, history of acromegaly, exposure to head or neck radiation, the growth rate of the neck mass, anterior neck pain, symptoms of dysphonia, dysphagia or dyspnea, signs of hyperthyroidism or hypothyroidism, use of iodine-containing medications or supplements, tobacco use, and stress [42].

The presence of certain risk factors may increase the potential for malignancy in thyroid nodules, summarized in **Table 2**. The prevalence of nodules increases with age, making them less common in children; however, the likelihood of malignancy in pediatric cases is twice that of adults [43]. Thyroid cancer rates in nodular patients, when viewed by gender, are found to be twice as high in men (8%) compared to women (4%). Additionally, the incidence of thyroid cancer is more common in adults under 30 or over 60 years compared to those between the ages of 30 and 60 [44]. Those with a history of head and neck radiation therapy or who have undergone bone marrow or solid organ transplantation have an increased incidence of cancer [45, 46].

Benign nodular goiter	Medullary carcinoma
Simple or hemorrhagic cysts	Anaplastic carcinoma
Follicular adenoma	Primary thyroid lymphoma
Focal thyroiditis areas	Rare primary malignancies (sarcoma, i.e.)
Papillary carcinoma	Metastatic tumors
Follicular carcinoma	Poorly differentiated carcinoma
Hurtle cell carcinoma	

Table 1.
Etiological causes of thyroid nodules.

Risk factors
Children
Adults under 30 and over 60 years
Male gender
History of head and neck radiation
Family history of medullary thyroid carcinoma, multiple endocrine neoplasia type 2, or papillary thyroid carcinoma
The rapid growth of the nodule
Hard and fixed nodule on palpation
Presence of cervical lymphadenopathy
Persistent dysphonia, dysphagia, or dyspnea

Table 2.
Risk factors increasing the potential for malignancy in thyroid nodules.

The physical examination of the thyroid is the simplest and most cost-effective method for detecting nodules, though its sensitivity is relatively low depending on the examiner's experience and the size of the palpable nodule [47]. If the thyroid gland is palpable, its size, the presence and number of nodules, irregularities in nodule borders, and consistency should be assessed [48]. Generally, nodules larger than 1 cm and anteriorly in the thyroid are palpable. During the examination, the cervical and supraclavicular lymphadenopathy should be assessed [30]. Rigid, fixed, palpable thyroid nodules, cervical lymphadenopathy, or symptoms such as hoarseness indicate malignancy. Physical findings, such as mucosal neuromas and a Marfanoid habitus, should raise suspicion for MEN 2B [49].

The most common and suitable method for grading goiter during a thyroid examination is the Pan American Health Organization (PAHO) grading system. This expanded section offers a comprehensive overview of the clinical assessment necessary for the management of thyroid nodules, detailing both the history to be gathered and the physical examination protocols:

- *Grade 0.* No goiter was detected visually or through palpation
- *Grade 1a.* No visible goiter, but palpable
- *Grade 1b.* Goiter is visible when the neck is slightly extended and palpable
- *Grade 2.* Goiter visible when the neck is in a normal position
- *Grade 3.* Goiter is visible from a distance and easily palpable

2.2.2 Laboratory assessment

In all patients diagnosed with a thyroid nodule, serum thyroid-stimulating hormone (TSH) levels must be measured without exception [37]. If the TSH level is low, particularly if the nodule exceeds 1.5 cm, a radionuclide thyroid scan should be conducted to determine the functionality of the nodule [29]. In cases where the nodule is identified as "hot," it can be assumed that the risk associated with these nodules is negligible; hence, FNAB is unnecessary [50]. In patients with high TSH levels, the thyroid nodule evaluation is similar to that in euthyroid patients, and assessments should be carried out accordingly [51]. Clinicians should consider the following algorithm when evaluating patients with thyroid nodules (**Figure 1**).

Thyroglobulin (Tg) should not be used as a tumor marker in evaluating thyroid nodules [50]. However, its utility becomes apparent in cases where suspicious lymphadenopathy is detected through neck ultrasound in the presence of a nodule [52]. High thyroglobulin washout values in FNAB washout fluids from lymph nodes are beneficial for detecting lymph node metastases of differentiated thyroid cancers [53]. Furthermore, preoperative Tg measurement may be prudent in patients scheduled for thyroid cancer surgery. In managing thyroid nodules, measuring calcitonin (CT) can be helpful in suspicious biopsies, repeatedly insufficient biopsies, or when the cytological diagnosis is unknown before thyroid surgery [54]. If there is suspicion of medullary thyroid carcinoma (MTC) or multiple endocrine neoplasia type 2, calcitonin measurement is imperative and should be repeated if initially found to be elevated [55, 56]. Elevated CT levels in the presence of symptoms such as diarrhea, lymph node metastasis, or flushing warrant further investigation [56]. Significantly high calcitonin levels are diagnostic of MTC, particularly when basal CT levels exceed 100 pg/ml, suggesting a high probability of MTC [57]. For CT levels between 10 and 100 pg/ml, a pentagastrin stimulation test is recommended after ruling out renal insufficiency and

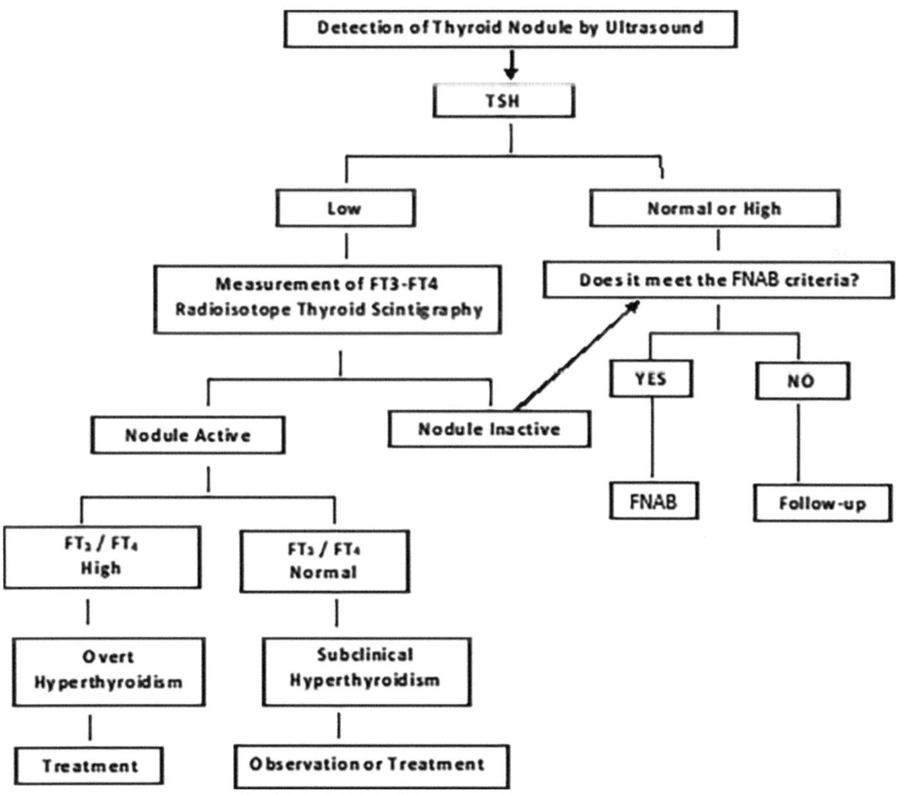

Figure 1.
Algorithm of thyroid nodule assessment.

using proton pump inhibitors [58]. Due to the difficulty of obtaining pentagastrin, some centers utilize long/short calcium stimulation tests as alternatives [59, 60].

2.2.3 Thyroid USG

Diagnostic thyroid ultrasound should be performed in patients suspected of having a thyroid nodule, those diagnosed with nodular goiter, or those with radiological findings indicating incidental nodules (detected in CT, MRI, or 18FDG-PET). High-resolution ultrasound is a noninvasive, cost-effective, universally applicable and repeatable imaging tool that provides a high accuracy rate with quality equipment and experienced operation [61]. Currently, it is critically essential in diagnosing and monitoring thyroid nodules [62]. Thyroid ultrasound offers the ability to confirm whether a palpable anomaly is indeed a nodule and assess its size, location, benign or suspicious characteristics, composition, and the presence of cervical lymph nodes [63]. When evaluating a thyroid nodule *via* ultrasound, the recommended reporting system includes:

- *Nodule size* (reported in three dimensions in millimeters) and its localization within the thyroid gland must always be specified.
- *Nodule composition* (solid, cystic, or mixed, i.e., complex)
- *Nodule echogenicity* (hyperechoic, isoechoic, hypoechoic, markedly hypoechoic)
- *Nodule margin* (well-defined and regular, indistinct and irregular)
- *Calcifications* (no calcifications, microcalcifications, macrocalcifications, linear, eggshell calcifications)
- *Halo* (a discernible rim around the nodule, either absent, thick or thin, continuous, or interrupted)
- *Doppler findings* (vascularity of the nodule) (Avascular—Type 1; Noticeable peripheral with minimal intra-nodular increase—Type 2; Prominent intra-nodular with minimal peripheral increase—Type 3)

The primary reason for evaluating a nodule with ultrasound is to investigate features that might predict the malignancy risk. General ultrasound characteristics of benign and malignant nodules are specified in **Table 3**. Additionally, certain cancer types may present characteristic features that can guide diagnosis.

For instance, papillary thyroid carcinoma (PTC) typically appears solid or predominantly solid and hypoechoic, often with infiltrative irregular margins and microcalcifications [64]. In contrast, follicular thyroid carcinoma (FTC) is generally isoechoic, rarely hyperechoic, features a thick and irregular halo, and lacks microcalcifications [65]. Certain sonographic appearances can be highly diagnostic for benign nodules. For example, a purely cystic nodule (less than 2% of all nodules) or a spongiform nodule—described as having more than half of its volume filled with multiple microcystic components—indicates a 99.7% likelihood of a benign thyroid nodule.

Malignant features	Benign features
Hypoechoicity	Hyper/Isoechoicity
Microcalcifications or interrupted rim calcifications	Continuous edge integrity with eggshell calcifications
Irregular margins	Spongy (spongiform) nodule
Absence of halo or incomplete halo	The presence of a halo or smooth border
Increased intra-nodular vascularity (Type 3)	Absence of vascularity (Type 1) or peripheral (Type 2) vascularity
Height greater than width (in transverse section)	Purely cystic nodule
Invasion into the anterior neck muscles	Decrease in nodule size over time, multiple coalescent nodules (merged nodules)
Presence of pathological cervical LAP	Reactive features in cervical LAP

Table 3.
Malignancy based on the USG characteristics of thyroid nodules.

The American College of Radiology (ACR) recently published a guide for managing thyroid nodules based on USG findings [66]. This guide introduces the ACR Thyroid Imaging Reporting and Data System (ACR-TIRADS), a five-tiered classification system [67]. ACR-TIRADS serves as a structured framework to standardize the reporting of thyroid ultrasound studies [68]. This system facilitates clear communication among healthcare providers by categorizing nodules according to their likelihood of malignancy, thereby assisting clinicians in making decisions about the need for biopsy or ongoing surveillance. The classification system ranges from TIRADS 1, suggesting no nodules are present, to TIRADS 5, indicating a high suspicion of malignancy [69]. Each level corresponds to a set of specific ultrasound characteristics, such as echogenicity, presence of microcalcifications, and nodule borders, among others, which collectively contribute to an overall risk score [70]. This score then guides the recommended clinical actions, balancing the benefits of early detection of thyroid cancer against the risks of unnecessary procedures [71]. It stratifies the risk of cancer within a thyroid nodule based on its ultrasonographic characteristics and size and also outlines the management of thyroid nodules—whether through FNAB or USG monitoring—dependent on these USG features (**Tables 4** and **5**).

While the EU-TIRADS, developed by the European Thyroid Association (ETA), is similar to the ACR-TIRADS, it is somewhat simpler [61, 68]. The EU-TIRADS system designates irregular shapes, margins, microcalcification, and marked hypoechoicity as high-risk criteria [61]. The recommendations are summarized in **Table 6**.

2.2.4 Thyroid fine-needle aspiration biopsy

Thyroid fine-needle aspiration biopsy is the decision-making tool in patients with nodules, guided by ultrasonographic and clinical findings [72]. It is the gold standard for distinguishing between benign and malignant thyroid nodules [73]. Sampling for cytological or histological examination from thyroid nodules can be performed using several techniques, including thick or fine-needle aspiration, Tru-cut biopsy needle, or fine-needle capillary sampling [74]. It is mandatory to obtain signed informed consent after providing the patient with the necessary information before the procedure.

Composition	P	Echogenicity	P	Shape	P	Margin	P	Echogenic foci	P
Cystic or almost completely cystic	0	Anechoic	0	Wider-than-tall	0	Smooth	0	None of the large comet-tail artifacts	0
Spongiform	0	Hyperechoic or isoechoic	1	Taller-than-wide	3	Ill-defined	0	Macrocalcifications	1
Mixed cystic and solid	1	Hypoechoic	2	—		Lobulated or irregular	2	Peripheral (rim) calcifications	2
Solid or almost completely solid	2	Very hypoechoic	3	—		Extrathyroidal extension	3	Punctate echogenic foci	3

Abbreviations. P: points.

Table 4.
ACR (2017)—TIRADS classification scheme for thyroid nodules.

TIRADS category	Total points	Malignancy risk (%)
TR1	0	0.3
TR2	2	1.5
TR3	3	4.8
TR4	4–6	9.1
TR5	7+	35

Abbreviations. TIRADS: Thyroid Imaging Reporting and Data System.

Table 5.
Risk stratification based on total points.

EU-TIRADS category	Sonographic pattern	Ultrasound characteristics
EU-TIRADS 1	Normal	No nodule
EU-TIRADS 2	Benign	Pure cystic or completely spongiform
EU-TIRADS 3	Low risk	Oval, well-defined isoechoic/hyperechoic, no high-risk features
EU-TIRADS 4	Intermediate risk	Oval, well-defined, hypoechoic, no high-risk features
EU-TIRADS 5	High risk	At least one of the following: non-oval shape, irregular margins, microcalcifications, marked hypoechogenicity (and solid)

Table 6.
EU-TIRADS classification.

The patient lies supine on a standard examination table with a pillow under the shoulders to increase neck extension. Patients are instructed not to swallow or speak during the procedure. The biopsy is usually performed with a 25-gauge needle (ranging from 23 to 27 gauge), with or without the use of local anesthesia (such as lidocaine cream or a jet injector). The skin over the nodule is cleansed with alcohol. The nodule is then identified under ultrasound guidance, and the needle is inserted parallel or at a slight angle to the skin, following visualization of the needle shaft on the ultrasound screen. The needle tip appears brightly on the ultrasound and is advanced and monitored as it enters the nodule. The needle is moved back and forth within the nodule 4–5 times, and if necessary, aspiration is performed using a 10 ml syringe. The aspirate from the nodule is then gently and swiftly spread onto microscope slides. Each nodule is accessed once or several times, depending on its size. Experienced physicians can achieve adequate sampling from solid nodules in 90–97% [75].

The risk of obtaining bloody cell aspirate increases in patients on anticoagulant or antiplatelet therapy due to the heightened risk of bleeding within the nodule [76]. Accordingly, the possibility of reporting the nodule as non-diagnostic increases as not enough cells will be found in the examination. There are views suggesting that in patients taking antiplatelet agents, the medication should ideally be discontinued 5–7 days before to be in a safe range, although there are also opinions that the procedure can be performed without stopping the medication. Some clinicians recommend performing biopsies on patients with an INR < 2 or within the normal range. After the procedure, applying pressure to the nodule for 5–10 minutes is recommended, and performing an ultrasound for bleeding control 15–30 minutes later. Discontinuing

Diagnostic category	Risk	Clinical approach
I. Nondiagnostic or unsatisfactory	5–10%	Repeat FNA under ultrasound guidance
II. Benign	0–3%	Follow-up with clinical and ultrasound assessment
III. Atypia of undetermined significance (AUS) or follicular lesion of undetermined significance (FLUS)	10–30%	Repeat FNA, molecular testing, or lobectomy
IV. Follicular neoplasm or suspicion of follicular neoplasm	25–40%	Molecular testing, lobectomy
V. Suspicious for malignancy	50–75%	Near-total thyroidectomy or lobectomy
VI. Malignant	97–99%	Near-total thyroidectomy or lobectomy

Table 7.
Bethesda diagnostic categories, malignancy risk, and clinical approach.

new-generation anticoagulants, such as rivaroxaban, apixaban, and dabigatran, is not recommended before the procedure [76, 77].

In the presence of multinodular goiter, rather than biopsy the dominant nodule, each nodule should be independently evaluated, and TFNAB should be performed on each nodule were indicated based on risk factors [37]. It is recommended that the TFNAB decision be based on the EU-TIRADS score. EU-TIRADS 3 nodules >20 mm (very low risk, malignancy risk 2–4%); EU-TIRADS 4 nodules >15 mm (low-medium risk, malignancy risk 6–17%); EU-TIRADS 5 nodules >10 mm (medium-high risk, malignancy risk 26–87%) should undergo TFNAB [36, 65]. The cytology of the thyroid nodule should be reported according to the diagnostic groups stated in the Bethesda system. Since its definition for reporting thyroid cytopathology in 2007, the Bethesda system has been applied extensively and yielded consistent results [78]. Practitioners must use a common language, which plays a significant role in standardizing follow-up and treatment. The Bethesda diagnostic categories, malignancy risk, and clinical approach are summarized in **Table 7**.

3. Clinical experience on thyroid nodules

We have performed two comprehensive published studies of thyroid nodules and their evaluation and management. One of these studies was about low-risk thyroid neoplasms. This study titled "investigation of preoperative demographic, biochemical, sonographic and cytopathological findings in low-risk thyroid neoplasms" explored various preoperative factors in low-risk thyroid neoplasms (LRTNs) [79]. Our research included a retrospective analysis of 2453 cases, narrowing down to 99 cases diagnosed as LRTNs. These were further divided into four subgroups, providing a rich analysis dataset. Most LRTNs were identified as noninvasive follicular thyroid neoplasm with papillary-like nuclear features, constituting 69.7% of the cases. The volume of the index nodule was significantly different among the subgroups, serving as a potential discriminative factor in sonographic evaluations. Well-differentiated carcinoma, which was not otherwise specified, had the smallest average volume, whereas follicular tumors of uncertain malignant potential displayed the largest.

Despite variations in nodule volume and other sonographic features, prognostic scores suggested similar outcomes across the groups, underscoring the complexity of predicting disease progression based solely on initial sonographic assessments. These observations suggest that while certain sonographic features like volume can aid in subgroup differentiation, the prognostic outcomes remain uncertain across different types of LRTNs.

The second study, "examining the impact of several factors including COVID-19 on thyroid fine-needle aspiration biopsy," focused on how the pandemic might have influenced the outcomes of thyroid fine-needle aspiration biopsies (TFNAB) [80]. This retrospective observational study involved 482 thyroid nodules and examined various factors, including COVID-19 history and vaccination status. The longitudinal diameter of thyroid nodules was significantly larger in nodules, yielding diagnostic results compared to nondiagnostic ones. This point suggests that smaller nodules are more challenging to diagnose accurately. No differences were observed concerning COVID-19 history or vaccination status. It indicates that, within the study's timeframe, these factors did not markedly affect the diagnostic yield of TFNAB.

These studies underscore the intricate balance required in thyroid nodule management, highlighting the challenges and the advancements in diagnostic techniques. The findings from the low-risk thyroid neoplasms study emphasize the nuanced differences in sonographic evaluations and the need for careful interpretation of such imaging results to guide clinical decisions. Meanwhile, the research on the impact of COVID-19 on thyroid fine-needle aspiration biopsy offers a reassuring indication that the pandemic has not significantly compromised the diagnostic effectiveness of TFNAB despite concerns to the contrary. Both strands of research collectively advance our understanding of thyroid pathology and the effects of external factors on medical diagnostics. As we continue to integrate these insights into clinical practice, they will improve the precision of diagnostic processes and enrich our strategies for managing thyroid conditions in a world where medical and societal variables are constantly evolving. This knowledge is invaluable in refining our approaches and ensuring that patient care remains informed and adaptable.

4. Conclusion

In addressing the complexities of thyroid nodule management, this chapter has illuminated the strides made in refining diagnostic procedures and therapeutic approaches. Using FNA, supplemented by advanced USG and molecular diagnostics, has dramatically enhanced our capacity to discern between benign and malignant thyroid nodules, thereby steering clinical decision-making toward more targeted and conservative treatments even though the challenges posed by indeterminate cytology and the inherent limitations of FNA, innovations in diagnostic techniques such as integrating core needle biopsy and applying refined cytological classification systems such as the Bethesda system have facilitated a more precise characterization of thyroid nodules. Moreover, the development of imaging protocols, such as ACR and EU-TIRADS, has standardized the assessment and management of thyroid nodules, contributing to a more uniform approach across clinical settings.

Our clinical experience, supported by studies on the demographic, biochemical, and sonographic variables influencing the prognosis of low-risk thyroid neoplasms as well as the resilience of thyroid diagnostics in the face of global challenges, such as the COVID-19 pandemic, emphasizes the evolving landscape of thyroid nodule management. These insights highlight the critical importance of individualized patient care and the need for continuous refinement of diagnostic and therapeutic strategies. We must continue to harness these diagnostic advancements while focusing on patient outcomes. As the field of thyroidology progresses, integrating emerging technologies and interdisciplinary approaches will be essential in addressing the nuanced needs of patients with thyroid nodules, thereby enhancing both the efficacy and safety of thyroid nodule management. This holistic and adaptive approach will undoubtedly contribute to better clinical outcomes and optimize patient care in the dynamic context of modern medicine.

Conflict of interest

The author declared no conflict of interest.

Nomenclature

Thyroid-stimulating hormone (TSH)	A hormone produced by the pituitary gland that regulates the production of hormones by the thyroid gland.
Fine-needle aspiration biopsy (FNA)	A diagnostic procedure for investigating lumps or masses. In this context, it is used to sample cells from thyroid nodules.
Sonographic risk assessment	Using ultrasound features to estimate the risk of a thyroid nodule being malignant.
Medullary thyroid carcinoma (MTC)	A type of thyroid cancer that originates from the parafollicular cells (C cells) that produce the hormone calcitonin.
Thyroglobulin (Tg)	A protein produced by the thyroid gland, used as a tumor marker for certain types of thyroid cancers.
Calcitonin (CT)	A hormone produced by the thyroid gland that helps regulate calcium levels in the blood.
Pentagastrin stimulation test	A diagnostic test used to measure calcitonin levels to screen for medullary thyroid carcinoma, particularly when basal levels are moderately elevated.
ACR-TIRADS	Thyroid Imaging Reporting and Data System developed by the American College of Radiology to standardize the reporting and diagnosis of thyroid nodules based on ultrasound characteristics.
EU-TIRADS	A similar system developed by the European Thyroid Association for the same purpose as ACR-TIRADS, using slightly different criteria.

Appendix A: diagnostic imaging and ultrasound characteristics

This appendix provides detailed information on diagnostic imaging techniques, particularly ultrasound characteristics crucial in assessing thyroid nodules. It includes a reference guide for ultrasound markers associated with benign and malignant thyroid nodules, as in **Table 3** of the main text.

Appendix B: bethesda diagnostic categories

This appendix elaborates on the Bethesda system for reporting thyroid cytopathology. It provides a comprehensive breakdown of each diagnostic category, associated malignancy risk, and recommended clinical approaches as outlined in **Table 7** of the main text.

Appendix C: ACR and EU-TIRADS classification systems

Comparison and detailed descriptions of the American College of Radiology (ACR) Thyroid Imaging Reporting and Data System and the European Thyroid Association (EU-TIRADS). This appendix helps clinicians understand both systems' specific criteria and risk stratification methodologies.

Author details

Muzaffer Serdar Deniz
Department of Endocrinology, Sincan Education and Research Hospital, Ankara, Turkey

*Address all correspondence to: md.mserdardeniz@gmail.com

References

[1] Durski JM, Bogsrud TV. Nuclear medicine in evaluation and therapy of nodular thyroid. In: Thyroid Nodules. Springer International Publishing; 2017. pp. 35-62

[2] Alexander EK, Cibas ES. Diagnosis of thyroid nodules. The Lancet Diabetes & Endocrinology. 2022;**10**(7):533-539

[3] Dean DS, Gharib H. Epidemiology of thyroid nodules. Best Practice & Research Clinical Endocrinology & Metabolism. 2008;**22**(6):901-911

[4] Pellegriti G, Frasca F, Regalbuto C, Squatrito S, Vigneri R. Worldwide increasing incidence of thyroid cancer: Update on epidemiology and risk factors. Journal of Cancer Epidemiology. 2013;**2013**:965212

[5] Siegel RL, Miller KD, Jemal A. Cancer statistics, 2015. CA: A Cancer Journal for Clinicians. 2015;**65**(1):5-29

[6] Kitahara CM, Schneider AB. Epidemiology of thyroid cancer. Cancer Epidemiology, Biomarkers & Prevention. 2022;**31**(7):1284-1297

[7] Turkkan E, Uzum Y. Evaluation of thyroid nodules in patients with fine-needle aspiration biopsy. Cureus. 2023;**15**(9):e44569

[8] Rao SN, Bernet V. Indeterminate thyroid nodules in the era of molecular genomics. Molecular Genetics & Genomic Medicine. 2020;**8**(9):e1288

[9] Danese D, Sciacchitano S, Farsetti A, Andreoli M, Pontecorvi A. Diagnostic accuracy of conventional versus sonography-guided fine-needle aspiration biopsy of thyroid nodules. Thyroid. 1998;**8**(1):15-21

[10] Rosen IB, Azadian A, Walfish PG, Salem S, Lansdown E, Bedard YC. Ultrasound-guided fine-needle aspiration biopsy in the management of thyroid disease. The American Journal of Surgery. 1993;**166**(4):346-349

[11] Bongiovanni M, Bellevicine C, Troncone G, Sykiotis GP. Approach to cytological indeterminate thyroid nodules. Gland Surgery. 2019;**8**(Suppl 2):S98-S104

[12] Chang H, Lee E, Lee H, Choi J, Kim A, Kim B. Comparison of diagnostic values of thyroid aspiration samples using liquid-based preparation and conventional smear: One-year experience in a single institution. APMIS. 2012;**121**(2):139-145

[13] Nagarajan N, Schneider EB, Ali SZ, Zeiger MA, Olson MT. How do liquid-based preparations of thyroid fine-needle aspiration compare with conventional smears? An analysis of 5475 specimens. Thyroid. 2015;**25**(3):308-313

[14] Ooi LY, Nga ME. Atypia of undetermined significance/follicular lesion of undetermined significance: Asian vs. non-Asian practice, and the Singapore experience. Gland Surgery. 2020;**9**(5):1764-1787

[15] Bang Y, Back K, Kim J-H, Choe J, Kim JS. The incidence and clinicopathologic characteristics of patients who had false-positive fine-needle aspiration results for papillary thyroid cancer. Journal of Endocrine Surgery. 2019;**19**(4):136

[16] Hatch-McChesney A, Lieberman HR. Iodine and iodine deficiency: A comprehensive review of a re-emerging issue. Nutrients. 2022;**14**(17):3474

[17] World Health O, Unicef, International Council for Control of Iodine Deficiency D. Assessment of Iodine Deficiency Disorders and Monitoring their Elimination: A Guide for Programme Managers. Geneva: World Health Organization; 2007

[18] Song J, Zou SR, Guo CY, Zang JJ, Zhu ZN, Mi M, et al. Prevalence of thyroid nodules and its relationship with iodine status in Shanghai: A population-based study. Biomedical and Environmental Sciences. 2016;**29**(6):398-407

[19] AlSaedi AH, Almalki DS, ElKady RM. Approach to thyroid nodules: Diagnosis and treatment. Cureus. 2024;**16**(1):e52232

[20] Furlanetto TW, Peccin S, Schneider MAO, Zimmer AS, Reis PS, Genro SK, et al. Prevalência de nódulos de tireóide detectados por ecografia em mulheres após os 40 anos. Revista da Associação Médica Brasileira. 2000;**46**(4):331-334

[21] Bomeli SR, LeBeau SO, Ferris RL. Evaluation of a thyroid nodule. Otolaryngologic Clinics of North America. 2010;**43**(2):229-vii

[22] Uludag M, Unlu MT, Kostek M, Aygun N, Caliskan O, Ozel A, et al. Management of thyroid nodules. Sisli Etfal Hastanesi Tip Bülteni. 2023;**57**(3):287-304

[23] Youserm DM, Huang T, Loevner LA, Langlotz CP. Clinical and economic impact of incidental thyroid lesions found with CT and MR. AJNR. American Journal of Neuroradiology. 1997;**18**(8):1423-1428

[24] Nguyen XV, Choudhury KR, Eastwood JD, Lyman GH, Esclamado RM, Werner JD, et al. Incidental thyroid nodules on CT: Evaluation of 2 risk-categorization methods for work-up of nodules. AJNR. American Journal of Neuroradiology. 2013;**34**(9):1812-1817

[25] Vander JB. The significance of nontoxic thyroid nodules. Annals of Internal Medicine. 1968;**69**(3):537

[26] Burman KD, Wartofsky L. Thyroid nodules. New England Journal of Medicine. 2015;**373**(24):2347-2356

[27] Walsh JP. Managing thyroid disease in general practice. Medical Journal of Australia. 2016;**205**(4):179-184

[28] Zou B, Sun L, Wang X, Chen Z. The prevalence of single and multiple thyroid nodules and its association with metabolic diseases in Chinese: A cross-sectional study. International Journal of Endocrinology. 2020;**2020**:5381012

[29] Tan GH. Solitary thyroid nodule. Archives of Internal Medicine. 1995;**155**(22):2418

[30] Zamora EA, Khare S, Cassaro S. Thyroid nodule. In: StatPearls. Treasure Island (FL): StatPearls Publishing Copyright © 2024, StatPearls Publishing LLC; 2024

[31] Bellynda M, Kamil MR, Yarso KY. Radiofrequency ablation for benign thyroid nodule treatment: New solution in our center. International Journal of Surgery Case Reports. 2022;**97**:107418

[32] Hegedüs L. The thyroid nodule. New England Journal of Medicine. 2004;**351**(17):1764-1771

[33] Smith-Bindman R, Lebda P, Feldstein VA, Sellami D, Goldstein RB, Brasic N, et al. Risk of thyroid cancer based on thyroid ultrasound imaging characteristics: Results of a population-based study. JAMA Internal Medicine. 2013;**173**(19):1788-1796

[34] Rahimi M, Farshchian N, Rezaee E, Shahebrahimi K, Madani H. To differentiate benign from malignant thyroid nodule comparison of sonography with FNAC findings. Pakistan Journal of Medical Sciences. 2013;**29**(1):77-80

[35] Molina-Vega M, Rodríguez-Pérez CA, Álvarez-Mancha AI, Baena-Nieto G, Riestra M, Alcázar V, et al. Clinical and ultrasound thyroid nodule characteristics and their association with cytological and histopathological outcomes: A retrospective multicenter study in high-resolution thyroid nodule clinics. Journal of Clinical Medicine. 2019;**8**(12):2172

[36] Durante C, Hegedüs L, Czarniecka A, Paschke R, Russ G, Schmitt F, et al. 2023 European thyroid association clinical practice guidelines for thyroid nodule management. European Thyroid Journal. 2023;**12**(5):e230067

[37] Tamhane S, Gharib H. Thyroid nodule update on diagnosis and management. Clinical Diabetes and Endocrinology. 2016;**2**:17

[38] Rago T, Vitti P. Risk stratification of thyroid nodules: From ultrasound features to TIRADS. Cancers (Basel). 2022;**14**(3):717

[39] Alsalamah S, Albesher M, Alwabili M, Almutairy A. Spontaneous hemorrhagic thyroid nodule: A case report and review of the literature. Journal of Surgical Case Reports. 2024;**2024**(3):rjae124

[40] Hakeem AH, Chandramathyamma SK, Hakeem IH, Wani FJ, Gomez R. Riedel's thyroiditis mimicking as anaplastic thyroid carcinoma: Unusual presentation. Indian Journal of Surgical Oncology. 2016;7(3):359-362

[41] Kim EH, Kim JY, Kim T-J. Aggressive primary thyroid lymphoma: Imaging features of two elderly patients. Ultrasonography. 2014;**33**(4):298-302

[42] Romero-Velez G, Sehnem L, Noureldine SI, Plitt G, Panagiotis B, Shin J, et al. Progression of nodular thyroid disease in familial adenomatous polyposis syndrome: Refined surveillance recommendations. Endocrine Practice. 2024

[43] Sandy JL, Titmuss A, Hameed S, Cho YH, Sandler G, Benitez-Aguirre P. Thyroid nodules in children and adolescents: Investigation and management. Journal of Paediatrics and Child Health. 2022;**58**(12):2163-2168

[44] Belfiore A, La Rosa GL, La Porta GA, Giuffrida D, Milazzo G, Lupo L, et al. Cancer risk in patients with cold thyroid nodules: Relevance of iodine intake, sex, age, and multinodularity. The American Journal of Medicine. 1992;**93**(4):363-369

[45] Barsouk A, Aluru JS, Rawla P, Saginala K, Barsouk A. Epidemiology, risk factors, and prevention of head and neck squamous cell carcinoma. Medical Sciences. 2023;**11**(2)

[46] Curtis RE, Rowlings PA, Deeg HJ, Shriner DA, Socié G, Travis LB, et al. Solid cancers after bone marrow transplantation. New England Journal of Medicine. 1997;**336**(13):897-904

[47] Fresilli D, David E, Pacini P, Del Gaudio G, Dolcetti V, Lucarelli GT, et al. Thyroid nodule characterization: How to assess the malignancy risk. Update of the literature. Diagnostics (Basel). 2021;**11**(8):1374

[48] Hsiao V, Arroyo N, Fernandes-Taylor S, Chiu AS, Davies L, Francis DO. Letter to the editor: Sensitivity of palpation for detection of thyroid nodules with attention to size. Thyroid: Official Journal of the American Thyroid Association. 2022;**32**(5):599-601

[49] Keskin Ç, Canpolat AG, Canlar Ş, Bahçecioğlu Mutlu AB, Erdoğan MF. Men 2b cases with atypical presentation, unusual clinical course and a literature review. Acta Endocrinologica. 2023;**19**(2):260-266

[50] Haugen BR, Alexander EK, Bible KC, Doherty GM, Mandel SJ, Nikiforov YE, et al. 2015 American Thyroid Association management guidelines for adult patients with thyroid nodules and differentiated thyroid cancer: The American Thyroid Association guidelines task force on thyroid nodules and differentiated thyroid cancer. Thyroid: Official Journal of the American Thyroid Association. 2016;**26**(1):1-133

[51] Cappelli C, Pirola I, Gandossi E, Rotondi M, Lombardi D, Casella C, et al. Could serum TSH levels predict malignancy in euthyroid patients affected by thyroid nodules with indeterminate cytology? International Journal of Endocrinology. 2020;**2020**:7543930

[52] Duval MAS, Zanella AB, Cristo AP, Faccin CS, Graudenz MS, Maia AL. Impact of serum TSH and anti-thyroglobulin antibody levels on lymph node fine-needle aspiration thyroglobulin measurements in differentiated thyroid cancer patients. European Thyroid Journal. 2017;**6**(6):292-297

[53] Boi F, Baghino G, Atzeni F, Lai ML, Faa G, Mariotti S. The diagnostic value for differentiated thyroid carcinoma metastases of thyroglobulin (Tg) measurement in washout fluid from fine-needle aspiration biopsy of neck lymph nodes is maintained in the presence of circulating anti-Tg antibodies. The Journal of Clinical Endocrinology & Metabolism. 2006;**91**(4):1364-1369

[54] Ogmen BE, Ince N, Aksoy Altınboga A, Akdogan L, Polat SB, Genc B, et al. An old friend, a new insight: Calcitonin measurement in serum and aspiration needle washout fluids significantly increases the early and accurate detection of medullary thyroid cancer. Cancer Cytopathology. 2023;**132**(3):161-168

[55] Roy M, Chen H, Sippel RS. Current understanding and management of medullary thyroid cancer. The Oncologist. 2013;**18**(10):1093-1100

[56] Pacini F, Castagna MG, Cipri C, Schlumberger M. Medullary thyroid carcinoma. Clinical Oncology. 2010;**22**(6):475-485

[57] Toledo SPA, Lourenço DM Jr, Santos MA, Tavares MR, Toledo RA, Correia-Deur JEM. Hypercalcitoninemia is not pathognomonic of medullary thyroid carcinoma. Clinics (São Paulo, Brazil). 2009;**64**(7):699-706

[58] Niederle MB, Scheuba C, Gessl A, Li S, Koperek O, Bieglmayer C, et al. Calcium-stimulated calcitonin - The "new standard" in the diagnosis of thyroid C-cell disease - Clinically relevant gender-specific cut-off levels for an "old test". Biochemia Medica (Zagreb). 2018;**28**(3):030710

[59] Colombo C, Verga U, Mian C, Ferrero S, Perrino M, Vicentini L, et al. Comparison of calcium and pentagastrin tests for the diagnosis and follow-up of medullary thyroid cancer. The Journal of Clinical Endocrinology & Metabolism. 2012;**97**(3):905-913

[60] Băetu M, Olariu CA, Moldoveanu G, Corneci C, Badiu C. Calcitonin stimulation tests: Rationale, technical issues and side effects: A review. Hormone and Metabolic Research. 2021;**53**(06):355-363

[61] Russ G, Bonnema SJ, Erdogan MF, Durante C, Ngu R, Leenhardt L.

European thyroid association guidelines for ultrasound malignancy risk stratification of thyroid nodules in adults: The EU-TIRADS. European Thyroid Journal. 2017;**6**(5):225-237

[62] Rago T, Vitti P. Role of thyroid ultrasound in the diagnostic evaluation of thyroid nodules. Best Practice & Research Clinical Endocrinology & Metabolism. 2008;**22**(6):913-928

[63] Russell MD, Orloff LA. Ultrasonography of the thyroid, parathyroids, and beyond. HNO. 2022;**70**(5):333-344

[64] Limaiem F, Rehman A, Mazzoni T. Papillary thyroid carcinoma. In: StatPearls [Internet]. Treasure Island (FL): StatPearls Publishing. p. 2024

[65] Borowczyk M, Woliński K, Więckowska B, Jodłowska-Siewert E, Szczepanek-Parulska E, Verburg FA, et al. Sonographic features differentiating follicular thyroid cancer from follicular adenoma-A meta-analysis. Cancers (Basel). 2021;**13**(5):93

[66] Wright K, Brandler TC, Fisher JC, Rothberger GD, Givi B, Prescott J, et al. The clinical significance of the American College of Radiology (ACR) thyroid imaging reporting and data system (TI-RADS) category 5 thyroid nodules: Not as risky as we think? Surgery. 2023;**173**(1):239-245

[67] Tessler FN, Middleton WD, Grant EG, Hoang JK, Berland LL, Teefey SA, et al. ACR thyroid imaging, reporting and data system (TI-RADS): White paper of the ACR TI-RADS committee. Journal of the American College of Radiology. 2017;**14**(5):587-595

[68] Hoang JK, Middleton WD, Tessler FN. Update on ACR TI-RADS: Successes, challenges, and future directions, from the *AJR* special series on radiology reporting and data systems. American Journal of Roentgenology. 2021;**216**(3):570-578

[69] Nie W, Zhu L, Yan P, Sun J. Thyroid nodule ultrasound accuracy in predicting thyroid malignancy based on TIRADS system. Advances in Clinical and Experimental Medicine. 2022;**31**(6):597-606

[70] Jin Z, Pei S, Shen H, Ouyang L, Zhang L, Mo X, et al. Comparative study of C-TIRADS, ACR-TIRADS, and EU-TIRADS for diagnosis and management of thyroid nodules. Academic Radiology. 2023;**30**(10):2181-2191

[71] Hess JR, Van Tassel DC, Runyan CE, Morrison Z, Walsh AM, Schafernak KT. Performance of ACR TI-RADS and the bethesda system in predicting risk of malignancy in thyroid nodules at a large children's hospital and a comprehensive review of the pediatric literature. Cancers (Basel). 2023;**15**(15):3975

[72] Titton RL, Gervais DA, Boland GW, Maher MM, Mueller PR. Sonography and sonographically guided fine-needle aspiration biopsy of the thyroid gland: Indications and techniques, pearls and pitfalls. American Journal of Roentgenology. 2003;**181**(1):267-271

[73] Keskin L, Karahan D, Yaprak B. Comparison of thyroid fine needle aspiration biopsy and ultrasonography results. Medicine (Baltimore). 2023;**102**(26):e33822

[74] Gupta N, Gupta P, Rajwanshi A. Trucut/core biopsy versus FNAC: Who wins the match? Thyroid lesions and salivary gland lesions: An overview. Journal of Cytology. 2018;**35**(3):173-175

[75] Bahn RS, Castro MR. Approach to the patient with nontoxic multinodular Goiter. The Journal of Clinical Endocrinology & Metabolism. 2011;**96**(5):1202-1212

[76] Abu-Yousef MM, Larson JH, Kuehn DM, Wu AS, Laroia AT. Safety of ultrasound-guided fine needle aspiration biopsy of neck lesions in patients taking antithrombotic/anticoagulant medications. Ultrasound Quarterly. 2011;**27**(3):157-159

[77] Polyzos SA, Anastasilakis AD. A systematic review of cases reporting needle tract seeding following thyroid fine needle biopsy. World Journal of Surgery. 2010;**34**(4):844-851

[78] Cibas ES, Ali SZ. The 2017 bethesda system for reporting thyroid cytopathology. Thyroid. 2017;**27**(11):1341-1346

[79] Deniz MS, Özdemir D, İmga NN, Başer H, Çuhacı Seyrek FN, Altınboğa AA, et al. Investigation of pre-operative demographic, biochemical, sonographic and cytopathological findings in low-risk thyroid neoplasms. Clinical Endocrinology. 2023;**99**(5):502-510

[80] Deniz MS, Dindar M. Examining the impact of several factors including COVID-19 on thyroid fine-needle aspiration biopsy. Diagnostic Cytopathology. 2023;**52**(1):42-49

Section 5

Hypothyroidism in Children

Chapter 12

The Role of Nuclear Medicine in Congenital Hypothyroidism

Aisyah Elliyanti

Abstract

Nuclear medicine imaging techniques are known as molecular functional radioisotope imaging. It has been used for decades in endocrinology and pediatric clinical practice. Thyroid scintigraphy (TS) results in many cases of congenital hypothyroidism (CH) may not affect the management immediately. However, TS, either Technetium-99 m Pertechnetate (^{99m}Tc-O4) or Iodine-123 (^{123}I), can help establish an etiology for hypothyroidism, including CH that may affect treatment decisions, prognosis, and counseling. Congenital hypothyroidism has potentially devastating neurologic consequences when delayed to manage. Screening CH by measuring Thyroid-Stimulating Hormone (TSH) and or thyroxine hormone (T4) using Radioimmunoassay (RIA) technique will detect CH rapidly, and the case can be treated as soon as possible. This review discusses *in vivo* and *in vitro* nuclear medicine techniques and the benefits and limitations of nuclear medicine techniques in evaluating hypothyroidism.

Keywords: agenesis, dyshormonogenesis, radioimmunoassay, scintigraphy, iodine-123, thyroid-stimulating hormone

1. Introduction

The inadequate concentration of thyroid hormones present at birth may lead to hypothyroidism, which is known as congenital hypothyroidism (CH) [1]. The condition causes mental retardation and growth failure in newborns [2, 3]. Universal newborn screening has been highly effective in reducing the incidence of CH. However, in regions where prompt diagnosis or treatment may not be readily available, CH still poses a risk for preventable intellectual disability. It is crucial to ensure that all newborns are screened for CH, regardless of geographical location, to facilitate early diagnosis and treatment [4]. With prompt diagnosis and treatment, children with CH can lead healthy everyday lives.

The various forms of CH, including primary (permanent or transient) and secondary, have different etiologies and implications, which can significantly impact treatment planning. Accurate diagnosis and differentiation between the subtypes of CH are crucial for effective treatment planning [5]. Primary CH is caused by thyroid dysgenesis (agenesis, ectopic, hypoplasia), which is present at birth. Another potential cause of primary CH is thyroid dyshormonogenesis, which is a genetic disorder that disrupts the thyroid gland's ability to produce hormones. Secondary CH is a rare

IntechOpen

condition due to a deficiency in thyroid-stimulating hormone (TSH) production or secretion by the pituitary gland or hypothalamus. This condition can cause an underactive thyroid gland, leading to symptoms of hypothyroidism, which is known as central hypothyroidism. It is essential to identify the causes of primary congenital hypothyroidism to determine the appropriate treatment and management plan for affected individuals.

Newborn screening tests are commonly used to detect congenital hypothyroidism. The screening measures the levels of TSH in the blood. If TSH levels are elevated, additional testing, such as thyroxine (T4) or T4 initial and secondary TSH tests, is needed. Both screening strategies have similar accuracy in detecting severe primary hypothyroidism [6]. Moreover, thyroid scintigraphy (TS) s a gold standard diagnostic test for determining the etiology of CH, providing a more specific diagnosis [1, 7]. The etiology of CH may play a vital role in determining the disease severity at diagnosis, management therapy, and parents' counsel on the certainty of lifetime therapy and prognosis [8, 9]. Clinically, CH is divided into distinctive forms: primary (permanent or transient) and secondary. The exact diagnosis and differentiation between the CH subtypes are crucial to effective treatment planning [3, 5]. Thyroid scintigraphy is helpful for re-evaluation to uncover transient or permanent hypothyroidism and the decision to continue or discontinue thyroxine therapy replacement [10]. Additionally, re-evaluation, including thyroid hormone levels and functional thyroid imaging, is vital for those who are born prematurely due to the frequency of transient hypothyroidism to avoid unnecessary extended thyroxine therapy. This review elaborates on nuclear medicine's role in the screening and diagnosis of congenital hypothyroidism.

2. Incidence

The incidence of CH mostly depends on the newborn screening program [1]. Initially, the incidence was between 3000 and 4000 births when newborn screening was introduced in the 1970s [1, 4]. The incidence of congenital hypothyroidism has nearly doubled in the last decade, with 2000 births [4, 11, 12]. The elevation in the incidence is due primarily to increasing newborn screening and lowering the TSH threshold for diagnosis, which leads to an increasing number of mild cases [11, 13]. However, the incidence of severe congenital hypothyroidism has remained unchanged [4]. Changing demographics may also influence the apparent incidence of this disorder by increasing birth rates [4, 5].

3. Etiologies

Congenital hypothyroidism is a serious condition that demands immediate attention and treatment. An effective treatment should be based on the root cause. It is interesting to note that thyroid gland abnormalities are the most common culprit behind CH. Congenital hypothyroidism (80%) is due to thyroid abnormalities (dysgenesis 85–90%), which include agenesis (35–40%), ectopic (60–65%), or hypoplastic gland [11, 13–15]. Additionally, if the thyroid gland visualizes but does not function properly (15%), it can also lead to congenital hypothyroidism (dyshormonogenesis 10%) [3, 14, 15]. Interestingly, several studies reported that 30–40% of CH had an ectopic thyroid gland that showed consistency with a form of dyshormonogenesis [14, 16–18]. However, pathophysiologically, hypothyroidism can be caused by impaired thyroid gland function (primary hypothyroidism) and also be affected by hypothalamic and pituitary control of the thyroid (central/secondary hypothyroidism).

Thyroid dysgenesis is a relatively common condition that can hinder the thyroid gland's ability to produce sufficient thyroid hormones. Despite its incidence, the underlying mechanisms of this sporadic disease remain poorly understood [1, 14]. However, it is significant to acknowledge the possibility of a familial component, and genetic mutations or other factors may play a role in its development [14]. Several genes are involved in thyroid development and have been linked to thyroid dysgenesis in some cases [1, 4, 14, 19]. At least 12 genes involved in thyroid dysgenesis and the defects in the biosynthesis of thyroid hormones have been described. However, genetic causes of CH were identified to be only between 2 and 5% [1, 14]. On the other hand, the progressive development of molecular techniques such as next-generation sequencing (NGS) has recently increased the genetic defects associated with CH in the range from 33 to 61.5% [20].

The TSH receptor (TSHR) mutation can result in resistance to TSH and a spectrum of thyroid dysfunctions ranging from elevated TSH levels and normal thyroid hormone levels to congenital hypothyroidism with thyroid hypoplasia, that leads to either sub-clinical congenital hypothyroidism (SCH) or congenital hypothyroidism [21]. Mutations in (TSHR) or genes encoding transcription factors involved in thyroid development (TTF1/NKX2.1, PAX8, FOXE1, NKX2–5, and GLIS3) [1, 20]. Moreover, dyshormonogenesis frequently is caused by defects in the cellular signaling of thyroid hormone synthesis, mutations of thyroglobulin (TG), thyroid peroxidase (TPO), dual oxidase 2 (DUOX2) which associated protein (DUOXA2), the Sodium-Iodide Symporter (NIS) SLC5A5, the apical iodide transporter pendrin (SLC26A4), and iodotyrosine deiodinase (IYD) DEHAL1 [1, 3, 4, 14, 20]. A molecular study using NGS reported severe CH variants in dyshormonogenesis genes in 84.8%, and cases associated with thyroid dysgenesis genes were reported in 13.1% [20]. It contradicts the previously expected distribution of etiological forms. The other study has reported more frequent mutations in dyshormonogenesis genes than in thyroid dysgenesis genes [20]. Additionally, the condition due to the pituitary gland's inability to produce enough TSH, related to the IGSF1 gene, which is involved in regulating TSH production, and mutations in the IGSF1 gene leading to a deficiency of TSH and subsequent central hypothyroidism [22].

Thyroid hemi-agenesis is a rare clinical condition that entails the absence of one lobe of the thyroid gland while the other remains in a normal position. Research suggests that a unilateral growth defect causes this condition [19]. An early asymmetrical growth defect causes hemi-agenesis and not by regression of the lobe once formed [19]. Notably, the amount of thyroid tissue in hemi-agenesis cases is sufficient to produce normal TH levels, similar to those after a hemi-thyroidectomy. Therefore, this condition may go undiagnosed until the thyroid is examined morphologically for other reasons. Interestingly, the hypoplastic thyroid in the animal study reported that Nkx2-1/Pax8 double-heterozygous-null mice are mostly normal-shaped, but 30% of mutant embryos develop hemi-agenesis almost identical to that seen in the patients. However, functional modification of this gene contributes to asymmetrical thyroid growth in Nkx2-1, and Pax8 mouse embryos has not been elucidated [19].

Several extrinsic factors can cause hypothyroidism in newborns. Transplacental passage of antithyroid drugs for hyperthyroidism therapy can be the underlying cause of transient congenital hypothyroidism [4, 14]. Pregnancy-related complications such as hypo and hyperthyroidism during pregnancy, placental abruption, or insufficiency have been identified as related to thyroid disorders [5]. Iodine deficiency during pregnancy remains a common cause of neonatal hypothyroidism worldwide, even though iodized salt programs have been implemented. Iodine excess can also cause hypothyroidism, particularly in preterm infants. Additionally, amiodarone for treating maternal and fetal dysrhythmias, including iodinated contrast media, may cause adverse thyroid effects [5, 14]. An understanding of the pathophysiology of congenital hypothyroidism and the condition that affects newborn screening is required to identify, evaluate, and treat this condition in the early stage appropriately.

4. Diagnosis

Rapid detection and immediate management of hypothyroidism are essential for treatment and prevention of long-term health complications. Transient hypothyroidism is around 30% in newborns with the thyroid gland in place [7]. Additionally, determining CH's etiology at the time of diagnosis is vital. Thyroid scintigraphy and ultrasound tests provide an accurate etiologic diagnosis of differentiated dysgenesis or dyshormonogenesis [2, 7, 11].

Hypothyroidism is diagnosed by measuring the concentration of TSH and total or free thyroxine (T4) [1]. Thyroid hormones circulate and bind to plasma proteins, and their biological action is exerted only by the unbound fraction of the hormone (0.02–0.1%) [14]. The free T4 concentration can be assayed directly or estimated free T4 index [14, 23]. The direct free T4 assay is generally reliable in healthy ambulatory patients. However, it may be inaccurate in patients with severe systemic illness or abnormalities of protein binding, so caution is needed when interpreting such tests in this setting [14].

In the primary hypothyroid case, increasing TSH level is the first detectable abnormality. The free T4 levels fall when severe hypothyroidism occurs [14]. Thyroid stimulating hormone measurement is the most sensitive test for diagnosing primary hypothyroidism and monitoring the treatment. Central hypothyroidism should be suspected when free T4 is low and TSH is in the low or normal range (TSH level is an inappropriate increase in response to low free T4) [14, 23]. During hypothyroidism, T3 is maintained at normal levels until the late stages of the disease. So, measurement of serum T3 or free T3 is generally not helpful in the evaluation of hypothyroidism [14].

The normal TSH and free T4 levels in infants and children differ by age. Therefore, it is essential to use appropriate age-specific reference ranges in interpreting thyroid function tests [14]. However, sometimes, physiologic variations in thyroid hormone production in newborns lead to CH, which typically resolves when the endocrine system matures by age 2–3 years. For this reason, it is common for patients to be taken off treatment whose CH status is not clear at 3 years of age [14]. Moreover, evaluation of a patient's thyroid status may be affected by numerous medications and by nonthyroidal illness ("euthyroid sick syndrome") that can mimic true thyroid dysfunction [24].

Some newborns may have false-negative results during initial screening or have a risk for CH, such as preterm, low birth weight, and illness, and need a second screening at 10–14 days of age. Newborns with Down's syndrome are recommended for level TSH test at the end of the neonatal period [1]. On the other hand, primary T4-algorithms are often at the cost of false-positive referrals due to low T4 caused by nonthyroidal illness or T4-binding globulin (TBG) deficiency [23]. A complete history and physical examination are needed to identify potential confounding factors that influence the level of TSH or T4.

5. Radioimmunoassay

Radioimmunoassay (RIA) is a laboratory technique widely used in the medical field to measure the concentration of various substances in biological samples. The technique uses a mixture of radioisotopes of the measured substance and a specific antibody [25]. Radioimmunoassay has several advantages over other immunoassay techniques, and it is susceptible and specific [25]. The technique can measure various analytes, including hormones, enzymes, and drugs, and provide accurate and precise results. In diagnosing and monitoring CH, RIA can measure TSH and T4 levels. The disadvantage of RIA is the use of radioactive material, which requires special handling and disposal procedures to ensure the safety of laboratory workers and the environment. Additionally, the technique may only be readily available in some laboratory settings.

Shifting in screening methods for CH has occurred over time; it is reasonable to evaluate whether such changes might be associated with CH's observed increasing rate [26]. There was a trend to change the T4-screening method from RIA to the enzyme immunoradiometric assay (EIA) or fluoroimmunoassay (FIA). The change in the laboratory had the most significant impact on the incidence rate of CH because of variations in the sensitivity and specificity of the screening test. However, laboratories that used RIA or either FIA or EIA still increased the CH-incidence rate, indicating that factors other than the T4-screening method also contributed to the CH-incidence rate [26]. Moreover, screening for TSH by FIA resulted in a 20% higher CH-incidence rate than radiochemical methods (RIA/IRMA), and screening for T4 by EIA or FIA methods led to a 38 and 24% higher CH-incidence rate, respectively, than the RIA method [26].

5.1 Thyroid stimulating hormone

Universal newborn screening for congenital hypothyroidism generally begins with measuring TSH and/or T4 in a dried blood spot collected from each infant within a few days after birth [4, 14]. The elevation of TSH with or without low free T4 indicates the presence of congenital primary hypothyroidism. In the case of free T4, it is low, and TSH is normal or low, secondary/central hypothyroidism may be present, and the condition can be challenging to diagnose, particularly in ill or preterm infants [14].

Many variables influence newborn screening results, such as patients' characteristics and sample collection timing. Blood samples obtained within 24 hours after birth may give false positives due to the surge in TSH secretion (up to 60–80 mIU/L). Preterm Newborns with low birth weight or ill may have altered patterns of thyroid function that may affect newborn screening results, including low free T4 with normal or low TSH that mimics central hypothyroidism or primary hypothyroidism with a delayed rise in TSH that may be missed in early screening [14].

Preterm newborns (<37 weeks) and/or with low birth weight (<2500 g) have a distinct pattern of postnatal thyroid function from the standard weight of term newborns. In this condition, the TSH levels increase slightly and lower free T4 concentrations that may decrease during the first days of life. These conditions are due to multiple factors, including immaturity of the hypothalamic-pituitary-thyroid axis; loss of maternal T4 that would typically be transferred to the fetus in the third trimester; changes in thyroid hormone metabolism; frequent and often severe illness in these newborns; and exposure to medications that may affect thyroid function (such as dopamine, glucocorticoids, and iodine-contained antiseptics) [14]. Naturally, preterm infants frequently result in a state of low T4 (or free T4) without increasing TSH, which resembles central hypothyroidism or nonthyroidal illness [14]. It suggested that hypothyroidism screening is performed by measuring TSH on the second and fifth post-birth to avoid the initial physiological elevation of this hormone after birth [13, 15]. Moreover, the potential presence of TSH receptor-blocking antibodies should be considered in patients with an ectopic thyroid gland, even if there is no history of autoimmune thyroid disease. If TSH receptor antibodies are detected in maternal or newborn serum, they portend a transient condition of hypothyroidism that resolves within 3–4 months [14].

5.2 Thyroxine hormone

North American Newborn Screening (NBS) strategy programs have measured T4 as the initial screening, whereas other countries often measured the concentration of TSH [26]. Elevations in TSH level are a better predictor for CH. However, T4 levels are more stable to physiological variations shortly after birth. Therefore, the T4 measurement was more popular in the initial screening strategy in North American systems affected by early hospital discharge [26]. Initial T4 screening is usually accompanied by second-tier TSH screening to improve screening sensitivity and specificity.

The proportion of specimens with abnormal T4 results was around 10%, followed by retesting to determine the TSH concentrations, and the combined T4 and TSH results were used together to determine the need for early management. The strategies (TSH screening alone or T4 screening with second-tier TSH screening) have provided equivalent case detection [26]. On the other hand, laboratory results from 1991 to 2000 showed that the TSH assay as a newborn screening reported an incidence rate of CH 24% higher than that of laboratories that used a T4 assay [26].

6. Thyroid scintigraphy

Thyroid scintigraphy and Radioiodine uptake (RAIU) tests are functional imaging and widely used methods to evaluate morpho-functional aspects of the thyroid gland. The imaging can quantify the tracer's spatial distribution and measure thyroid glands' RAIU and the image results are correlated to the TSH, which shows whether the function is adapted to the physiological stimulus (normal status) or not (hyper- or hypo-function). The advantage of functional imaging is that it reports signals from structures that reflect the functional status of thyroid glands [27]. Therefore, TS remains an essential procedure to identify the etiology of congenital hypothyroidism and is the gold standard diagnostic test for determining the etiology of CH [1, 7].

Determining CH's etiology does not alter initial management, but it provides a prognosis, avoids unnecessary therapy, and optimizes thyroxine therapy [1, 3, 7]. However, it can help distinguish between thyroid agenesis, ectopia, hemigenesis, hypoplasia, and dyshormonogenesis [1, 2, 7, 15]. Visualization of the thyroid gland by scintigraphy depends on the presence and thickness of the functional thyroid tissue [27]. In CH cases, TS should be done under high levels of TSH, and the best time was done before or during the first week of thyroxine therapy [2, 7]. Suppose TS is not performed before the therapy; in that case, the scintigraphy should be done after 3 years, when treatment interruption no longer poses a risk (the critical period of neurocognitive development has passed), or using recombinant TSH to avoid replacement hormone therapy withdrawal [7]. Moreover, TS should never be allowed to delay treatment initiation.

Thyroid scintigraphy generally uses radionuclides such as Technetium-99 m-sodium pertechnetate ($^{99m}Tc\text{-}O_4$) and Iodine-123 (^{123}I). The $^{99m}Tc\text{-}O_4$ is taken up by follicular cells but is not organified, and it has a six-hour half-life, is a pure gamma emitter, and is cheaper than ^{123}I [27]. Normal TS image using $^{99m}Tc\text{-}O_4$, as shown in **Figure 1**. The false positive is caused by the salivary glands' uptake of $^{99m}Tc\text{-}O_4$, which may give a falsely positive image for ectopic thyroid (**Figure 1A**) [2, 3, 8]. On the other hand, Iodine transport via sodium-iodine symporter (NIS) forms extracellular to inside follicular thyroid cells and can be organified [28]. Therefore, ^{123}I can diagnose dysgenesis and dyshormonogenesis and identify organification defects [27]. Iodine-123 has higher accuracy, especially for diagnosing the ectopic thyroid gland [2, 3]. However, it is more expensive and available only in specific clinics, and requires pre-order [2].

6.1 Thyroid dysgenesis

Hypothyroidism due to dysgenesis includes agenesis (35–40%), ectopic (60–65%), or hypoplastic gland [11, 13–15]. Thyroid agenesis should be considered when no significant uptake of radionuclide appears on the scintigraphy, and the field of view includes the neck and the head, with elevated TSH level as shown in **Figure 1B**, and it confirmed with the ultrasound image [3]. Dysgenesis with agenesis is permanent hypothyroid. However, about 35% of patients with dysgenesis with a eutopic thyroid gland have transient disease and will not require lifelong therapy [4, 15].

Ectopic thyroid tissue may lie between the tongue, the thyroid bed, or the mediastinum [3, 29]. The relationship between thyroid ectopic and its dysfunction is poorly understood. In some cases, an ectopic thyroid may produce thyroid hormone, but in other cases, the condition may be dysgenic or show diminished thyroid function. The ectopic thyroid gland mainly causes dyshormonogenesis, and in most cases, the thyroid gland is enlarged due to an over-stimulation by increasing TSH levels [2, 3]. Thyroid scintigraphy shows an increasing uptake [2]. Both $^{99m}Tc\text{-}O_4$ and ^{123}I of TS can detect ectopic glands, but when the ectopic tissue is situated near the mouth, it can be hidden or impeded by oral activity when using $^{99m}Tc\text{-}O_4$. To accurately pinpoint the molecular defect's location, identifying eutopic tissue and dyshormonogenesis is best achieved using ^{123}I [3].

Thyroid hypoplasia cases are considered relatively uncommon, and their diagnosis requires a combination of scintigraphy and ultrasound imaging. Scintigraphy results typically indicate a low uptake of radionuclides and a smaller thyroid gland. At the same time, ultrasound imaging can reveal a modified shape, such as round-shaped lobes, unilobed, or asymmetry in the location of the lobes, as well as a reduction in glandular volume. It is important to note that hypoplasia in permanent hypothyroid cases may present with a customarily located gland in 15% of cases. However, relying on a single imaging technique can result in false-positive or false-negative results. Therefore, a comprehensive approach using complementary techniques is recommended for a more accurate diagnosis [3].

6.2 Dyshormonogenesis

Dyshormonogenesis accounts for about 10% of cases of CH and reflects a defect in any of the steps in thyroid hormone synthesis [3]. The non-visualized thyroid gland in TS, but displayed in ultrasound, maybe a dyshormonogenesis due to the presence of thyroid-blocking antibodies (maternal autoimmune thyroid disease), a genetic change in the TSH-gene and loss of NIS function that caused a defect of iodide uptake (**Figure 2**) [1, 13, 15, 30]. Other causes of iodine defect uptake can be thyroid gland prematurity, prior medication of thyroid hormone, or a central type of congenital

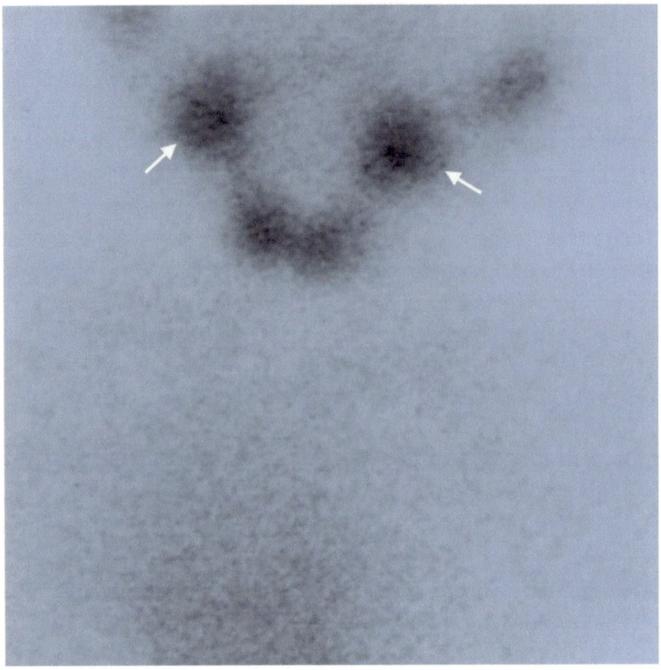

(A)

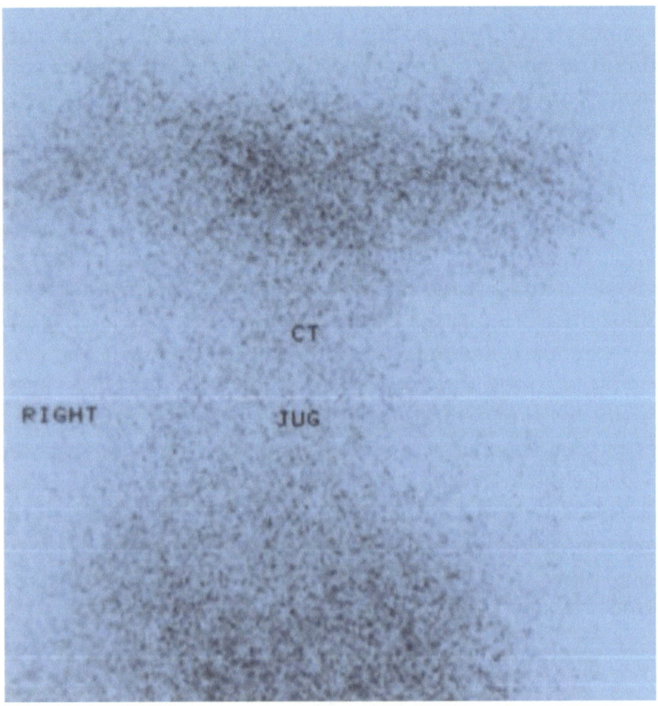

(B)

Figure 1.
A 17-month-old girl with a history of growth retardation. (A) Thyroid scintigraphy ($^{99m}Tc-O_4$) showed a normal thyroid gland and the uptake of $^{99m}Tc-O_4$ by salivary glands (white arrow). (B) Thyroid agenesis, non-visualized TS, and it confirmed ultrasound image.

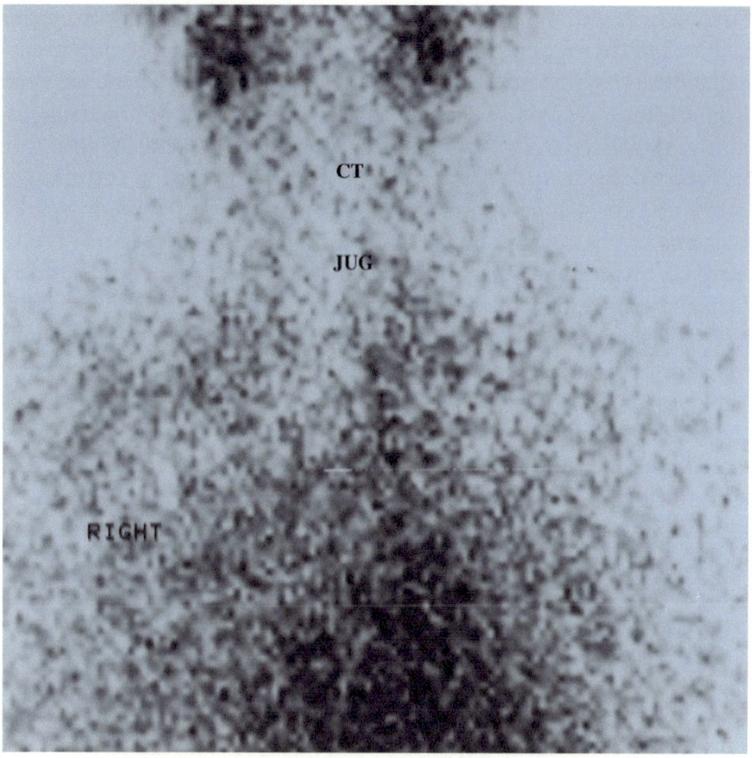

(A)

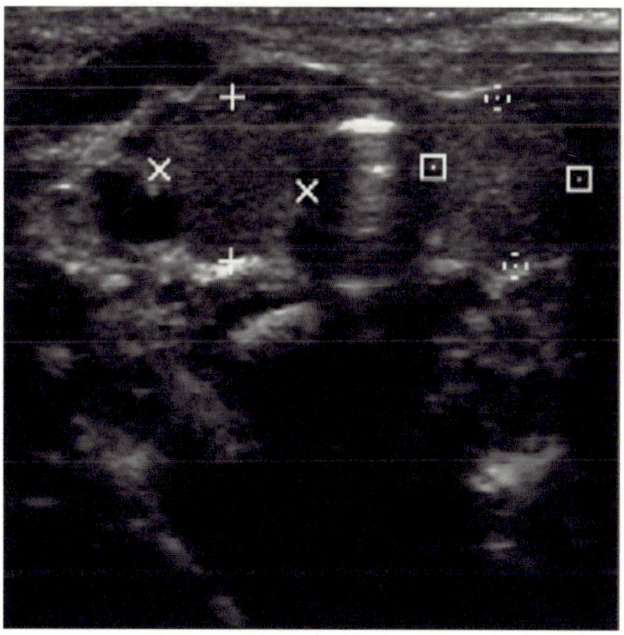

(B)

Figure 2.
A 10-year-old boy was diagnosed with dyshormonogenesis with an elevation of TSH level (>100 μIU/mL) and a low level of FT4 (0.4 ng/dL). (A) Thyroid scintigraphy is non-visualized of the thyroid gland. (B) The image of ultrasonography showed normal thyroid glands in the thyroid bed.

hypothyroidism in addition to thyroid aplasia [11]. The thyroid may be eutopic in cases of a partial block of thyroid hormonogenesis, and auditory evoked potentials may be needed to diagnose some forms of thyroid dyshormonogenesis (Pendred syndrome, Hollander syndrome), especially when there is a family history of hearing loss [15].

The scintigraphy thyroid in dyshormonogenesis can be classified into three types of defects. Type 1 defects are characterized by impaired function at the basal membrane/loss of NIS expression, resulting in low to blunted radionuclide uptake despite high TSH plasma levels. Late ^{123}I images are more often positive than ^{99m}Tc-O_4 images. The defective thyrotropin receptor (R-TSH) is often associated with thyroid hypoplasia or reflects maternal autoantibodies' transient blockade of the thyrotropin receptor. Defective (R-TSH) or abnormal NIS expression yields no radionuclide uptake at the thyroid and stomach level. Type 2 defects are characterized by impaired function at the apical membrane, responsible for reduced iodide organification. Both scintigraphy and uptake are high and rise quickly in an enlarged thyroid. The perchlorate discharge test is positive with a washout value >10% (partial) and > 50% (complete) organification defect [3, 31]. Total organification defects are most often due to a mutation in the TPO gene. Partial defects occur in minor thyroid peroxidase (TPO) abnormalities and Pendred syndrome (abnormal pendrin) [3, 31]. Type 3 defects are post-organification defects, including a goiter with pre-served uptake and a normal organification process (negative per-chlorate discharge test). Indeed, iodide, which has entered the organification process, cannot be chemically displaced by perchlorate. Mutations in the thyroglobulin (Tg) gene are more common than other abnormalities, such as defective pinocytic resorption of the Tg. Finally, DEHAL1 produces a secondary iodine-deficient state due to excessive renal losses of Iodine in MIT and DIT [3].

6.3 Radiopharmaceutical administration and image acquisition

Scintigraphy images provide the function of thyroid glands by using ^{99m}Tc-O_4 or ^{123}I [1, 7]. The image acquisition was 15 minutes after administration of ^{99m}Tc-O_4 intravenous. It is inexpensive and well tolerated; no complications have been reported [7, 10]. Other centers preferred to use ^{123}I, a more physiologic agent that addresses the thyroid gland's global function and can be administered intravenously or orally. The image acquisition can occur within 0.5–24 hours after ^{123}I administration [3, 7, 10]. We should not use ^{99m}Tc-O4 for uptake measurement because it is not organified. So, it is not suitable to quantify the radionuclide uptake.

It is essential to determine the appropriate radiopharmaceutical dose examinations. High doses may lead to increased radiation exposure without improving diagnostic sensitivity or accuracy, while low doses may not allow for adequate examination. In that case, the minimum amount of activity necessary for a satisfactory diagnosis is administered in the shortest possible time. Adhering to this principle will avoid unnecessary radiation exposure in newborns/infants. The activity dose radionuclides for thyroid examination are 1.1 MBq (0.03 mCi)/kg, with a minimum dose of 7.5 MBq (0.2 mCi) for 99mTc-O4, and 0.025–0.03 mCi (0.9–1.1 MBq) for ^{123}I. The average thyroid dose is less than 5 mSv/MBq (18.5 rem/mCi) [7, 29].

The image acquisition is taken in an immobilized supine position with head extension, which can use a particular design mattress or the newborn/infant in sleep [29]. A low-energy, high-resolution for ^{99m}Tc-O_4 and a high- or medium-energy collimator are available for imaging ^{123}I [7, 10, 29]. A medium-energy collimator produces a superior image quality than the high-sensitivity or ultra-high-resolution collimators for ^{123}I [29]. The best image is obtained with a pinhole collimator [29].

7. Perchlorate discharge test

Iodine is captured at the basal pole by active transport using NIS as a co-transporter, and then transported to the apical pole of thyrocytes, where it is fixed (organified) to thyroglobulin tyrosine residues, leaving no free iodide in the thyrocyte [28]. Iodide accumulates in the thyrocytes if organification is defective. In this case, sodium perchlorate, which is also captured by thyroid cells but not organified, competes with iodide and chases it out of the cells [2, 7]. Perchlorate discharge tests and genetic mutation studies might be helpful for the identification of the type of dyshormonogenesis [2, 3].

The effect of sodium perchlorate is evaluated before and 1 hour after its administration. Perchlorate does not alter iodine uptake in the normal newborn; therefore, the test is negative. The test is positive when iodine uptake is reduced by defective organification. Iodine uptake is measured before and after perchlorate. A 10% iodine uptake change is considered significant [7]. It can reach 98% in children with no iodide or ganification. Defective organification is usually permanent because of a defect in a gene involved in organification (the TPO and DUOX2/DUOXA2 genes in 470% of cases) [7]. However, it can also be transient following iodine overload due to povidone-iodine disinfection before maternal surgery (e.g., cesarean). Monitoring of thyroid function and thyroxine dose adjustment is recommended in all forms of hypothyroidism associated with an ectopic thyroid gland. In a French study of 71 neonates with CH with a positive result for the perchlorate test, CH was transient in 11 cases. Only one of the 11 children had a discharge showing a change exceeding 90% [7].

8. Ultrasonography

Thyroid scintigraphy and ultrasound are complementary for the evaluation of CH. Thyroid scintigraphy is highly sensitive for detecting ectopic thyroid tissue, and ultrasound helps assess gland size and morphology. Ultrasound may be beneficial for confirming the presence of non-functioning thyroid tissue [29]. Detecting the causes of thyroid dysgenesis and differentiating them from dyshormonogenesis can be effectively achieved through ^{123}I scintigraphy and ultrasonography [13, 29]. The absence of radionuclide uptake and ultrasound result confirms thyroid aplasia.

Meanwhile, ultrasound may help ensure the presence of non-functioning thyroid tissue due to TSHb gene mutations, TSH receptor inactivating mutation, defected iodide trapping, or maternal TRB-Ab [13, 29]. An abnormal positioning and larger-than-normal thyroid gland in ultrasound may indicate dyshormonogenesis [2, 13]. Additionally, a study reported that utilizing thyroid ultrasound with color Doppler flow can identify up to 90% of cases of ectopic thyroid [32].

9. Conclusion

Nuclear medicine offers a range of advantages, such as *in-vitro* and *in-vivo* diagnostic tools. However, using radionuclides can be limiting as they are only sometimes widely available. RIA for newborn screening is a relatively simple and susceptible method. Additionally, TS can assist in identifying the cause of congenital hypothyroidism and differentiating types of dyshormonogenesis. This safe and clinically meaningful procedure maximizes the information available for accurate diagnosis and optimal treatment. The scintigraphy provides insight into the relationship between clinical and genetic factors in CH, and it can help clinicians determine the certainty of lifetime therapy for children with a dysplastic thyroid or the possibility of later discontinuing therapy for children with an ectopic thyroid. If the thyroid gland is absent or ectopic, parents can be advised that the newborn will require lifetime thyroid therapy. However, suppose the thyroid gland is in the normal position. In that case, permanent treatment may not be necessary if the condition is transient, as demonstrated by controlled withdrawal of the thyroid at an older age.

Author details

Aisyah Elliyanti
Faculty of Medicine, Radiology Department, Division of Nuclear Medicine, Universitas Andalas, Padang, Indonesia

*Address all correspondence to: aelliyanti@med.unand.ac.id

References

[1] van Trotsenburg P, Stoupa A, Léger J, Rohrer T, Peters C, Fugazzola L, et al. Congenital hypothyroidism: A 2020-2021 consensus guidelines update-an ENDO-European reference network initiative endorsed by the European Society for Pediatric Endocrinology and the European Society for Endocrinology. Thyroid. 2021;**31**(3):387-419. DOI: 10.1089/thy.2020.0333

[2] Volkan-Salancı B, Kıratlı PÖ. Nuclear medicine in thyroid diseases in pediatric and adolescent patients. Molecular Imaging and Radionuclide Therapy. 2015;**24**(2):47-59. DOI: 10.4274/mirt.76476

[3] Clerc J, Monpeyssen H, Chevalier A, Amegassi F, Rodrigue D, Leger FA, et al. Scintigraphic imaging of paediatric thyroid dysfunction. Hormone Research. 2008;**70**(1):1-13. DOI: 10.1159/000129672

[4] Wassner AJ. Congenital hypothyroidism. Clinics in Perinatology. 2018;**45**(1):1-18. DOI: 10.1016/j.clp.2017.10.004

[5] Klosinska M, Kaczynska A, Ben-Skowronek I. Congenital hypothyroidism in preterm newborns—The challenges of diagnostics and treatment: A review. Frontiers in Endocrinology (Lausanne). 2022;**18**(13):860862. DOI: 10.3389/fendo.2022.860862

[6] Cherella CE, Wassner AJ. Update on congenital hypothyroidism. Current Opinion in Endocrinology, Diabetes, and Obesity. 2020;**27**(1):63-69. DOI: 10.1097/MED.0000000000000520

[7] Keller-Petrot I, Leger J, Sergent-Alaoui A, de Labriolle-Vaylet C. Congenital hypothyroidism: Role of nuclear medicine. Seminars in Nuclear Medicine. 2017;**47**(2):135-142. DOI: 10.1053/j.semnuclmed.2016.10.005. Epub 2016 Dec 16

[8] Schoen EJ, Clapp W, To TT, Fireman BH. The key role of newborn thyroid scintigraphy with isotopic iodide (123I) in defining and managing congenital hypothyroidism. Pediatrics. 2004;**114**(6):e683-e688. DOI: 10.1542/peds.2004-0803

[9] Hanukoglu A, Perlman K, Shamis I, Brnjac L, Rovet J, Daneman D. Relationship of etiology to treatment in congenital hypothyroidism. The Journal of Clinical Endocrinology and Metabolism. 2001;**86**(1):186-191. DOI: 10.1210/jcem.86.1.7124

[10] Sfakianakis GN, Ezuddin SH, Sanchez JE, Eidson M, Cleveland W. Pertechnetate scintigraphy in primary congenital hypothyroidism. Journal of Nuclear Medicine. 1999;**40**(5):799-804

[11] Chun S, Lee YS, Yu J. Thyroid imaging study in children with suspected thyroid dysgenesis. Annals of Pediatric Endocrinology and Metabolism. 2021;**26**(1):53-59. DOI: 10.6065/apem.2040120.060

[12] Ford G, LaFranchi SH. Screening for congenital hypothyroidism: A worldwide view of strategies. Best Practice & Research Clinical Endocrinology & Metabolism. 2014;**28**(2):175-187

[13] Al-Qahtani M. Congenital hypothyroidism. The Journal of Maternal-Fetal & Neonatal Medicine. 2022;**35**(19):3761-3769. DOI: 10.1080/14767058.2020.1838480

[14] Wassner AJ. Pediatric hypothyroidism: Diagnosis and

treatment. Paediatric Drugs. 2017;**19**(4):291-301. DOI: 10.1007/s40272-017-0238-0

[15] Rodríguez Sánchez A, Chueca Guindulain MJ, Alija Merillas M, Ares Segura S, Moreno Navarro JC, et al. Diagnosis and follow-up of patients with congenital hypothyroidism detected by neonatal screening. Anales de Pediatria (English Edition). 2019;**90**(4):250.e1-250.e8. Spanish. DOI: 10.1016/j.anpedi.2018.11.002

[16] Deladoey J, Ruel J, Giguere Y, Van Vliet G. Is the incidence of congenital hypothyroidism really increasing? A 20-year retro- spective population-based study in Quebec. The Journal of Clinical Endocrinology and Metabolism. 2011;**96**(8):2422-2429

[17] Olivieri A, Fazzini C, Medda E, Collaborators. Multiple factors influencing the incidence of congenital hypothyroidism detected by neonatal screening. Hormone Research in Pædiatrics. 2015;**83**(2):86-93

[18] Chiesa A, Prieto L, Mendez V, Papendieck P, Calcagno Mde L, Gruneiro-Papendieck L. Prevalence and etiology of congenital hypothyroidism detected through an argentine neonatal screening program (1997-2010). Hormone Research in Pædiatrics. 2013;**80**(3):185-192

[19] Nilsson M, Fagman H. Mechanisms of thyroid development and dysgenesis: An analysis based on developmental stages and concurrent embryonic anatomy. Current Topics in Developmental Biology. a2013;**106**:123-170. DOI: 10.1016/B978-0-12-416021-7.00004-3

[20] Makretskaya N, Bezlepkina O, Kolodkina A, Kiyaev A, Vasilyev EV, Petrov V, et al. High frequency of mutations in 'dyshormonogenesis genes' in severe congenital hypothyroidism. PLoS One. 2018;**13**(9):e0204323. DOI: 10.1371/journal.pone.0204323

[21] Schoenmakers N, Chatterjee V. TSHR mutations and subclinical congenital hypothyroidism. Nature Reviews. Endocrinology. 2015;**11**:258-259. DOI: 10.1038/nrendo.2015.27

[22] Sun Y, Bak B, Schoenmakers N, van Trotsenburg AS, Oostdijk W, Voshol P, et al. Loss-of-function mutations in IGSF1 cause an X-linked syndrome of central hypothyroidism and testicular enlargement. Nature Genetics. 2012;**44**(12):1375-1381. DOI: 10.1038/ng.2453

[23] Stroek K, Visser A, van der Ploeg CPB, Zwaveling-Soonawala N, Heijboer AC, et al. Machine learning to improve false-positive results in the Dutch newborn screening for congenital hypothyroidism. Clinical Biochemistry;**116**:7-10. DOI: 10.1016/j.clinbiochem.2023.03.001

[24] Fliers E, Bianco AC, Langouche L, Boelen A. Thyroid function in critically ill patients. The Lancet Diabetes and Endocrinology. 2015;**3**(10):816-825

[25] Sharma A, Pillai MRA, Gautam S. |S.N. Immunological techniques for detection and analysis in mycotoxin. In: Batt CA, Tortorello ML, editors. Encyclopedia of Food Microbiology (Second Edition). Academic Press; 2014. pp. 869-879. DOI: 10.1016/B978-0-12-384730-0.00233-0

[26] Hertzberg V, Mei J, Therrell BL. Effect of laboratory practices on the incidence rate of congenital hypothyroidism. Pediatrics. 2010;**125**(Suppl. 2):S48-S53. DOI: 10.1542/peds.2009-1975E

[27] Giovanella L, Petranović OP. Functional and molecular thyroid

imaging. The Quarterly Journal of Nuclear Medicine and Molecular Imaging. 2022;**66**(2):86-92. DOI: 10.23736/S1824-4785.22.03428-8

[28] Elliyanti A. Radioiodine for graves' disease therapy. In: Gensure R, editor. Graves' Diseas. 1st ed. London: Intechopen; 2021. DOI: 10.5772/intechopen.91498

[29] Treves ST, Baker A, Fahey FH, Cao X, Davis RT, Drubach LA, et al. Nuclear medicine in the first year of life. Journal of Nuclear Medicine. 2011;**52**(6):905-925. DOI: 10.2967/jnumed.110.084202

[30] Citterio CE, Targovnik HM, Arvan P. The role of thyroglobulin in thyroid hormonogenesis. Nature Reviews. Endocrinology. 2019;**15**(6):323-338. DOI: 10.1038/s41574-019-0184-8

[31] Rastogi MV, LaFranchi SH. Congenital hypothyroidism. Orphanet Journal of Rare Diseases. 2010;**10**(5):17. DOI: 10.1186/1750-1172-5-17

[32] Ohnishi H, Sato H, Noda H, et al. Color Doppler ultra- sonography: Diagnosis of ectopic thyroid gland in patients with congenital hypothyroidism caused by thyroid dysgenesis. The Journal of Clinical Endocrinology and Metabolism. 2003;**88**(11):5145-5149

Chapter 13

Congenital Hypothyroidism

Adina Mariana Ghemigian and Nicoleta Dumitru

Abstract

Congenital hypothyroidism is considered the most common neonatal endocrine disorder, with an incidence of 1/3000–1/4000 newborns. It is defined by insufficient synthesis of thyroid hormones from the newborn thyroid. The hormonal deficiency can vary from a slightly low level to a severe deficiency, also called myxedema. It is often a chronic condition caused mainly by thyroid dysgenesis or a defect in the thyroid hormones synthesis (dyshormonogenesis). Less often, it is secondary to abnormal pituitary or hypothalamic control of thyroid function. Considering the major role played by thyroid hormones in the early development of the central nervous system, congenital hypothyroidism is considered the most common condition involved in the etiology of mental retardation in children. Thus, early detection through neonatal screening programs and initiation the earliest possible of thyroid hormone replacement treatment prevent irreversible neurodevelopmental delay and optimize developmental outcome of affected newborns.

Keywords: congenital hypothyroidism, myxedema, central hypothyroidism, newborn screening, hormone therapy

1. Introduction

Congenital hypothyroidism (CH) is defined as dysfunction of the hypothalamic-pituitary-thyroid (HPT) axis present at birth, which will generate an insufficient production of thyroid hormones (TH). Axis dysfunction can be of varying degrees, as a result of which the hormonal deficit can vary from mild to severe [1]. It is considered the most common endocrine disorders, reported to occur in 1 in 3000–4000 newborns worldwide [2, 3].

Thyroid hormones play a crucial role in neuronal differentiation, myelination, and synapsis development in the prenatal and newborn periods, regulating early central nervous system development [2, 4, 5]. Thereby, severe undiagnosed and untreated CH is associated with neurological and psychiatric deficits, intellectual disability, spasticity, and impaired gait and coordination [2, 4]. Thyroid hormones are also important for growth during childhood and for normal metabolic functions throughout life [5]. These negative effects of thyroid hormone deficiency on metabolism and growth are reversible by therapy, regardless of when it is initiated. The situation is not the same in the case of cerebral tissue; if the treatment is not initiated as early as possible, the brain damage becomes irreversible [5]. There are studies that have shown the inverse relationship between age at the initiation of treatment (before 3 months)

IntechOpen

and the intelligence quotient (IQ) level later in life [6]. Despite all that, CH is one of the most common preventable causes of mental retardation [4].

2. Epidemiology

The overall incidence of CH ranges from 1 in 3000 to 1 in 4000 live births, with variation worldwide by geographic location or ethnicity [2, 7]. Before the 1970s, prior to the onset of newborn screening programs, when the diagnosis of CH was made based on clinical manifestations, the incidence ranges between 1;7000 and 1:10,000 [7, 8].

Among racial groups, the incidence is higher in Hispanic, Native American, and Asian population and lower in White and Black infants [2, 7, 8]. Besides, almost all screening programs report a female preponderance, of nearly 1.5 or 2 to 1 female to male ratio, and is also higher in twin births, multiple births, and preterm infants [2, 7].

Over the past few decades, a trend of increasing incidence is observed based on newborn screening programs, with an incidence reported of 1:2000 in ~2000 [2, 8]. The reasons for this rise in the overall incidence of CH are multifactorial: lowering of TSH screening cutoffs in TSH-based screening programs, leading to increased detection of milder cases; earlier discharge from the hospital with screening specimen obtained earlier, closer to the TSH surge after birth; changes in the population demographics (increased births of Asians and Hispanic babies); or increased screening of preterm or low-birth weight infants by improvements in neonatal medicine [2, 8].

3. Etiopathogeny

The HPT axis is a complex neuroendocrine regulatory loop involved in tight regulation of the thyroid function for maintaining a stable level of circulating TH (T4—thyroxine and T3—triiodothyronine) and thus the euthyroid state [9]. At the central level, hypothalamic thyrotropin-releasing hormone (TRH) stimulates the synthesis and secretion of pituitary thyrotropin (thyroid-stimulating hormone, TSH). The latter acts at the thyroid level to stimulate all steps of TH biosynthesis and secretion [9]. Conversely, TH controls the TRH and TSH secretion by negative feedback, maintaining physiological levels of central hormones of the HPT axis. In conclusion, reduction of circulating TH levels results in increased TRH and TSH production, whereas the opposite occurs when circulating TH are in excess. It is considered that serum thyroid parameters show substantial interindividual variability and thus that every individual has a unique hypothalamus-pituitary-thyroid axis set point, mainly determined by genetic factors [9].

As we mentioned in the introduction, CH represents a condition characterized by dysfunction of the HPT axis. CH is classified based on [2, 4, 7]:

- Origin—in primary or central/secondary hypothyroidism.
- Severity—in compensated (FT4 levels within the normal range for age) or decompensated (subnormal FT4 levels).
- Duration—in permanent and transient congenital hypothyroidism. In contrast to the permanent form, the transient CH is characterized by a temporary deficiency of thyroid hormones diagnosed at birth, with the possibility of recovery and restoration of euthyroidism in the first months or years of life [7].

Primary CH is caused by damage of the thyroid gland, thereby is characterized biochemical by low TH levels with elevated TSH concentrations [5, 9]. Instead, in central CH, the cause for inadequate TH production is located at the central level (hypothalamus or pituitary) and is defined biochemically by low thyroid hormone concentrations, while TSH is normal, low, or slightly elevated [5, 9]. The slightly elevated TSH concentrations observed in central hypothyroidism can be partly explained by intact immunoactivity but decreased bioactivity [9].

With these in mind, we can conclude that diagnosis of primary hypothyroidism is based on finding of an elevated TSH concentration [9]. Instead, central hypothyroidism may be more difficult to diagnose. It relies on correct interpretation of FT4 concentration using age-specific reference intervals and to recognize when FT4 is too low [9].

3.1 Primary congenital hypothyroidism

Primary CH is caused by a defect in thyroid gland and is the most common form of CH [2, 4, 5]. The majority of primary CH is due to thyroid dysgenesis, summing approximately 80–85% of cases [2, 3, 5]. The remaining 15–20% of cases are due to inborn errors of thyroid hormones biosynthesis, the so-called thyroid dyshormonogenesis [3, 5].

Thyroid dysgenesis encompasses a group of entities including thyroid agenesis (absence of the gland), thyroid ectopy (misplacement of the gland), and thyroid hypoplasia (underdevelopment of the thyroid gland) [2, 3, 5]. Thyroid dysgenesis is almost always sporadic or nonhereditary [2, 10]. However, in 2–5% of cases, mutations in a variety of genes responsible for thyroid gland development have been described [3, 5, 10]. Thus, thyroid dysgenesis can be associated with PAX8 (paired box 8), NKX2–1 (thyroid transcription factor-1), FOXE1 (thyroid transcription factor-2), NKX2–5 (NK2 homeobox 5), HHEX (hematopoietically expressed homeobox), and TSHR (thyroid-stimulating hormone receptor) mutations [2, 3, 5]. Some of these patients have extrathyroidal complications like benign chorea for those with an NKX2–1 variant or urogenital tract malformations in those with a PAX8 variant [7, 10].

Thyroid dyshormonogenesis can also be associated with multiple genetic defects interfering with encoding components of the thyroid hormone biosynthesis machinery like SLC5A5 (sodium/iodide symporter—NIS), TPO (thyroid peroxidase), DUOX2 (Dual oxidase 2), DUOXA2 (Dual oxidase maturation factor 2), SLC26A4 (Pendrin), Tg (Thyroglobulin), and DEHAL1 (Iodotyrosine dehalogenase 1) [3, 5, 10]. These variants cause loss of function, resulting in inadequate thyroid hormone synthesis with or without compensatory goiter [10]. In most of these cases, the CH is isolated. An exception to this in the Pendred syndrome (SLC26A4 variant), in which patients experience sensorineural hearing loss [10]. The genetic defects are often transmitted in an autosomal recessive manner in most cases, but autosomal dominant inheritance has also been reported [3, 10].

Next-generation sequencing (NGS) has brought a major change in understanding the molecular basis of CH, but it also allowed demonstrating a significant overlap in the genetic etiologies in the thyroid dysgenesis and dyshormonogenesis subgroups [10].

While thyroid dysgenesis and dyshormonogenesis cause permanent CH, in a small number of cases (5%), we can have a transient primary CH caused by extrinsic factors [2, 5]. Thus, transplacental passage of maternal anti-thyroid medications (methimazole or propylthiouracil), maternal TSH receptor-blocking antibodies (from a mother with autoimmune thyroid disease), or iodine deficiency or excess can be the causes for transient primary CH factors [2, 5]. Of all these factors, an important role is attributed to iodine, a mineral essential for thyroid hormone biosynthesis [5, 11]. It is worth noting that iodine deficiency remains an important cause of congenital hypothyroidism globally [2, 11]. Compared to an adult, the neonatal thyroid is much more susceptible to iodine deficiency as thyroidal iodide content at birth is extremely low and the daily neonatal iodide turnover is accelerated [11]. Although considerable efforts have been made to reduce the number of iodine-deficient countries in the last 20–25 years, especially through salt iodization, there are still many iodine-deficient areas, including in Europe [7, 11]. On the other hand, exposure of newborns to excess iodine can also result in transient hypothyroidism by interfering with thyroid hormone synthesis *via* the Wolff-Chaikoff effect [2, 11]. In general, a normofunctional thyroid is capable to "escapes" from the Wolff-Chaikoff effect after around 2 weeks by downregulation of its sodium-iodide symporter from the basolateral membrane and so to decrease its intracellular iodide concentration [11]. Instead, both fetal and neonatal thyroid, especially in preterm infants, cannot escape from the Wolf-Chaikoff effect, making them extremely susceptible to iodine excess [10, 11]. Exposure to excess iodine in this age group, through either iodine-containing antiseptics, radiographic contrast agents, iodine-rich food products (seaweed), iodine-rich supplements, or drugs like amiodarone, can result in blockade of thyroidal iodine transport for weeks to months [2, 7, 10, 11].

Another rare form of transient CH can be found in infants with hepatic hemangiomas [7, 12]. Congenital liver hemangiomas are benign vascular tumors affecting 5–10% of infants. These tumors, which can be unifocal, multifocal, or diffuse, can generate a rare form of hypothyroidism also called consumptive hypothyroidism. The pathogenic mechanism involved includes overexpression of deiodinase type 3 by vascular endothelium, a thyroid hormone-inactivating enzyme that converts T4 to reverse triiodothyronine (rT3) and T3 to diiodothyronine [7, 11, 12]. Medical treatment and reduction in tumor burden lead to consumptive hypothyroidism resolution in most cases [11, 12].

3.2 Central or secondary congenital hypothyroidism

This is a less frequently encountered cause of CH [4]. It is generated by insufficient hypothalamic or pituitary stimulation of an otherwise normal thyroid gland, which will result in secondary low serum level of thyroid hormones concentrations [4, 5]. Normally, thyrotropin-releasing hormone (TRH) from the hypothalamus stimulates anterior pituitary thyrotropes cells to secrete TSH. Congenital defects in this system, either from abnormal hypothalamic or pituitary development or from genetic alterations that impair TRH or TSH function, will lead to central congenital hypothyroidism [13]. Based on this, it is classified as central hypothyroidism with isolated TSH deficiency (one-third of cases), or more commonly TSH deficiency associated with other pituitary hormone deficiencies [4, 5, 9, 13]. Through combination of basal and dynamic endocrine investigation, genetic testing, and high-resolution magnetic resonance imaging, it was possible to obtain increasing knowledge about the etiology of central CH [9].

3.2.1 Central congenital hypothyroidism as part of multiple pituitary hormone deficiency

The anterior pituitary lobe or adenohypophysis consists of five specialized cell types involved in secreting of six hormones: thyrotrophs producing TSH, somatotrophs producing growth hormone (GH), corticotrophs producing adrenocorticotropic hormone (ACTH), gonadotrophs producing luteinizing hormone (LH) and follicle-stimulating hormone (FSH), and lactotrophs producing prolactin (PRL) [5, 9]. Multiple pituitary hormone deficiency is an inborn shortage of at least two anterior pituitary hormones, so beside central congenital hypothyroidism, we can meet GH deficiency or ACTH deficiency or central hypogonadism, or all together [5, 14].

Developmental or structural anomalies of the hypothalamus and/or pituitary usually lead to multiple deficits in pituitary hormones [13]. Some of these cases have a genetic basis being attributed to mutations in one of several genes critical for the normal early development of these structures like HESX1, LHX3, LHX4, SOX3, and OTX2 [13, 14]. These genes encodes a series of transcription factors essential for early embryonic brain development [9, 13]. Mutation of these genes are responsible for syndromic features that combine multiple pituitary hormone deficiency with cerebral and extra-cerebral abnormalities [9, 13, 14]. The cerebral structures interested in these conditions are midline brain, eye, inner ear, and the craniofacial structures. So, the newborn can present with holoprosencephaly, septo-optic dysplasia (SOD), absence of corpus callosum, cerebellar malformations, Arnold Chiari malformation, pituitary stalk interruption syndrome (PSIS), cleft lip, or palate and dental malformations [9]. The extra-cerebral structures involved are heart, urinary or gastrointestinal tract, and axial skeleton [9]. When the genetic defects affect transcription factors involved in the final steps of pituitary cellular differentiation, like POU1F1, PROP1, the child will have milder combined pituitary hormone deficiency without other syndromic malformation [9, 13].

Obvious neurological and developmental birth defects will usually lead to an early diagnosis of syndromic multiple pituitary hormone deficiency [9]. In their absence, other neonatal signs that can lead to the diagnosis are hypoglycemia, lethargy, feeding problems, poor weight gain, persistent jaundice, as well as potentially life-threatening adrenal crises due to ACTH deficiency [5]. Also, the male neonates can present with undescended testicles or a micropenis in case of central hypogonadism [5]. It should be mentioned that not all these symptoms are present from birth. So, without screening for central CH, the diagnosis is often delayed until childhood when developmental delay from thyroid hormones deficiency, poor growth secondary to GH deficiency, and delayed pubertal development due to LH/FSH deficiency triggers the diagnosis [5, 9, 14].

3.2.2 Isolated central congenital hypothyroidism

This form is characterized by the presence of an isolated TSH deficiency that leads to the appearance of central congenital hypothyroidism, with an estimated frequency of 1 in 40,000 newborns [5, 9, 15].

Until 2012, only TSH β-subunit (TSHB) and TRH receptor (TRHR) gene variants were reported as causes of isolated central CH [4, 5, 15]. In the last decade, with the help of NGS techniques, three new X-linked genetic causes of isolated central CH were discovered: Immuno Globulin Super-Family member 1 (IGSF1 in 2012), transducing-beta-like 1 gene (TBL1X in 2016), and insulin receptor substrate-4 gene (IRS4 in 2018) [4, 5, 9, 15]. Of these last three genetic defects identified, IGSF1 gene variants seem to be the most frequent cause of isolated central CH followed by variants in TBL1X and IRS4 [5, 13].

It is considered that this pure form of congenital isolated TSH deficiency has a variant type, namely, combined TSH/prolactin (PRL) deficiency, because TRH receptor signaling affects not only TSH secretion but also PRL secretion in both physiological and pathological conditions [15].

3.2.2.1 TSH β-subunit gene (TSHB)

Thyroid-stimulating hormone or TSH is a glycoprotein hormone consisting of two chains: an alpha and a beta chain. Its structure is very similar to the other glycoprotein hormones produced by the anterior pituitary, LH and FSH, and to human chorionic gonadotropin (hCG), all sharing the same alpha subunit. The β subunit is different for all these hormones, being the one who confers them the biological specificity. TSHB encodes the β subunit of TSH and its mutations cause severe central CH with neonatal onset [5, 9]. Patients shows an elevated α-subunit concentrations, an impaired TSH response to TRH, a normal or high PRL level, and a hyperplastic pituitary gland on MRI [5, 15].

3.2.2.2 TRH receptor gene (TRHR)

A far less common genetic cause of central CH with isolated TSH deficiency is mutations in the TRHR gene. Despite the absence of TRH signaling in the pituitary, patients with mutations in the TRHR gene have normal TSH concentrations but low PRL circulating levels and a blunted TSH/PRL responses to exogenous TRH [5, 14, 15].

3.2.2.3 IGSF1 gene

The IGSF1 gene lies on the X chromosome and encodes a hypothalamic plasma membrane glycoprotein whose functions are not fully known [5]. IGSF1 is expressed at high levels in testes and the pituitary, specifically in thyrotrophs, somatotrophs, and lactotrophs [9]. Mutations in IGSF1 gene are considered the most common genetic cause of isolated central CH [5, 9]. Numerous studies, both *in vivo* and *in vitro*, support that IGSF1 deficiency causes central hypothyroidism by impairing expression and downstream signaling of the TRH receptor in pituitary thyrotropes [13]. For this reason, the affected individuals will have a blunted response to exogenous TRH stimulation [13, 14].

The boys with inactivating mutation of IGSF1 will have delayed pubertal rise in testosterone levels, besides central hypothyroidism. As adults, the plasma testosterone levels will remain in the low-normal range and will also have macroorchidism (although testicular enlargement can begin before the onset of puberty), variable hypoprolactinemia and transient growth hormone deficiency [5, 13, 14]. Even if the IGSF 1 deficiency is X-linked, women carrying the mutation can also present with central hypothyroidism and prolactin deficiency but with an apparently normal lactation and late menarche in a minority of cases [13, 14].

3.2.2.4 Neonatal screening

Because thyroid hormone deficiency early in life is harmful to brain, growth, and development and in many cases difficult to recognize shortly after birth, newborn screening (NBS) programs for CH were implemented in many countries worldwide since the 1970s [1, 9]. The introduction of neonatal screening was justified by the fact that the costs of screening and diagnosis are much lower than those necessary for the care of children with intellectual disabilities, during their lifetime [4]. In addition, neonatal screening programs allow early diagnosis, soon after birth, much faster than the moment when signs and symptoms of hypothyroidism become clinically evident [4]. In this way, NBS for CH should be performed in all infants [16]. Prompt diagnosis by NBS leads to an early and adequate treatment, preventing hypothyroidism morbidity and ensuring a grossly normal neurocognitive outcomes in adulthood [4, 16]. Nevertheless, it is estimated that only 25% of the worldwide birth population undergoes screening for CH [7, 8]. A significant percentage of infants worldwide are born in areas that do not have access to neonatal screening, and so, the diagnosis will be made after development of clinical manifestations of hypothyroidism [1, 7, 8, 16]. Furthermore, many of these infants are born in areas of iodine deficiency, increasing their risk of thyroid hormone deficiency [1].

There are different screening strategies for CH worldwide [17], and these are based on [8]:

- Primary determination of TSH, followed by subsequent dosing of T4, when TSH exceeds certain values.

- Initial determination of blood thyroxine (T4) concentrations, with subsequent TSH dosing, when T4 is below certain limits (usually less than the 10th percentile for a given day).

- Simultaneous determination of TSH and T4 values (combined method), this represents the ideal screening approach but involves higher costs.

Each program must develop its own T4 and TSH cutoff for recall of infants with abnormal test results and to use age-related cutoffs, considering rapid changes in TSH and T4 in the first few days of life [7].

The strategy for selecting neonatal screening tests focuses on detecting all forms of primary CH, mild, moderate, and severe, as early as possible because disability due to primary CH is greatest in patients not treated before 3 months of age [1, 4].

Early in the neonatal screening, when radioimmunoassays developed and made possible measurement of T4 levels from dried blood spots, most programs undertook an initial T4 test, with a follow-up TSH test on infants below a specified T4 cutoff [4, 5, 7]. Unfortunately, T4-based screening is not very specific in detecting central CH and some mild cases of primary CH [4, 5]. Low blood T4 concentrations are also found in premature and sick neonates, as well as in thyroxine-binding globulin (TBG) deficiency [5]. TBG deficiency is an X-linked recessive disorder that occurs in approximately 1:4000 infants, primarily males [7]. It is considered a harmless condition. The infants are usually euthyroid, and treatment is not necessary but can generate a high number of false-positive NBS results [5, 7].

With increasing accuracy of TSH measurement, most countries worldwide changed their screening program from initial T4 test to primarily TSH-based NBS for CH [5, 7]. Nowadays, many screening programs carry out an initial TSH test to detect congenital hypothyroidism [7]. For this reason, TSH levels are determined from blood collected after the first 24 hours and should be the single most important test in any screening program [4]. More accurate and the best "window" for TSH testing for full-term infants is 48–72 hours of age [4, 16]. Blood is spotted onto filter paper after heel prick, allowed to dry, and sent to a centralized laboratory for TSH analysis [4]. The report result may vary according to the NBS program. Thus, some programs report TSH value in serum units while others in whole blood units. TSH results in whole blood unit are approximately one-half of the corresponding serum value. Thereby, the infant whose TSH is >30 mU/L serum (>15 mU/L whole blood) will be recalled for clinical evaluation and serum testing [7]. The reason that the filter paper screening test cutoff is approximately 30 mU/L is because of the TSH surge that occurs shortly after birth [7]. Later, after the first to 2 weeks of life, the TSH range falls to approximately 10 mU/L [7].

There are some programs that use an upper percentile TSH cutoff, for instance, > 97th percentile [7].

As we already mentioned, it is important to use a TSH cutoff adjusted for the infant's age to avoid false-negative results in those with mild hypothyroidism [16]. And this is important to know especially if a screening sample is collected after the 4 days of life, since TSH decreases sharply during the first week of life [7].

There is a category of neonates, namely, preterm neonates (less than 37 weeks of gestational age); low birth weight (LBW) and very low birth weight, under 1500 grams (VLBW) neonates; infants with Down syndrome; ill neonates admitted to neonatal intensive care; and multiple births, particularly in case of monozygotic twins, that are at risk of transient or permanent CH [4, 16]. The initial screening tests in these newborns may be inappropriate, providing false-negative or false-positive results due to [4]:

- suppression of TSH caused by drug administration,
- hypothalamic-pituitary immaturity,
- fetal blood mixing in multiple births,
- other effects of serious neonatal illnesses

In many centers, for this category, a second screening strategy will be applied, with remeasurement of dried blood spot TSH at about 2–4 weeks of age or as they approach discharge from hospital [4, 7, 16].

It should also be emphasized that while TSH-based NBS effectively detects primary CH, it does not detect central CH [5, 13]. Even though it is a less common condition than primary CH, there are enough evidence to support that neonatal screening for central CH fulfills the criteria for disease screening:

- Central CH is a relatively frequent disease, with an incidence similar to phenylketonuria, condition for which newborn screening was introduced since the 1960s [4, 13].
- Central CH is unlikely to be diagnosed during the neonatal period, without a neonatal screening [5].
- Most central CH patients have moderate-to-severe hypothyroidism instead of mild, based on pre-treatment serum FT4 concentrations [5].
- Screening tests and treatment are available, inexpensive, and effective [4].
- The risks in cases of delayed diagnosis are in for an unfavorable outcome [4, 5].

According to European Society of Pediatric Endocrinology (ESPE) guidelines, the screening strategies for central CH detection are based on two approaches [4]:

- a combination of primary T4 and TSH screening or
- a combination of primary T4 screening with secondary TSH testing followed by thyroxine binding globulin (TBG) determination.

The three-step T4-reflex TSH-reflex TBG NBS program, currently used by the Dutch national health system as a diagnostic strategy, led to an improved detection of central CH with an approximate incidence of 1:16,000, which is much higher than reported in countries with T4-reflex TSH or TSH-based strategies [5, 14].

4. Diagnosis

Diagnosis and treatment should not be based on screening test results alone. That is why all newborns with an abnormal NBS result must be referred to an expert center for immediate measurement of TSH and FT4 in a serum sample, to confirm the diagnosis of CH as soon as possible, preferably within 24 hours [1, 7, 16]. Besides TSH and FT4, it can also measure total T4 and triiodothyronine (T3) uptake to determine the type of hypothyroidism and establish the management approach. Measuring a TBG concentration when T4 is low but FT4 is normal may assist in distinguishing central hypothyroidism from TBG deficiency [16].

If the NBS TSH is >40 mIU/L, levothyroxine (L-T4) treatment should be initiated immediately after drawing the confirmatory serum sample, without waiting for the results [1, 16]. Such a value is highly suggestive of moderate-to-severe primary CH [1]. CH severity can be also assessed clinically (symptomatic hypothyroidism), biologically, respectively, based on knee X-ray and thyroid imaging results [4].

The infant with abnormal NBS result should be evaluated by a physician (primary care provider or pediatric endocrinologist) that should [16]:

- Obtain a complete history, including prenatal maternal thyroid status, maternal medications, and family history
- Perform a complete physical examination of the newborn.

The clinical symptoms and signs of symptomatic CH include sleepiness and not waking for feeds, poor and slow feeding, cold extremities, prolonged neonatal jaundice, lethargy, hypotonia, macroglossia, umbilical hernia, and dry skin with or without a puffy face [4]. Persistence of the posterior fontanelle, a large anterior fontanelle, and a wide sagittal suture all reflect delayed bone maturation, which can be further documented by knee X-ray [4]. The absence of one or both knee epiphyses is a reliable index for the severity of intrauterine hypothyroidism [1, 4]. Also, it has been shown to be related to T4 concentration at diagnosis and neurodevelopmental and IQ outcome [1, 4].

Biologically, based on plasma FT4 concentrations, it possible to construct a scale of CH severity in [4]:

- Severe—FT4 levels <5 pmol/l,
- Moderate—FT4 levels between 5 and < 10 pmol/l, or
- Mild—FT4 levels >10–15 pmol/l

Although it does not change initial treatment, it is recommended to determine the etiology of CH at the time of diagnosis using thyroid radionuclide uptake and scan, ultrasonography, serum thyroglobulin, and test for thyroid autoantibodies or urinary iodine excretion [1]. However, this approach should never delay the start of treatment in newborns with CH [1, 8, 16].

1. Thyroid scintigraphy—using Technetium-99 m (^{99m}Tc) or iodine-123 (^{123}I) is the most accurate diagnostic test for determining the etiology of CH, allowing to define the size and location of any thyroid tissue [1, 8]. ^{131}I delivers a higher dose to the thyroid and total body and should not be used [7]. For an accurate scintigraphic examination, it should only be performed when the TSH is elevated and thus before or within the first 2–3 days after initiating of L-T4 treatment [16].

   ^{99m}Tc is more widely available, less expensive, faster in use (image acquisition after 15 minutes), and has a shorter half-live than ^{123}I but is not organified and the images are of lower quality than with ^{123}I [1]. The latter isotope adds more information about organification process and exposes infants to a lower dose of whole-body irradiation than ^{99m}Tc (3–10 uCi/kg vs. 50–250 uCi/kg body weight) [1]. Radionuclide uptake and scanning identify thyroid aplasia, hypoplasia (decreased uptake, small gland in a eutopic location), or an ectopic gland (small gland located somewhere between the foramen cecum and over the thyroid cartilage) [8].

   A large gland with increased uptake is compatible with a dyshormonogenesis, one of the inborn errors of thyroid hormone production beyond trapping of iodide [7, 8]. In such cases, ^{123}I uptake can be followed by a perchlorate discharge test [1, 7]. The test consists in administration of sodium perchlorate with thyroid activity measured before and 1 hour afterward [1]. The perchlorate discharge test is considered positive when discharge of ^{123}I is more than 10% of the administered dose [1].

   Absence of uptake can be seen in thyroid aplasia and also with TSHβ gene mutations, TSH receptor-inactivating mutations, iodide-trapping defects, or with maternal thyrotropin receptor-blocking antibodies (TRB-Ab) [7].

2. Thyroid ultrasonography—it is an important diagnostic tool for determining the presence of the thyroid gland, its location, size, and echotexture, but it is less accurate than radionuclide scan for detection of an ectopic thyroid gland [1, 8]. Identifying a large gland on thyroid ultrasonography can guide the diagnostic towards a case of dyshormonogenesis [7].

3. Serum Tg determination—it reflects the amount of thyroid tissue, and it is generally elevated with increased thyroid activity [7]. It can be helpful in further evaluation of infants with absent radionuclide uptake [7, 8]. In cases of true

thyroid aplasia, serum thyroglobulin levels are absent [7]. Together with the perchlorate discharge test, it provides useful information for targeted genetic testing to diagnose the various forms of CH caused by dyshormonogenesis [1].

4. Serum TRB-Ab determination—it may be useful in case of absent radionuclide uptake and a small or normal eutopic gland determined by ultrasonography, in an infant born to a mother with autoimmune thyroid disease [8]. TRB-Ab can cross the placenta and block TSH binding, inhibiting fetal thyroid gland development and function [7].

5. Urinary iodine determination—it a measure that approximates iodine intake [7]. It can be useful in an infant with CH born in an area of endemic iodine deficiency or if there is a history of excess iodine exposure [7, 8].

5. Management

As we mentioned in the introduction, CH is one of the most common treatable causes of mental retardation [2, 7]. Also, there are studies that have shown that the timing of therapy is crucial to neurologic outcome [6, 7]. But even when it is diagnosed early, neurologic development may suffer if treatment is not optimized in the first 3 years of life [7].

According to the ESPE consensus guidelines, treatment of infants with severe primary CH should be with L-T4 in dose of 10–15 μg/kg per day [4]. Treatment should be started as soon as possible, no later than the first 2 weeks of life or immediately after confirmatory serum test results [1, 4]. The goal of L-T4 treatment is to obtain a rapid normalization of serum FT4 and TSH levels, preferably within 2–4 weeks from initiation, to improve neurocognitive outcomes [16]. Infants with moderate primary CH should be treated with an initial dose of ~10 μg/kg per day, and for infants with mild form, we can use even a lower starting dose (5–10 μg/kg) [1].

Oral L-T4 administration is preferred, either in the form of tablets that are crushed and suspended in 2–5 milliliters of water, breast milk/nonsoy-containing formula or as an oral solution [4, 16]. It can be taken in the morning or evening, either before feeding or with food, and it should be administered in the same way every day [4, 16]. The bioavailability of oral L-T4 is about 50–80% [1, 4]. It is mainly absorbed in the proximal small intestine, and this process can be influenced by food presence (soy, fiber) or minerals (calcium, iron). For this reason, simultaneously administration should be avoided [1, 4, 16]. In cases where oral administration is not an option, L-T4 can be administered intravenously in a smaller dose, approx. 75–80% of the enteral dose [4, 16].

The newborn's family must receive verbal and written instructions from the endocrinologist or their primary care provider regarding appropriate method for administering L-T4, the substances that can interfere with L-T4 absorption, and the importance of adherence to the treatment plan, including regular follow-up, to ensure a normal neurocognitive development and growth [1, 4, 16].

The follow-up evaluation (clinical evaluation and TSH, FT4 measurements) should take place 1–2 weeks after the start of L-T4 treatment with subsequent evaluation every 2 weeks until complete normalization of serum TSH [1]. Thereafter, the evaluations can be made [1]:

- Every 1–3 months until the age of 12 months.
- Every 2–4 months between 12 months and 3 years,
- Every 3–6 months until growth is completed.

Monitoring is important being useful in avoiding under or overdosing [1, 10, 16]. It should be mentioned that the collection of TSH and FT4 must be performed before, or at least 4 hours after the last L-T4 administration [1]. The therapeutic targets are [16]:

- Maintaining a serum TSH in the age-specific reference range, usually between 0.5 and 5 mIU/L after 3 months of life;
- Maintaining a serum FT4 levels in the upper half of the age-specific reference range.

Regardless of the etiopathogenic form of CH (primary or central), the treatment consists of hormone replacement with L-T4. The biggest differences between the two forms are the L-T4 starting dose and how the treatment is monitored [1]. Although central CH can be a severe condition, most cases are classified as mild to moderate with an FT4 at diagnosis between 5 and 15 pmol/L [1, 5]. For this reason, the usual recommended dose of L-T4 is 5–10 μg/kg, but it can be increased to 10–15 μg/kg in severe cases [1, 17]. Once the replacement therapy is started, patients should be monitored based on FT4 levels at the same intervals as done with primary hypothyroidism [1, 9], the goal being the maintenance of FT4 levels in the reference ranges for age [1, 9, 14]. When FT4 is around the lower limit of the reference interval, especially when is associated with a TSH >1.0 mU/L, undertreatment should be considered. Inversely, when serum FT4 is around or above the upper limit of the reference interval, particularly if associated with clinical signs of thyrotoxicosis, or a high T3 concentration then overtreatment should be considered, excluding the situation in which L-T4 was administered just before blood withdrawal [1].

Considering that central HC is most often associated with other pituitary hormone deficits, it must be taken into account that L-T4 initiation should be start after exclusion of a concomitant cortisol deficit [14, 17]. In those with concomitant adrenal insufficiency or when its presence cannot be excluded, L-T4 supplementation should be started after adequate glucocorticoid supplementation, to prevent induction of an adrenal crisis [14]. Also, both estrogens and GH influence thyroid hormone transport and metabolism; this is why sex steroid and GH deficiencies can mask an underlying central CH, while the introduction of these replacement therapies often requires an uptitration of L-T4 dose [14]. Taking all these data into account, particular attention should be given to patients with central CH as part of multiple pituitary hormone deficiency whenever new replacement therapies are added or modified [14].

As we mentioned before, some patients with a positive NBS for CH have transient congenital hypothyroidism and will receive hormone replacement treatment. Predictive factors that increase the likelihood of a transient or permanent disease are listed in **Table 1** [1, 17].

If the diagnosis has not been fully confirmed at the time of the initial evaluation of the newborn, a trial of L-T4 therapy should be considered at 3 years of age, particularly if the patient is adequately treated with a low dose of L-T4 (<2 mcg/kg/day) [16].

Transient CH	Permanent CH
Sex (more often in boys) Low birthweight Neonatal morbidity requiring intensive care Race/ethnicity (more often in nonwhite patients) Less severe CH at diagnosis (assessed by screening or diagnostic TSH or FT4)	Prematurity Other congenital abnormalities A family history of thyroid disease Abnormal thyroid morphology (thyroid hypoplasia at diagnosis) TSH elevation >10 mU/L after the age of 1 year A higher L-T4 dose requirement

Table 1.
Predictive factors that increase the likelihood of a transient or permanent CH.

At that time, the serum levels of TSH and FT4 will be determined after 4 weeks of stopping L-T4 treatment [1, 16, 17]:

- If TSH and FT4 levels remain in the age-specific reference range, then transient CH is confirmed.
- If the TSH >10 mIU/L and/or FT4 is low, permanent CH is confirmed and L-T4 therapy should be reinstituted.
- If TSH is mildly elevated (greater than the age-specific reference range, but <10 mIU/L) and FT4 is normal, TSH and FT4 levels should be repeated in another 4–8 weeks.

According to the ESPE guide, it is considered that there is sufficient evidence to support early treatment withdrawal to assess the necessity of further treatment and this can be considered and done from the age of 6 months onward, particularly in patients with a gland *in situ*, a negative first-degree family history of CH, or in those requiring a low L-T4 dose [1]. And thus, it will be an early identification of children who do not require long-term treatment.

6. Prognosis

Most children with CH identified early and treated appropriately will have a normal level of neurocognitive development and school performance, with a significant reduction/even disappearance of intellectual disability (defined by an IQ <70) [1]. However, subtle cognitive and motor deficits and low school performance may persist in patients with severe CH despite early and appropriate treatment. These may reflect prenatal brain damage caused by thyroid hormone deficiency in utero, damage that is not fully recovered by postnatal treatment [1]. These children may exhibit reduced hippocampal volume and abnormal cortical morphology, which may account for subtle and specific deficits in memory, language, sensorimotor, and visuospatial function [1]. In addition, thyroid hormones play an important role in the development of cochlear and auditory function; thus, subjects with CH have a three times higher risk of developing a hearing deficit, compared to the general population, a fact that can negatively affect the development of speech, school performance, and quality of life [1]. So, it is estimated than 20–25% of adolescents with CH will associate mild and subclinical hearing loss, despite early and appropriate L-T4 treatment [1].

It is also worth mentioning that poor socioeconomic status with poor adherence to treatment or excessive treatment in the first months of life, considered a critical period for brain development, may also affect cognitive outcome and can be associated with school-age attention deficit and lower IQ scores.

Children and adolescents with primary CH due to dyshormonogenesis may have an increased risk of developing goiter and thyroid nodules and may even have an increased risk of malignancy [1]. These cancers can develop at various ages but are most common in middle-aged individuals and can be aggressive [10]. The mechanisms implicated in the development of thyroid cancer in patients with thyroid dyshormonogenesis are not fully understood; presumably, constant and prolonged stimulation by TSH, a growth factor for thyroid epithelial cells, may result in goiter, thyroid nodules, or thyroid cancer [10]. Thus, they will require periodic follow-up with physical examination and ultrasound evaluation, especially in patients with poorly controlled disease, to identify nodules that will require fine needle biopsy to exclude thyroid carcinoma [1, 10].

We previously mentioned that patients with severe hypothyroidism associate delayed skeletal maturation, however, in the first months of life, treatment with L-T4 rapidly normalizes bone maturation. Nevertheless, excessive L-T4 treatment can increase bone turnover with greater bone resorption than formation, resulting in progressive bone loss [1].

Body mass index and composition are generally normal in children and adults with CH; still about 40% of young adults have a tendency and increased risk of being overweight or obese. Therefore, lifestyle interventions including diet and exercise and good adherence to treatment should be encouraged to avoid metabolic abnormalities and maintain an optimal cardiovascular health [1].

7. Conclusions

The neurodevelopmental outcome in children with CH is highly dependent on early diagnosis and therapy. Newborn screening for CH has been a great success story, and it is desirable it will continue to expand worldwide. And so, by its extension to a larger birth population that undergoes comprehensive screening, it will be possible to identify new mechanisms involved in the etiopathogenesis of this condition. Besides an early identification, we should also keep in mind that compliance with hormonal substitution and the therapeutic regimen can influence the long-term prognosis; this is why the maintenance of treatment adherence should be promoted throughout life.

DOI: http://dx.doi.org/10.5772/intechopen.1005825

Author details

Adina Mariana Ghemigian and Nicoleta Dumitru*
C.I Parhon National Institute of Endocrinology, "Carol Davila" University of Medicine and Pharmacy, Bucharest, Romania

*Address all correspondence to: nicoleta3fan@gmail.com

References

[1] van Trotsenburg P, Stoupa A, Léger J, Rohrer T, Peters C, Fugazzola L, et al. Congenital hypothyroidism: A 2020-2021 consensus guidelines update-an ENDO-European reference network initiative endorsed by the European society for pediatric endocrinology and the European society for endocrinology. Thyroid. 2021;**31**(3):387-419. DOI: 10.1089/thy.2020.0333

[2] Bowden SA, Goldis M. Congenital hypothyroidism. In: StatPearls. Treasure Island (FL): StatPearls Publishing; 2024

[3] Kollati Y, Akella RRD, Naushad SM, Patel RK, Reddy GB, Dirisala VR. Molecular insights into the role of genetic determinants of congenital hypothyroidism. Genomics and Informatics. 2021;**19**(3):e29. DOI: 10.5808/gi.21034. Epub: 2021 Sep 30

[4] Léger J, Olivieri A, Donaldson M, Torresani T, Krude H, van Vliet G, et al. European society for paediatric endocrinology consensus guidelines on screening, diagnosis, and management of congenital hypothyroidism. The Journal of Clinical Endocrinology and Metabolism. 2014;**99**(2):363-384. DOI: 10.1210/jc.2013-1891. Epub: 2014 Jan 21

[5] Boelen A, Zwaveling-Soonawala N, Heijboer AC, van Trotsenburg ASP. Neonatal screening for primary and central congenital hypothyroidism: Is it time to go Dutch? European Thyroid Journal. 2023;**12**(4):e230041. DOI: 10.1530/ETJ-23-0041

[6] Klein AH, Meltzer S, Kenny FM. Improved prognosis in congenital hypothyroidism treated before age three months. The Journal of Pediatrics. 1972;**81**(5):912-915. DOI: 10.1016/s0022-3476(72)80542-0

[7] Rastogi MV, LaFranchi SH. Congenital hypothyroidism. Orphanet Journal of Rare Diseases. 2010;**5**:17. DOI: 10.1186/1750-1172-5-17

[8] LaFranchi SH. Approach to the diagnosis and treatment of neonatal hypothyroidism. The Journal of Clinical Endocrinology and Metabolism. 2011;**96**(10):2959-2967. DOI: 10.1210/jc.2011-1175

[9] Lauffer P, Zwaveling-Soonawala N, Naafs JC, Boelen A, van Trotsenburg ASP. Diagnosis and management of central congenital hypothyroidism. Frontiers in Endocrinology. 2021;**12**:686317. DOI: 10.3389/fendo.2021.686317

[10] Itonaga T, Hasegawa Y, Higuchi S, et al. Knowns and unknowns about congenital hypothyroidism: 2022 update. Clinical Pediatric Endocrinology: Case Reports and Clinical Investigations: Official Journal of the Japanese Society for Pediatric Endocrinology. 2023;**32**(1):11-25. DOI: 10.1297/cpe.2022-0016

[11] Peters C, Schoenmakers N. Mechanisms in endocrinology: The pathophysiology of transient congenital hypothyroidism. European Journal of Endocrinology. 2022;**187**(2):R1-R16. DOI: 10.1530/eje-21-1278

[12] Siano MA, Ametrano O, Barbato F, Sammarco E, Ranucci G, Pietrobattista A, et al. Consumptive hypothyroidism due to hepatic hemangiomas: A case series and review of the literature. JPGN Reports. 2022;**3**(4):e270. DOI: 10.1097/PG9.0000000000000270

[13] Cherella CE, Wassner AJ. Congenital hypothyroidism: Insights into pathogenesis and treatment. International Journal of Pediatric Endocrinology. 2017;**2017**:11. DOI: 10.1186/s13633-017-0051-0

[14] Persani L, Cangiano B, Bonomi M. The diagnosis and management of central hypothyroidism in 2018. Endocrine Connections. 2019;**8**(2):R44-R54. Available from: April 10, 2024. DOI: 10.1530/EC-18-0515

[15] Sugisawa C, Takamizawa T, Abe K, Hasegawa T, Shiga K, Sugawara H, et al. Genetics of congenital isolated TSH deficiency: Mutation screening of the known causative genes and a literature review. The Journal of Clinical Endocrinology and Metabolism. 2019;**104**(12):6229-6237. DOI: 10.1210/jc.2019-00657

[16] Rose SR, Wassner AJ, Wintergerst KA, Yayah-Jones NH, Hopkin RJ, Chuang J, et al. Congenital hypothyroidism: Screening and management. Pediatrics. 2023;**151**(1): e2022060419. DOI: 10.1542/peds.2022-060419

[17] Hashemipour M, Rabbani A, Rad AH, Dalili S. The consensus on the diagnosis and management of congenital hypothyroidism in term neonates. International Journal of Preventive Medicine. 2023;**14**:11. DOI: 10.4103/ijpvm.ijpvm_535_21

Section 6

Therapy

Chapter 14

Optimizing Levothyroxine Replacement in Primary Care Practice

Kalaipriya Gunasekaran and Ngiap Chuan Tan

Abstract

Individuals with hypothyroidism will require lifelong thyroxine replacement therapy to alleviate symptoms and prevent long-term consequences. Levothyroxine (LT4), a synthetic form of thyroxine (T4), is the standard and most prescribed medication for managing hypothyroidism. Triiodothyronine (T3) is another thyroid hormone that can be used in replacement therapy, but it is not typically used as a first-line treatment. However, a combination of T4 and T3 may be considered in uncommon situations when T4 to T3 conversions are reduced. Optimal replacement therapy is individualized, and factors such as age, weight, etiology, comorbidities, and medication interactions must be considered while determining LT4 dose. In addition, individuals on LT4 replacement therapy (TRT) require regular monitoring with thyroid function tests (TFT) and dose adjustments to maintain optimal thyroid function. Individualizing LT4 dosing based on specific factors such as age, weight, comorbidities, and concomitant medications is crucial to achieving optimal thyroid hormone levels and improving patient outcomes. The chapter also explores potential factors that can interfere with LT4 absorption and metabolism, including gastrointestinal conditions, dietary supplements, and drug interactions. Various LT4 formulations are discussed, highlighting differences in bioavailability and their impact on treatment efficacy.

Keywords: levothyroxine, drug formulation, drug food interactions, liothyronine, primary care

1. Introduction

Levothyroxine (LT4) has long been the established standard for treating hypothyroidism, demonstrating effective resolution of symptoms through daily oral administration. Despite its overall efficacy, a subset of hypothyroid patients undergoing LT4 therapy experiences dissatisfaction with the treatment's perceived ineffectiveness in restoring optimal health. Furthermore, several studies show a risk of being over- and under-replacement, ranging from 1.3–19.8% to 3.0–27.5%, respectively [1–6]. Factors such as poor medication adherence and those interfering with thyroxine absorption and bioavailability like gastrointestinal (GI) comorbidities or concurrent use of

IntechOpen

supplements like iron and calcium, may result in under-replaced thyroid function [7–10]. Estimates from various literature indicate poor adherence to LT4 falls between 23.9 and 54.9% [11–14]. Furthermore, genetic variations in thyroid hormone transporters are implicated in fatigue and despair among treated hypothyroid patients. These revelations underscore the importance of recognizing individual variations in thyroid function and genetic factors, urging a more personalized approach to hypothyroidism management to attain optimal health outcomes.

2. LT4 replacement

2.1 LT4 absorption and metabolism

Levothyroxine (LT4) has a narrow therapeutic index, indicating that even small changes in dose or blood levels can affect therapeutic efficacy or cause adverse reactions [15]. The intraluminal digestion of LT4 tablets involves disintegration and dissolution in the presence of an acidic environment in the stomach and absorption primarily in the small intestine [16]. In a fasting state, approximately 70–80% of orally administered LT4 is absorbed, primarily in the jejunum and ileum with minimal uptake in the duodenum and none in the large intestine [17, 18]. Absorption involves transport via the Organic Acid Transporting Polypeptide 2B1 (OATP2B1) transporter. In contrast, oral T3 is almost entirely absorbed from intestine and disappears faster from serum than intravenous T3 [19]. LT4 is metabolized to T3 by deiodinases DIO 1 and DIO 2, while DIO 3 deactivates thyroid hormones. Polymorphisms in deiodinases may hinder this conversion, explaining incomplete symptom resolution in some hypothyroid patients. The elimination half-life of LT4 is close to 7.5 days in hypothyroid patients, slightly lower in euthyroid subjects, whereas T3 has a shorter half-life of 1–1.4 days [17].

2.2 LT4 dose requirement

The primary goal of thyroxine replacement therapy (TRT) is to resolve symptoms and signs of hypothyroidism, normalize biochemical abnormalities, and prevent both undertreatment and overtreatment. Successful management relies on factors, such as experience with LT4 efficacy, its favorable side effect profile, ease of administration, and stable T3 levels it produces [16]. Upon diagnosis, lifelong LT4 therapy is usually initiated, except in cases of transient thyroiditis or reversible causes like drug induced where LT4 therapy can be discontinued after recovery [15].

The initial dose of LT4 depends on factors, such as residual endogenous thyroid function and the patient's weight, body mass index (BMI), or lean body mass [20]. For patients younger than 60 years, a starting dose of 1.5–1.8 μg/kg/day is recommended, while for those 60 years or older or with known/suspected heart disease, a lower starting dose of 12.5–50 μg/day is suggested [21]. The mean daily thyroxine dose for adults with hypothyroidism varies globally, with Asian patients requiring lower doses (1.1–1.2 μg/kg/day) compared to Western populations (1.36 μg/kg/day) [1, 5, 6]. The reason for the lower LT4 dose requirement compared to the American Academy of Family Physician (AAFP) recommendations is because the guidelines rely on the ideal body weight (weight for height) or lean body mass instead of actual body weight, preventing over-replacement in overweight or obese individuals [20, 22].

The dosage requirement for LT4 in adults with hypothyroidism varies depending on factors, such as TSH goal (normal versus suppression), degree of TSH elevation, pregnancy, and age [16]. The etiology of hypothyroidism also plays a role, likely reflecting the amount of residual thyroid function [16]. Patients with thyroid malignancies requiring TSH suppression typically need higher doses. Likewise, thyroidectomized (athyreotic) patients require higher doses than those with Hashimoto's thyroiditis [23]. Radioiodine therapy for Graves' hyperthyroidism may lead to variable LT4 requirement, depending on the remaining functional autonomous thyroid tissue [16, 24]. Pre-treatment serum TSH levels can also predict dosage requirements accurately in four out of five patients with primary hypothyroidism [25].

2.3 LT4 dose administration and monitoring

Oral LT4 should be taken once daily, preferably 30–60 minutes before food and at least 4 hours before or after medications that might interfere with its absorption [21]. Switching between different LT4 products (such as generic or different brand names) may lead to variations in administered doses and altered TSH values [16]. Therefore, it is generally recommended to avoid such switches to maintain stability in thyroid hormone levels.

For non-pregnant individuals, TSH levels should be monitored every 6–8 weeks until they normalize, and subsequently every 6–12 months, unless there is a change in clinical status [21]. In cases where TSH levels remain stable and symptoms are well managed with a daily thyroxine dose below 75 μg, extending monitoring interval beyond 1 year is reasonable. Dosages are adjusted based on TSH levels; a decrease of 12.5–25 μg per day is recommended for low TSH levels indicating over-replacement, while an increase of 12.5–25 μg per day is advised for high TSH levels indicating under-replacement. If TSH levels or symptoms do not improve after two to three cycles of dose adjustments, referral to an endocrinologist may be considered after reassessing differential diagnoses, medication adherence, and potential interactions with other drugs or food.

2.4 Factors influencing LT4 dose

2.4.1 Medication adherence and LT4 replacement

Inadequate adherence to LT4 replacement presents a significant global burden, impacting the management of hypothyroidism, quality of life, and healthcare costs worldwide. Globally, the prevalence of poor adherence to LT4 replacement ranges from 23.9 to 54.9% [11–14]. Poor adherence to LT4 replacement therapy can result from the combination of intentional and non-intentional actions. Understanding these underlying factors is essential for healthcare providers to develop tailored interventions and support strategies.

Intentional poor adherence can arise when individuals deliberately skip doses due to fear or concerns regarding potential adverse effects of LT4. They may omit the TRT because of inadequate comprehension about the relevance and importance of LT4 therapy stemming from limited health literacy. Additionally, some patients intentionally opt for alternative treatment over LT4 replacement.

Non-intentional poor adherence can result from failure to adhere to complex LT4 dosage regimens and forgetfulness due to aging and cognitive impairment.

Improving adherence to LT4 replacement involves educational programs, simplifying medication regimens, implementing reminder systems, and addressing patient concerns. Patient decision aids (PDA) facilitate shared decision-making by providing information about the treatment options and outcomes, and by clarifying their concerns [26]. Integrating PDAs into clinical practice can effectively optimize patient outcomes and improve adherence to LT4 replacement in the management of hypothyroidism. PDAs have been shown to improve medication adherence across different chronic diseases like osteoporosis and prevention of coronary heart diseases with aspirin yet are lacking for hypothyroidism [27, 28]. Further research is required to determine their effectiveness in improving adherence and outcomes in hypothyroidism management.

2.4.2 LT4-food interactions

Oral LT4 is absorbed within 20–30 minutes after ingestion, with complete absorption taking about 3 hours. Ingesting LT4 with food can delay absorption and decrease peak absorption value by 15–40%. Lamson et al. and Seechurn et al. [29, 30]. demonstrated significant reductions in LT4 absorption and efficacy when taken with food. Coadministration with dietary fiber, soy products, and milk products has also been shown to impair absorption [7, 16, 31–33]. However, the recent systematic review by Otun et al. [34] concluded that soy supplementation had no effect on the thyroid hormones, but it can lead to a slight increase in TSH levels, the clinical significance of which remains unclear.

Food intake can interfere with LT4 absorption, underpinning the commonly recommended practice of taking it on an empty stomach before breakfast. Alternative dosing times such as at bedtime, has shown promise in some studies [32, 35–37]. The GI tract's circadian rhythms, like reduced bowel movement at night, can improve LT4 absorption by allowing more time for contact with the intestinal wall. Besides, the basal gastric acid secretion is highest during the evening, which can help LT4 absorption [38]. It is recommended to consistently take LT4 either 60 minutes before breakfast or at bedtime, as timing significantly influences serum TSH levels [16, 31]. On the other hand, adherence and patient preference should also be considered in deciding on the timing of LT4 dosing. While fasting LT4 may promote optimal absorption, it might not be the most suitable for selected patients due to social factors such as shift work or rushing to work in the morning. Balancing between adherence and absorption efficiency in TRT is part of the shared decision-making process between the healthcare providers and their patients [16].

2.4.3 Coadministration with other drugs

Several medications and supplements can interfere with the absorption of LT4, including calcium carbonate, ferrous sulfate, aluminum hydroxide, sucralfate, proton pump inhibitors (PPIs), bile acid sequestrants, and some multivitamins [7, 16, 31–33]. Some antibiotics like ciprofloxacin also interrupt LT4 absorption, as their concomitant administration is associated with a significantly lower area under the plasma T4 concentration-time curve [7, 38]. These interactions can lead to increased serum TSH and decreased serum free thyroxine (fT4) levels, necessitating dose adjustments or separation of administration by 2–4 hours. Switching to an oral liquid form of LT4 may be beneficial, as it bypasses potential absorption issues associated with tablet formulations [33]. Nevertheless, liquid LT4 is not widely available in the community. Patient education, monitoring thyroid function tests regularly, and titrating their LT4 doses accordingly are essential to ensure optimal thyroid hormone levels in these patients taking these medications or supplements concurrently.

Vitamin C may enhance LT4 absorption by lowering gastric pH and can be considered in patients with impaired LT4 absorption [7, 38]. Rifampicin affects LT4 absorption differently depending on its duration of use. Long-term use of rifampicin induces enzymes, decreasing LT4 effectiveness over time. Conversely, immediate inhibition of enzymes upon single-dose administration may increase LT4 bioavailability [38]. **Table 1** summarizes LT4 interactions with other medications through the mechanism and recommended actions.

2.4.4 Concomitant diseases and genetic conditions

In patients requiring higher than expected doses of LT4, gastrointestinal disorders, such as *Helicobacter pylori*-related gastritis, atrophic gastritis, or celiac disease should be considered [16, 18]. Gastric disorders like *H. pylori* infection and autoimmune gastritis reduce LT4 efficacy due to hypochlorhydria, while gastroparesis delays stomach emptying, affecting LT4 absorption [16, 18, 32, 42]. Bariatric surgery, particularly procedures involving gastric restriction, can also impact LT4 dosage due to changes in gastric pH, impaired absorption due to concurrent medications use, and supplements and altered anatomical absorption sites [42, 43]. In contrast, some evidence suggests weight loss post-surgery may decrease the required LT4 dose due to improved drug pharmacokinetics. A meta-analysis reported significant decrease in LT4 dose post-bariatric surgery, particularly with longer follow-up periods [43].

Medication	Effects on LT4	Mechanism	Suggestion
Calcium supplements	↑ in TSH; ↓ in LT4 absorption	LT4 adsorbs to calcium carbonate in an acidic environment, which may reduce its bioavailability [39].	Calcium supplements should be taken 6–8 hours after LT4 or switch to a liquid LT4 formulation can be considered.
Iron supplements	↑ in TSH; ↑ in LT4 dose requirements to achieve euthyroid state	Phenolic, carboxylate, and amine functional groups of LT4 can bind with ferrous salts, potentially affecting drug absorption.	Screen for the use of iron or calcium supplements and a switch to a liquid LT4 formulation can be considered, similar to calcium.
Antacids, H_2 blockers and PPIs	↑ in TSH; ↓ in LT4 absorption	Alkalization of gastric environment impairs dissolution of LT4 tablet; an optimum gastric acidic environment is a prerequisite for effective absorption.	Consider switching from tablets to liquid form/gel capsules and monitor thyroid parameters more frequently.
Bile acid sequestrants	↓ in serum T4	LT4 malabsorption due to binding with cholestyramine and colesevelam in the intestine [38].	There should be a time interval of 4–6 hours between these two drugs [40].
Ciprofloxacin	↓ in plasma T4	Coadministration significantly reduced LT4 absorption [41].	Consider increasing LT4 dose.
Vitamin C	↓ in TSH; ↑ in FT4 and TT3	Vitamin C helps LT4 absorption by lowering gastric pH.	Vitamin C supplementation can be considered in patients with malabsorption.

Table 1.
Concomitant medications interfering LT4 absorption and metabolism [7, 16, 31, 33, 37–41].

In addition to gastric conditions, disorders affecting the intestinal mucosa, such as celiac disease, lactose intolerance, and parasitic infestations like intestinal giardiasis, can impair LT4 absorption [16, 42]. Short bowel syndrome, resulting from surgical resection of the small intestine, can also lead to LT4 malabsorption due to reduced absorptive surface and altered transit time [42]. Moreover, solid organ disorders like cystic fibrosis, pancreatic insufficiency, and liver cirrhosis, affecting organs involved in digestion, may also interfere with LT4 efficacy (**Figure 1**) [32, 42]. Treatment approaches include addressing underlying diseases, switching to alternative LT4 formulations or administration routes, and adjusting LT4 dosage.

The intestinal absorption of LT4 involves the Organic Acid Transporting Polypeptide 2B1 (OATP2B1) transporter, which transports T4 and T3. Variations in OATP2B1 gene transcription and translation might alter the pharmacodynamics of thyroid hormones including their tissue distribution [44]. Deiodinases (DIO 1 and DIO 2) are enzymes responsible for converting T4 into its more active form T3. Genetic conditions affecting DIO 1 and DIO 2 genes show inconsistent associations with thyroid hormone levels and treatment preferences. Additionally, indirect effects on deiodinases, such as interleukin-6 induced inhibition of T3 and rT3 deiodination, and genetic variations in enzymes and transporters like UGT1A and MCT10, also contribute to the complexity. Furthermore, factors like selenium deficiency and oxidative stress may influence deiodinase activity and thyroid hormone levels, although their exact effects remain unclear [7].

2.5 Weekly LT4 replacement

One of the most common reasons for poor response to LT4 replacement is non-compliance to the medication, due to the need to take the drug daily on an empty stomach. Various strategies like bi-weekly, alternate day and once-weekly replacement have been proposed to address poor compliance. Since LT4 has a longer elimination half-life ($t_{1/2}$) of about 7 days, weekly dosing appears a feasible alternative [45].

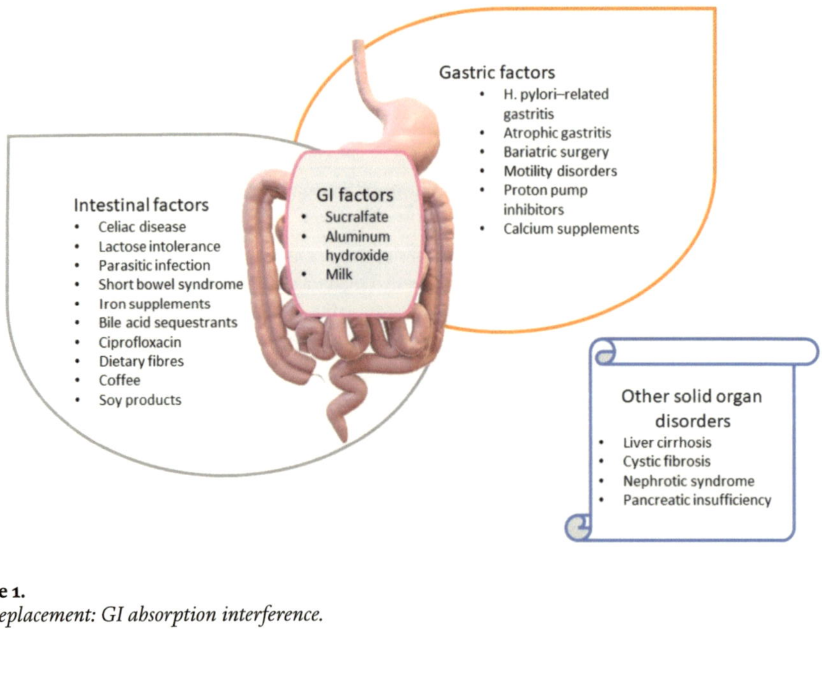

Figure 1.
LT4 Replacement: GI absorption interference.

Weekly LT4 replacement is reported to be as effective as daily regimen though T3 and T4 level decreases slightly with increased TSH before the next weekly dose [46–48]. A meta-analysis reported that weekly LT4 dosing led to a slightly higher TSH levels than daily dosing, but still within the normal range and did not observe any cardiac adverse events, symptoms of overtreatment, as well as symptoms of hypothyroidism [48]. However, further research is needed to determine cardiac safety, especially in the elderly, and to understand long-term effects.

2.6 Other LT4 formulations

Persistently high TSH despite a daily LT4 dose of more than 1.9 μg/kg/day indicates refractory hypothyroidism [32]. Though LT4 tablets are most frequently prescribed, various factors like concomitant medications and many conditions can undermine the LT4 tablet's effectiveness as mentioned above. In such circumstances, an LT4 absorption test helps to distinguish between malabsorption and pseudo-malabsorption (treatment noncompliance) [49]. The LT4 absorption test is defined as the ingestion of a high dose of LT4 (ranging from 600 to 1000 μg) in a fasted state followed by hourly thyroid function monitoring for 2–5 h [32, 50, 51]. In cases where malabsorption is diagnosed through the LT4 absorption test, novel LT4 formulations including liquid and soft gel capsules, as well as alternative routes like per rectum and intramuscular (IM) injection may be considered.

2.6.1 Liquid solutions

Liquid formulation is primarily made of ethanol, glycerol, and other ingredients. Ethanol containing formulations should be used cautiously in certain patients like pregnant and lactating women and patients with epilepsy and liver disease. It is also forbidden in patients due to religious reasons. Some alternatives free from ethanol, like propylene glycol exist for liquid formulations [52]. Lower doses of LT4 are generally required with liquid and soft gel formulations compared with traditional tablets.

Various studies underscore the potential use of liquid LT4 solution over tablets in managing refractory hypothyroidism [32, 52–57]. Liquid formulations have shown better absorption rates, rapid onset of action, and more stable TSH levels. These are particularly beneficial in patients with malabsorption, including those with gastrointestinal conditions, or taking interfering medications like calcium supplements or PPIs. Liquid LT4 also improves patient compliance, especially for those with difficulty in swallowing like pediatric patients. Infants with congenital hypothyroidism showed improved TSH levels with liquid LT4. The formulation also appeared effective and easy to handle in patients fed by enteric tube [56]. The timing of liquid LT4 intake with breakfast does not affect thyroid function. Despite these advantages, liquid preparations are more expensive and may have taste issues for some patients which prompt them to resume tablet intake [32].

2.6.2 Soft gel capsules

Soft gel capsules containing LT4 offer a convenient and effective alternative to traditional tablets and liquid solutions [32]. These capsules dissolve LT4 powder in glycerine solvent, encased in a soft gelatin shell, demonstrating pharmacokinetic equivalence with tablets in healthy volunteers [58]. Clinical studies show that soft gel capsules effectively overcome malabsorption associated with concomitant ingestion of milk products and coffee, etc. [53]. These soft gel capsules result in a significant decrease in mean TSH levels compared to tablets. The improved TSH levels after switching to soft gel capsules suggest enhanced bioavailability, particularly in patients with impaired gastric acidic output. Soft gel and liquid LT4 formulations prove to be beneficial to patients with various conditions, such as hypo-achlorhydria, polypharmacy, bariatric surgery, and gastroesophageal reflux disease, among others [53, 59–61].

Patients taking soft gel capsules experienced fewer dose adjustments and improved symptoms compared to those taking tablets. Although liquid solutions offer convenience, capsules are easier to administer and carry, making them a more practical option. Despite being more expensive, soft gel LT4 may be more cost-saving for patients requiring frequent dose adjustments. However, it is important to note that some excipients in soft gel capsules may cause oral mucositis. Overall, soft gel capsules are considered ideal second-line therapy for hypothyroidism, offering superior efficacy and convenience compared to tablets.

2.6.3 Powder form

The powder formulation of LT4 presents a promising solution for patients with lactose intolerance (LI), who experience treatment-resistant hypothyroidism. Despite the minimal lactose content in L-T4 tablets, LI-induced malabsorption can compromise therapeutic efficacy. Recent findings from a case study demonstrate that switching to the powder formulation of L-T4, which lacks lactose, successfully restored euthyroidism in a patient with LI and severe hypothyroidism unresponsive to high doses of tablets. This suggests improved absorption compared to tablets, as similar responses were observed when tablets were crushed into powder before administration, a process known as pulverized [62]. Further research is needed to confirm its effectiveness and safety in this patient population.

2.6.4 Injectable preparations

Injectable preparations of LT4 offer alternative routes of administration for patients with specific needs or circumstances. Intravenous (IV) injection is reserved for thyroid emergencies or instances where oral administration is not feasible, such as myxoedema crisis or presurgical preparation [63]. The appropriate IV equivalent dose of LT4 is estimated to be between 48 and 74% of a previously adequate oral LT4 dose [64]. Consequently, the American Thyroid Association recommends administering an IV LT4 dose equivalent to 75% of the oral dose [16]. However, parenteral administration is not recommended for routine use in primary care due to its rapid and potent effects, which can lead to adverse events like cardiac arrest [32].

Intramuscular (IM) injection provides a sustained-release option, beneficial for patients with myxoedema or swallowing difficulties [32]. IM injection has been shown to maintain thyroid function in patients with athyreosis, with weekly doses ranging from 400 to 1000 μg. Subcutaneous (SC) injection, similar to IM, offers sustained release but with smaller fluctuations in TH levels and slower release into circulation [32, 65]. SC injection may be suitable for patients with malabsorption issues, with weekly doses of 500 μg reported to achieve euthyroidism.

Intra-amniotic (IA) injection is utilized in rare cases of fetal goiters induced by maternal thyroid dysfunction, necessitating careful monitoring and individualized dosing to prevent fetal complications [32, 66]. For IA injection, which is performed by trained specialists or obstetricians, a recommended dose ranging from 10 to 150 pg./kg/day is suggested, with intervals between injections varying from 1 to 4 weeks. The specific dose and frequency depend on factors such as the size of the goiter and fetal serum thyroid hormone levels. It is important to note that fetal goiters induced by mutations affecting T4 transport and metabolism may exhibit poorer responses to LT4 supplementation. Each injectable route offers unique advantages and considerations, providing tailored options for patients with specific needs or conditions.

2.6.5 Suppositories

Rectal administration of LT4 suppositories serves as an alternative route for treating hypothyroidism in patients unable to take oral formulations due to conditions like short bowel syndrome or gastrointestinal tract obstruction. However, rectal administration requires a higher dose of LT4, typically 100% or more, to achieve normalization of plasma thyroid hormone levels [67, 68]. This increased demand may be attributed to rectal pH impairing LT4 absorption and differences in TH transporter expression between the small intestine and rectum. Despite its challenges, rectal administration provides a viable option for patients with specific gastrointestinal conditions, offering an alternative route for LT4 delivery [32].

2.6.6 Other routes of administration

In the oral cavity, liquid solutions administered sublingually can help manage refractory hypothyroidism, with ethanol aiding permeation through the mucosal epithelium [32]. The respiratory tract presents a potential avenue for noninvasive delivery, with studies showing promising permeability of LT4 through the respiratory mucosa cells, although further testing in animal models is necessary [32, 69]. External application on the skin, particularly in creams, aims to reduce adipose tissue deposits, but challenges like low transfer through the epidermis and enzymatic degradation in the skin require refinement in sustained-release profiles, possibly through encapsulation in nanoparticles or microemulsion systems [32, 70].

2.6.7 LT4 and nanomaterials

Nanomaterials offer a promising avenue for the development of sustained-release systems for LT4 delivery. Nanomaterials are supposed to minimize the inconvenience of daily administration and enhance patient compliance. Various approaches have been explored, including subcutaneous (SC) implants, coated nanoparticles for oral solutions, and injectable preparations with thermosensitive polymers [32]. For SC implants, researchers have utilized porous silicon membranes and biodegradable polymers to achieve controlled release profiles lasting up to several weeks or even years. Coating LT4 nanoparticles with materials like PEG stearate or chitosan aims to enhance intestinal absorption and prolong release. Injectable preparations with thermosensitive polymers form in situ implants in the SC space, offering gradual release over extended periods. Microneedle patches have also been investigated for transdermal delivery, although current doses show no superiority over oral preparations [32, 71]. While these approaches hold potential, challenges such as burst release, low drug load, and chemical instability need to be addressed before clinical application. Further research, including animal and human studies, is essential to evaluate pharmacokinetics, biocompatibility, and efficacy, paving the way for the clinical use of LT4-combined nanomaterials.

Table 2 provides a comparison of various LT4 formulations, outlining their absorption, dosing, and potential interactions.

2.6.8 Therapies other than LT4

A significant proportion of patients with LT4 replacement still experience residual symptoms because of an imbalance in serum TH levels (high T4/lower T3). Studies in thyroidectomized rats suggest that tissue euthyroid state requires normalization of serum T3 levels [73]. While alternative treatments such as LT4/liothyronine (LT3) combination therapy or thyroid extract therapy have been explored, no consistent evidence supports their superiority over monotherapy with LT4 in improving health outcomes, possibly due to concerns with LT3 preparations, including rapid absorption and metabolism [74]. Trials investigating such therapies have produced varied results regarding patient preference and perceived benefits.

The Thr92Ala D2 polymorphism has been suggested to influence the response to combine LT4/LT3 therapy [75]. However, studies evaluating this polymorphism in large population cohorts did not find associations with thyroid function, metabolic syndrome, or quality of life [74]. Nevertheless, emerging findings in rodents suggest

LT4 formulations	Absorption and bioavailability	Dosing factors	Interaction with food and drugs
Tablet (Oral)	Dissolution and disintegration – Abdomen; Absorption- Small intestine	LT4 dose varies with age: adults require 1.5–1.8 μg/kg/day; newborns require 10–15 μg/kg/day.	Certain foods and medications (as mentioned above) can interfere with absorption.
Liquid (Oral, sublingual)	No dissolution required; Absorption- Small intestine. No FT4 change after switch from tablet; however, LT4 liquid has a greater TSH lowering effect [54].	Liquid LT4 can be given in slightly lower doses than tablets with an observed mean dose of 1.33 μg/kg/day [72].	Liquid LT4 formulations offer advantages in overcoming impaired intestinal absorption induced by drug or food interference and gastrointestinal diseases.
Soft gel capsule (Oral)	LT4 is pre-dissolved in glycerol within the gelatin shell which melts in gastric fluid; Absorption- Small intestine. A more pronounced TSH lowering effect indicates that soft gel capsules are 109.1% more bioavailable than LT4 tablets [54].	Soft gel capsule requires lower doses than tablets to reach the target TSH levels, with better absorption.	Soft gel capsules overcome impaired absorption due to food and drug interactions, making them a more effective option than tablets in managing hypothyroidism.
Injectables (IM, IV, SC)	IV injection is primarily used for emergencies while IM and SC injection, on the other hand, can be an alternative for sustained release, administered once or twice weekly.	IV injection dose typically being 75% of the oral dose.	LT4 injections, bypass the digestive system and are directly absorbed into the bloodstream. Therefore, interactions with other medications that affect absorption are generally not a concern with injections.

Table 2.
Comparison of LT4 formulations: absorption, dosing, and interactions.

that carriers of this polymorphism may exhibit diminished thyroid hormone signaling, potentially impacting treatment response.

Controversies persist regarding the efficacy and preference for alternative treatments beyond LT4 monotherapy, highlighting the need for continued research to inform treatment decisions and improve patient outcomes.

2.6.9 Accessibility to LT4 formulations and T3 in primary care and tertiary care

Accessibility of LT4 formulations, as well as triiodothyronine T3, varies significantly between primary care and tertiary care settings globally. In primary care, LT4 is typically widely accessible, offering various oral formulations, including tablets, liquid solutions, and soft gel capsules, making it convenient for most patients with hypothyroidism. However, the availability of T3 formulations may be limited in primary care settings, with some regions relying solely on LT4 therapy due to cost considerations or healthcare provider preferences. In contrast, tertiary care centers often has broader access to a range of LT4 formulations and T3 options, including combination therapies, which may be utilized for more complex cases or patients requiring specialized management.

Additionally, over-the-counter purchase of LT4 is regulated differently across countries, with some allowing it under certain conditions, such as low-dose formulations or with a prescription exemption, while others strictly restrict its availability without a prescription. Primary care providers, including physicians, pharmacists, nurses, and others, play integral roles in facilitating access to LT4 replacement, promoting adherence, and optimizing patient care across primary and tertiary care settings.

2.7 Levothyroxine in specific subpopulations

2.7.1 Pregnancy and lactation

During pregnancy and lactation, maintaining adequate thyroid hormone levels is crucial for both maternal health and fetal development. Hypothyroidism during pregnancy has been associated with adverse outcomes such as miscarriage, preterm birth, low birth weight, and impaired cognitive development in the offspring [76]. Therefore, ensuring optimal thyroid hormone levels is essential to minimize these risks. LT4 is considered safe for use during pregnancy and lactation. Several studies have demonstrated its effectiveness in improving maternal thyroid function and preventing adverse pregnancy outcomes when administered to pregnant women with hypothyroidism [77, 78]. Research article by Maraka et al. [79] showed that LT4 treatment in pregnant women with subclinical hypothyroidism improved maternal thyroid function and reduced the risk of adverse pregnancy outcomes.

LT4 monotherapy is the recommended treatment for hypothyroidism during pregnancy due to the inability of triiodothyronine (T3) to cross the placenta. Consequently, the use of T3, T3/T4 combination therapy, or desiccated thyroid may result in insufficient thyroid hormone availability to the fetus despite normal maternal thyroid function [80].

During pregnancy, there is a significant increase in LT4 requirements due to higher thyroxine-binding globulin concentrations and increased plasma volume. Approximately 50–85% of pregnant women require increased LT4 doses, with the need for an increase occurring early in the first trimester. The percentage increase in dosage can be as high as 30–50%, especially in cases of thyroidectomy or thyroid gland ablation [74, 81]. A study by Alexander et al. investigated the timing and magnitude of increases in LT4 requirements during pregnancy in women with hypothyroidism. The study revealed that pregnant women with hypothyroidism may require an increase in their LT4 dosage as early as the first trimester [78]. The increment is greater in those without residual functional thyroid tissue (following radioiodine ablation, total thyroidectomy) than in those with residual thyroid tissue (Hashimoto's thyroiditis).

The dosage of LT4 should be adjusted to achieve and maintain serum TSH concentrations below specific trimester-specific ranges, aiming for less than 2.5 mIU/L in the first trimester or 3 mIU/L in the second and third trimesters. TFT should be rechecked within 30–40 days and then every 4–6 weeks. Additionally, women with thyroid autoimmunity who are initially euthyroid during early pregnancy should be monitored for TSH elevation above the normal pregnancy range every 4–6 weeks. After delivery, most hypothyroid women usually need to reduce their T4 dosage to the pre-pregnancy level [81].

Similarly, LT4 replacement therapy is considered safe during lactation. Evidence suggests that LT4 does not pose a risk to breastfeeding infants, as it does not accumulate in breast milk and has not been associated with adverse effects on infant thyroid function or growth [80]. Adequate LT4 replacement during lactation may normalize milk production in hypothyroid mothers [82]. Consequently, breastfeeding mothers should also undergo regular thyroid function testing to monitor their thyroid status and adjust their LT4 dosage if necessary.

2.7.2 Elderly

Treating hypothyroidism in the elderly is challenging because of various factors like associated health conditions and medications that can affect thyroid function like lithium, antiarrhythmic drug amiodarone, and glucocorticoids, which can inhibit thyroid hormone synthesis and metabolism and may cause transient reversible elevation of serum TSH [83]. Assessing the patients' cardiac status before initiating LT4 replacement is vital as hypothyroidism has a profound negative effect on cardiac performance leading to reduced exercise capacity. However, normalizing thyroid function through LT4 replacement eventually benefits cardiac health, emphasizing the importance of treatment compliance, despite initial challenges.

Studies have shown a decreased LT4 requirement in older individuals, although this may be influenced by changes in weight accompanying aging [80]. It's important to consider age adjusted TSH reference ranges and avoid over-replacement in older individuals to prevent exacerbating other medical conditions. While a TSH level above 10 mIU/L may warrant treatment, other factors such as symptoms and comorbidities should also be considered [84]. A randomized controlled trial (2017) reported no significant improvement in symptoms with LT4 therapy in older patients with subclinical hypothyroidism, but further research is needed to confirm these findings [85]. In addition, the choice of LT4 formulation should be tailored to the patient's needs and circumstances, with liquid and soft gel formulations potentially offering advantages in certain situations. Combined therapy with T3 and LT4 is still debated and should be considered only in specific cases after educating patients about the treatment's chronic nature and potential risks.

DOI: http://dx.doi.org/10.5772/intechopen.1005906

2.7.3 Pediatric group

Thyroid hormones play a crucial role in early neurocognitive development and overall growth in children. Hypothyroidism can occur at birth (congenital) due to thyroid dysgenesis or dyshormonogenesis or later in life (acquired) [86]. Early treatment with LT4 is crucial for children with hypothyroidism to ensure normal growth, development, and cognitive function.

Newborns, children, and adolescents typically require higher LT4 doses compared to adults [74]. LT4 dose required in children varies with age, with newborns typically need 10–15 μg/kg/day, one-year-old children requiring 4–6 μg/kg/day, and adolescents needing 2–4 μg/kg/day [16]. Treatment aims to maintain TSH levels below 5 mIU/L and keep free T4 or total T4 within the upper half of the age-specific reference range, while eliminating hypothyroidism symptoms. Subclinical hypothyroidism (SH) in children refers to elevated TSH levels with normal free T4 concentrations. While treating SH with TSH levels above 10 mIU/L is generally agreed upon, managing mild cases (TSH between 4.5 and 10 mIU/L) is debated [87]. Children with mild SH typically have normal growth and cognitive development, although slight metabolic and cognitive deficits may occur. Treatment decisions for mild SH in children should consider individual factors.

2.7.4 Thyroid malignancies

Thyroidectomy remains the treatment of choice for those with benign and malignant thyroid disorders. LT4 is commonly prescribed post-thyroidectomy to replace thyroid hormone production, particularly in cases of thyroid malignancy where TSH-suppressive therapy may be required based on cancer staging [88]. According to the latest Italian Consensus on Diagnosis and Treatment of DTC, patients in the high-risk category should aim for TSH suppression below 0.1 mIU/L, unless contraindicated by age or comorbidities. Intermediate-risk patients should maintain TSH levels between 0.1 and 0.5 mIU/L, while low-risk patients with undetectable thyroglobulin should aim for TSH levels between 0.5 and 2 mIU/L, or 0.1–0.5 mIU/L if thyroglobulin is low. In cases of comorbidities or advanced age, both low- and intermediate-risk categories should maintain TSH levels between 0.5 and 2 mIU/L [89]. However, recent studies cast doubt on the benefits of suppressive therapy, even in high-risk patients [90, 91].

Various dosing methods exist for LT4 dosing after thyroidectomy based on patient's body weight and lean body mass estimated using regression equation incorporating factors like body weight, age, or BMI. Most commonly, the initial dose is based on the patient's body weight, generally 1.6–1.7 μg/kg. Despite proper administration and compliance, a significant proportion of patients require a prolonged period of dose adjustment before achieving euthyroidism [92]. Atruktsang et al. [93] reported that achieving euthyroidism after thyroidectomy may take up to 4 months.

Acknowledgements

The publication cost is supported by SingHealth Polyclinics - Centre Grant CG21APR3006 (NMRC/CG3/001/2022-SHP).

Conflict of interest

The authors declare no conflict of interest.

Author details

Kalaipriya Gunasekaran[1] and Ngiap Chuan Tan[1,2]*

1 SingHealth Polyclinics, Singapore

2 SingHealth Duke-NUS Family Medicine Academic Clinical Program, Singapore

*Address all correspondence to: tan.ngiap.chuan@singhealth.com.sg

References

[1] Tan NC, Chew RQ, Koh YL, et al. Primary hypothyroidism in the community: Lower daily dosages of levothyroxine replacement therapy for Asian patients. Medicine. 2017;**96**(7):e6145. DOI: 10.1097/MD.0000000000006145

[2] Thayakaran R, Adderley NJ, Sainsbury C, et al. Thyroid replacement therapy, thyroid stimulating hormone concentrations, and long term health outcomes in patients with hypothyroidism: Longitudinal study. BMJ. 2019;**366**:l4892. DOI: 10.1136/bmj.l4892

[3] La Cour JL, Medici BR, Grand MK, et al. Risk of over-and under-treatment with levothyroxine in primary care in Copenhagen, Denmark. European Journal of Endocrinology. 2021;**185**(5):673-679. DOI: 10.1530/EJE-21-0485

[4] Kostev K. Frequency of over-and under-treatment with levothyroxine in primary care in Germany. European Journal of Endocrinology. 2022;**186**(3):L5. DOI: 10.1530/EJE-21-0916

[5] Okosieme OE, Belludi G, Spittle K, et al. Adequacy of thyroid hormone replacement in a general population. QJM. 2011;**104**(5):395-401. DOI: 10.1093/qjmed/hcq222

[6] Yavuz DG, Yazıcı D, Keskin L, et al. Out-of-reference range thyroid-stimulating hormone levels in levothyroxine-treated primary hypothyroid patients: A multicenter observational study. Frontiers in Endocrinology (Lausanne). 2017;**8**:215. DOI: 10.3389/fendo.2017.00215

[7] Caron P, Grunenwald S, Persani L, et al. Factors influencing the levothyroxine dose in the hormone replacement therapy of primary hypothyroidism in adults. Reviews in Endocrine & Metabolic Disorders. 2021;**23**:463-483. DOI: 10.1007/s11154-021-09691-9

[8] Chakera AJ, Pearce SH, Vaidya B. Treatment for primary hypothyroidism: Current approaches and future possibilities. Drug Design, Development and Therapy. 2012;**6**:1-11. DOI: 10.2147/DDDT.S12894

[9] McMillan M, Rotenberg KS, Vora K, et al. Comorbidities, concomitant medications, and diet as factors affecting levothyroxine therapy: Results of the CONTROL surveillance project. Drugs RD. 2016;**16**:53-68. DOI: 10.1007/s40268-015-0116-6

[10] Hueston WJ. Treatment of hypothyroidism. American Family Physician. 2001;**64**(10):1717-1724. Erratum in: Am Fam Physician 2002;65(12):2438

[11] El Helou S, Hallit S, Awada S, et al. Adherence to levothyroxine among patients with hypothyroidism in Lebanon. Eastern Mediterranean Health Journal. 2019;**25**(3):149-159. DOI: 10.26719/emhj.18.022

[12] Vezzani S, Giannetta E, Altieri B, et al. An Italian survey of compliance with major guidelines for l-thyroxine of primary hypothyroidism. Endocrine Practice. 2018;**24**(5):419-428. DOI: 10.4158/EP-2017-0159

[13] Bocale R, Desideri G, Barini A, et al. Long-term adherence to levothyroxine replacement therapy in thyroidectomized patients. Journal of Clinical Medicine. 2022;**11**(15):4296. DOI: 10.3390/jcm11154296

[14] Shakya Shrestha S, Risal K, Shrestha R, et al. Medication adherence to levothyroxine therapy among hypothyroid patients and their clinical outcomes with special reference to thyroid function parameters. Kathmandu University Medical Journal (KUMJ). 2018;**16**(62):129-137

[15] Chiovato L, Magri F, Carlé A. Hypothyroidism in context: Where we've been and where we're going. Advances in Therapy. 2019;**36**(Suppl. 2):47-58. DOI: 10.1007/s12325-019-01080-8. Epub 2019

[16] Jonklaas J, Bianco AC, Bauer AJ, et al. American Thyroid Association task force on thyroid hormone replacement. Guidelines for the treatment of hypothyroidism: Prepared by the American Thyroid Association task force on thyroid hormone replacement. Thyroid. 2014;**24**(12):1670-1751

[17] Lipp HP. Administration and pharmacokinetics of levothyroxine. In: Kahaly GJ, editor. 70 Years of Levothyroxine [Internet]. Cham (CH): Springer; 2021. DOI: 10.1007/978-3-030-63277-9_2. Available from: https://www.ncbi.nlm.nih.gov/books/NBK585644/

[18] Virili C, Brusca N, Capriello S, et al. Levothyroxine therapy in gastric malabsorptive disorders. Frontiers in Endocrinology (Lausanne). 2021;**11**:621616. DOI: 10.3389/fendo.2020.621616

[19] Hays MT. Absorption of triiodothyronine in man. The Journal of Clinical Endocrinology and Metabolism. 1970;**30**(5):675-676. DOI: 10.1210/jcem-30-5-675

[20] Jonklaas J. Optimal thyroid hormone replacement. Endocrine Reviews. 2022;**43**(2):366-404. DOI: 10.1210/endrev/bnab031

[21] Wilson SA, Stem LA, Bruehlman RD. Hypothyroidism: Diagnosis and treatment. American Family Physician. 2021;**103**(10):605-613

[22] Muncie HL Jr. Weight-based levothyroxine dosage adjustment for hypothyroidism. American Family Physician. 2022;**105**(1):6-7

[23] Ramírez Stieben LA, Pustilnik E, Feldman R, et al. Optimal levothyroxine dose to achieve euthyroidism in patients with primary hypothyroidism: Analysis according to etiology. Revista de la Facultad de Ciencias Médicas de Córdoba. 2022;**79**(4):353-357. DOI: 10.31053/1853.0605.v79.n4.35157

[24] Mathiphanit S, Yenseung N, Chatchomchuan W, et al. Profile of levothyroxine replacement therapy in Graves' disease patients with hypothyroidism post-radioactive iodine ablation: Focus on different weight-based regimens. Journal of the ASEAN Federation of Endocrine Societies. 2022;**37**(1):62-68. DOI: 10.15605/jafes.037.01.19. Epub 2022 May 7

[25] Nair A, Chellamma J, Gopi A, et al. Efficacy of a levothyroxine dosage regimen based on serum thyrotropin level, for primary hypothyroidism. An open label dose finding study. Journal of Family Medicine and Primary Care. 2024;**13**(1):70-76. DOI: 10.4103/jfmpc.jfmpc_654_23

[26] The Ottawa Hospital Research Institute. Patient Decision Aids [Internet]. Ottawa: The Ottawa Hospital Research Institute; c2024. [updated 2024; cited 2024]. Available from: https://decisionaid.ohri.ca

[27] Montori VM, Shah ND, Pencille LJ, et al. Use of a decision aid to improve treatment decisions in osteoporosis: The osteoporosis choice randomized trial.

The American Journal of Medicine. 2011;**124**(6):549-556. DOI: 10.1016/j.amjmed.2011.01.013

[28] Sheridan SL, Draeger LB, Pignone MP, et al. A randomized trial of an intervention to improve use and adherence to effective coronary heart disease prevention strategies. BMC Health Services Research. 2011;**11**:331. DOI: 10.1186/1472-6963-11-331

[29] Lamson MJ, Pamplin CL, Rolleri RL, et al. Quantitation of a substantial reduction in levothyroxine (T4) absorption by food. Thyroid. 2004;**14**(10):873-876

[30] Seechurn S, Sharma S, Oyibo S. Administration of levothyroxine 45-60 minutes before breakfast improves biochemical availability as evidenced by reduced thyrotropin levels. Open Journal of Endocrine and Metabolic Diseases. 2012;**2**(03):36-39

[31] Wiesner A, Gajewska D, Paśko P. Levothyroxine interactions with food and dietary supplements-a systematic review. Pharmaceuticals (Basel). 2021;**14**(3):206. DOI: 10.3390/ph14030206

[32] Liu H, Li W, Zhang W, et al. Levothyroxine: Conventional and novel drug delivery formulations. Endocrine Reviews. 2023;**44**(3):393-416. DOI: 10.1210/endrev/bnac030

[33] Gatta E, Bambini F, Buoso C, Gava M, Maltese V, Anelli V, et al. Liquid levothyroxine formulations in patients taking drugs interfering with L-T4 absorption. Frontiers in Endocrinology (Lausanne). 2022;**13**:1080108. DOI: 10.3389/fendo.2022.1080108

[34] Otun J, Sahebkar A, Östlundh L, et al. Systematic review and meta-analysis on the effect of soy on thyroid function. Scientific Reports. 2019;**9**(1):3964. DOI: 10.1038/s41598-019-40647-x

[35] Pang X, Pu T, Xu L, et al. Effect of l-thyroxine administration before breakfast vs at bedtime on hypothyroidism: A meta-analysis. Clinical Endocrinology. 2020;**92**(5):475-481. DOI: 10.1111/cen.14172. Epub 2020

[36] de Mello RB, Giassi K, Stahl G, et al. Evaluation of bedtime vs. morning levothyroxine intake to control hypothyroidism in older patients: A pragmatic crossover randomized clinical trial. Frontiers in Medicine (Lausanne). 2022;**9**:828762. DOI: 10.3389/fmed.2022.828762

[37] Liu H, Lu M, Hu J, et al. Medications and food interfering with the bioavailability of levothyroxine: A systematic review. Therapeutics and Clinical Risk Management. 2023;**19**:503-523. DOI: 10.2147/TCRM.S414460

[38] Skelin M, Lucijanić T, Amidžić Klarić D, et al. Factors affecting gastrointestinal absorption of levothyroxine: A review. Clinical Therapeutics. 2017;**39**(2):378-403. DOI: 10.1016/j.clinthera.2017.01.005. Epub 2017 Jan 30

[39] Singh N, Singh PN, Hershman JM. Effect of calcium carbonate on the absorption of levothyroxine. Journal of the American Medical Association. 2000;**283**(21):2822-2825. DOI: 10.1001/jama.283.21.2822

[40] Liwanpo L, Hershman JM. Conditions and drugs interfering with thyroxine absorption. Best Practice & Research. Clinical Endocrinology & Metabolism. 2009;**23**(6):781-792. DOI: 10.1016/j.beem.2009.06.006

[41] Goldberg AS, Tirona RG, Asher LJ, et al. Ciprofloxacin and rifampin have opposite effects on levothyroxine

absorption. Thyroid. 2013;**23**(11):1374-1378. DOI: 10.1089/thy.2013.0014. Epub 2013 Oct 16

[42] Virili C, Antonelli A, Santaguida MG, et al. Gastrointestinal malabsorption of thyroxine. Endocrine Reviews. 2019;**40**(1):118-136. DOI: 10.1210/er.2018-00168

[43] Azran C, Hanhan-Shamshoum N, Irshied T, et al. Hypothyroidism and levothyroxine therapy following bariatric surgery: A systematic review, meta-analysis, network meta-analysis, and meta-regression. Surgery for Obesity and Related Diseases. 2021;**17**(6):1206-1217. DOI: 10.1016/j.soard.2021.02.028. Epub 2021

[44] Meyer Zu Schwabedissen HE, Ferreira C, Schaefer AM, Oufir M, et al. Thyroid hormones are transport substrates and transcriptional regulators of organic anion transporting polypeptide 2B1. Molecular Pharmacology. 2018;**94**(1):700-712. DOI: 10.1124/mol.117.111161. Epub 2018

[45] Toro-Diez AD, Solá-Sánchez E, Mangual-García M. Effect of once weekly oral levothyroxine therapy. Endocrinology, Diabetes & Metabolism Case Reports. 2021;**2021**:21-0045. DOI: 10.1530/EDM-21-0045. Epub ahead of print

[46] Rajput R, Pathak V. The effect of daily versus weekly levothyroxine replacement on thyroid function test in hypothyroid patients at a tertiary care centre in Haryana. European Thyroid Journal. 2017;**6**(5):250-254. DOI: 10.1159/000477348. Epub 2017

[47] Jayakumari C, Nair A, Puthiyaveettil Khadar J, et al. Efficacy and safety of once-weekly thyroxine for thyroxine-resistant hypothyroidism. Journal of the Endocrine Society. 2019;**3**(12):2184-2193. DOI: 10.1210/js.2019-00212

[48] Chiu HH, Larrazabal R Jr, Uy AB, et al. Weekly versus daily levothyroxine tablet replacement in adults with hypothyroidism: A meta-analysis. Journal of the ASEAN Federation of Endocrine Societies. 2021;**36**(2):156-160. DOI: 10.15605/jafes.036.02.07. Epub 2021

[49] Caron P, Declèves X. The use of levothyroxine absorption tests in clinical practice. The Journal of Clinical Endocrinology and Metabolism. 2023;**108**:1875-1888

[50] Ghosh S, Pramanik S, Biswas K, et al. Levothyroxine absorption test to differentiate pseudomalabsorption from true malabsorption. European Thyroid Journal. 2020;**9**:19-24

[51] Balla M, Jhingan RM, Rubin DJ. Rapid levothyroxine absorption testing: A case series of nonadherent patients. International Journal of Endocrinology and Metabolism. 2015;**13**:e31051

[52] Benvenga S, Carlé A. Levothyroxine formulations: Pharmacological and clinical implications of generic substitution. Advances in Therapy. 2019;**36**(Suppl. 2):59-71. DOI: 10.1007/s12325-019-01079-1. Epub 2019

[53] Antonelli A, Elia G, Ragusa F, et al. The stability of TSH, and thyroid hormones, in patients treated with tablet, or liquid levo-thyroxine. Frontiers in Endocrinology (Lausanne). 2021;**12**:633587. DOI: 10.3389/fendo.2021.633587

[54] Nagy EV, Perros P, Papini E, et al. New formulations of levothyroxine in the treatment of hypothyroidism: Trick or treat? Thyroid. 2021;**31**(2):193-201. DOI: 10.1089/thy.2020.0515. Epub 2020

[55] Trimboli P, Scappaticcio L, De Bellis A, et al. Different formulations of levothyroxine for treating

hypothyroidism: A real-life study. International Journal of Endocrinology. 2020;**2020**:4524759. DOI: 10.1155/2020/4524759

[56] Gietka-Czernel M, Hubalewska-Dydejczyk A, Kos-Kudła B, et al. Expert opinion on liquid L-thyroxine usage in hypothyroid patients and new liquid thyroxine formulation - Tirosint SOL (Opinia ekspertów dotycząca stosowania płynnej postaci lewotyroksyny oraz nowego preparatu Tirosint SOL u chorych na niedoczynność tarczycy). Endokrynologia Polska. 2020;**71**(5):441-465. DOI: 10.5603/EP.a2020.0065

[57] Cherchir F, Oueslati I, Mouelhi Y, et al. Levothyroxine liquid oral substitution as an alternative treatment for refractory hypothyroidism due to gastrointestinal malabsorption: A case report. SAGE Open Medical Case Reports. 2023;**11**:2050313X231209229. DOI: 10.1177/2050313X231209229

[58] Colucci P, D'Angelo P, Mautone G, et al. Pharmacokinetic equivalence of a levothyroxine sodium soft capsule manufactured using the new Food and Drug Administration potency guidelines in healthy volunteers under fasting conditions. Therapeutic Drug Monitoring. 2011;**33**(3):355-361

[59] Virili C, Capriello S, Stramazzo I, et al. Daily requirement of softgel thyroxine is independent from gastric juice pH. Frontiers in Endocrinology (Lausanne). 2022;**13**:1002583. DOI: 10.3389/fendo.2022.1002583

[60] Trimboli P, Mouly S. Pharmacokinetics and clinical implications of two non-tablet oral formulations of L-thyroxine in patients with hypothyroidism. Journal of Clinical Medicine. 2022;**11**(12):3479. DOI: 10.3390/jcm11123479

[61] Benvenga S. Liquid and softgel capsules of l-thyroxine results lower serum thyrotropin levels more than tablet formulations in hypothyroid patients. Journal of Clinical & Translational Endocrinology. 2019;**18**:100204. DOI: 10.1016/j.jcte.2019.100204

[62] Jojima T, Shinzawa T, Ohira E, et al. Switching from the tablet to the powder formulation of levothyroxine corrects severe hypothyroidism in a patient with lactose intolerance. Endocrine Journal. 2022;**69**(8):941-945. DOI: 10.1507/endocrj.EJ21-0656. Epub 2022

[63] Avichal D, Kravets I. Intravenous levothyroxine during hemodialysis in a patient with hypothyroidism and non-adherence to oral medications. AACE Clinical Case Reports. 2020;**6**(5):e230-e233

[64] Ritter MJ, Gupta S, Hennessey JV. Alternative routes of levothyroxine administration for hypothyroidism. Current Opinion in Endocrinology, Diabetes, and Obesity. 2020;**27**(5):318-322

[65] Naman A, Delemer B, Marot D, et al. Efficacy of subcutaneous levothyroxine in a case of refractory hypothyroidism: A case report. Medicine (Baltimore). 2022;**101**(26):e29690. DOI: 10.1097/MD.0000000000029690

[66] Nemescu D, Tanasa IA, Stoian DL, et al. Conservative *in utero* treatment of fetal dyshormonogenetic goiter with levothyroxine, a systematic literature review. Experimental and Therapeutic Medicine. 2020;**20**(3):2434-2438. DOI: 10.3892/etm.2020.8794. Epub 2020

[67] Ybarra M, dos Santos TJ, Cabido Pinheiro CT, et al. Rectal levothyroxine for the treatment of hypothyroidism: A case study. Pediatrics. 2018;**142**(2):e20173317

[68] Obeidat KA, Saadeh NA, As'ad A, et al. Successful management of hypothyroidism in gastric outlet obstruction using levothyroxine rectal enemas: A case report. American Journal of Case Reports 2018;19: 903-905.

[69] Agu RU, Mactavish J, Yeung PK, et al. Thyroid hormone (levothyroxine) replacement via the respiratory route by inhalation: in vitro exploratory studies. Expert Opinion on Drug Delivery. 2016;**13**(2):195-205

[70] Padula C, Nicoli S, Santi P. Innovative formulations for the delivery of levothyroxine to the skin. International Journal of Pharmaceutics. 2009;**372**(1-2):12-16

[71] Ghazi RF, Al-Mayahy MH. Levothyroxine sodium loaded dissolving microneedle arrays for transdermal delivery. ADMET DMPK. 2022;**10**(3):213-230

[72] Negro R, Valcavi R, Agrimi D, et al. Levothyroxine liquid solution versus tablet for replacement treatment in hypothyroid patients. Endocrine Practice. 2014;**20**(9):901-906. DOI: 10.4158/EP13378.OR

[73] Werneck de Castro JP, Fonseca TL, Ueta CB, et al. Differences in hypothalamic type 2 deiodinase ubiquitination explain localized sensitivity to thyroxine. Journal of Clinical Investigation. 2015;**125**(2):769-781

[74] Duntas LH, Jonklaas J. Levothyroxine dose adjustment to optimise therapy throughout a patient's lifetime. Advances in Therapy. 2019;**36**(Suppl. 2):30-46. DOI: 10.1007/s12325-019-01078-2. Epub 2019

[75] Concepción-Zavaleta MJ, Ildefonso-Najarro SP, Paz-Ibarra JL, et al. Liothyronine use in primary hypothyroidism - current concepts. Endokrynologia Polska. 2021;**72**(6):650-660. DOI: 10.5603/EP.a2021.0093. Epub 2021 Dec 2

[76] Casey BM, Leveno KJ. Thyroid disease in pregnancy. Obstetrics and Gynecology. 2006;**108**(5):1283-1292. DOI: 10.1097/01.AOG.0000244103.91597.c5

[77] Abalovich M, Gutierrez S, Alcaraz G, et al. Overt and subclinical hypothyroidism complicating pregnancy. Thyroid. 2002;**12**(1):63-68. DOI: 10.1089/105072502753451986

[78] Alexander EK, Marqusee E, Lawrence J, et al. Timing and magnitude of increases in levothyroxine requirements during pregnancy in women with hypothyroidism. The New England Journal of Medicine. 2004;**351**(3):241-249. DOI: 10.1056/NEJMoa040079

[79] Maraka S, Mwangi R, McCoy RG, et al. Thyroid hormone treatment among pregnant women with subclinical hypothyroidism: US national assessment. BMJ. 2017;**356**:i6865. DOI: 10.1136/bmj.i6865

[80] Lee SY, Pearce EN. Testing, monitoring, and treatment of thyroid dysfunction in pregnancy. The Journal of Clinical Endocrinology and Metabolism. 2021;**106**(3):883-892. DOI: 10.1210/clinem/dgaa945

[81] De Groot L, Abalovich M, Alexander EK, et al. Management of thyroid dysfunction during pregnancy and postpartum: An Endocrine Society clinical practice guideline. The Journal of Clinical Endocrinology and Metabolism. 2012;**97**(8):2543-2565. DOI: 10.1210/jc.2011-2803. Erratum in: J Clin Endocrinol Metab. 2021;106(6):e2461

[82] National Institute of Child Health and Human Development; Levothyroxine - Drugs and Lactation Database (LactMed®) [Internet]. Bethesda (MD): National Institute of Child Health and Human Development; 2006. [Updated 2023 Sep 15]. Available from: https://www.ncbi.nlm.nih.gov/books/NBK501003/ [Accessed: March 8, 2024]

[83] Effraimidis G, Watt T, Feldt-Rasmussen U. Levothyroxine therapy in elderly patients with hypothyroidism. Frontiers in Endocrinology (Lausanne). 2021;**12**:641560. DOI: 10.3389/fendo.2021.641560

[84] Calsolaro V, Niccolai F, Pasqualetti G, et al. Hypothyroidism in the elderly: Who should be treated and how? Journal of the Endocrine Society. 2018;**3**(1):146-158. DOI: 10.1210/js.2018-00207

[85] Stott DJ, Rodondi N, Kearney PM, et al. Thyroid hormone therapy for older adults with subclinical hypothyroidism. The New England Journal of Medicine. 2017;**376**(26):2534-2544. DOI: 10.1056/NEJMoa1603825. Epub 2017

[86] Leung AKC, Leung AAC. Evaluation and management of the child with hypothyroidism. World Journal of Pediatrics. 2019;**15**(2):124-134. DOI: 10.1007/s12519-019-00230-w. Epub 2019

[87] Salerno M, Improda N, Capalbo D. Management of endocrine disease subclinical hypothyroidism in children. European Journal of Endocrinology. 2020;**183**(2):R13-R28. DOI: 10.1530/EJE-20-0051

[88] Stramazzo I, Capriello S, Antonelli A, et al. Seeking optimization of LT4 treatment in patients with differentiated thyroid cancer. Hormones (Athens, Greece). 2022;**21**(4):537-543. DOI: 10.1007/s42000-022-00376-9. Epub 2022 Jun 2

[89] Pacini F, Basolo F, Bellantone R, et al. Italian consensus on diagnosis and treatment of differentiated thyroid cancer: Joint statements of six Italian societies. Journal of Endocrinological Investigation. 2018;**41**(7):849-876. DOI: 10.1007/s40618-018-0884-2. Epub 2018

[90] Tian T, Huang R, Liu B. Is TSH suppression still necessary in intermediate- and high-risk papillary thyroid cancer patients with pre-ablation stimulated thyroglobulin <1 ng/mL before the first disease assessment? Endocrine. 2019;**65**(1):149-154. DOI: 10.1007/s12020-019-01914-z. Epub 2019

[91] Klubo-Gwiezdzinska J, Auh S, Gershengorn M, et al. Association of thyrotropin suppression with survival outcomes in patients with intermediate- and high-risk differentiated thyroid cancer. JAMA Network Open. 2019;**2**(2):e187754. DOI: 10.1001/jamanetworkopen.2018.7754

[92] Ojomo KA, Schneider DF, Reiher AE, et al. Using BMI to predict optimal thyroid dosing following thyroidectomy. Journal of the American College of Surgeons. 2013;**216**(3):454-460

[93] Atruktsang TS, Zaborek NA, Imbus JR, et al. Identifying predictors of prolonged levothyroxine dose adjustment after thyroidectomy. The Journal of Surgical Research. 2019;**242**:166-171. DOI: 10.1016/j.jss.2019.03.049. Epub 2019 May 9